Mechanisms of Transdermal Drug Delivery

DRUGS AND THE PHARMACEUTICAL SCIENCES

Executive Editor

James Swarbrick

AAI, Inc.
Wilmington, North Carolina

Advisory Board

DRUGS AND THE PHARMACEUTICAL SCIENCES

A Series of Textbooks and Monographs

Mechanisms of Transdermal Drug Delivery

edited by

Russell O. Potts
Cygnus, Inc.
Redwood City, California

Richard H. Guy
Centre Interuniversitaire de Recherche et d'Enseignement
Archamps, France

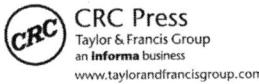

CRC Press
Taylor & Francis Group
an **informa** business
www.taylorandfrancisgroup.com

6000 Broken Sound Parkway, NW
Suite 300, Boca Raton, FL 33487
711 Third Avenue
New York, NY 10017
2 Park Square, Milton Park
Abingdon, Oxon OX14 4RN, UK

FIRST INDIAN REPRINT, 2015

Library of Congress Cataloging-in-Publication Data

Mechanisms of transdermal drug delivery / edited by Russell O. Potts, Richard H. Guy.
    p. cm. — (Drugs and the pharmaceutical sciences 83)
   Includes bibliographical references and index.
   ISBN 0-8247-9863-5 (hardcover : alk. paper)
   1. Transdermal medication. 2. Transdermal medication—Research—Methodology.
I. Potts, Russell O. II. Guy, Richard H. III. Series.
   [DNLM: 1. Administration, Cutaneous. 2. Skin—metabolism. 3. Skin—anatomy &
histology. W1 DR893B v.83 1997 / WB 340 M486 1997]
   RM151.M43 1997
   615'.6—dc21
   DNLM/DLC
   for Library of Congress   97-20470
                                                           CIP

Cover illustration by Dr. Jim McKie

The publisher offers discounts on this book when ordered in bulk quantities. For more information, write to Special Sales/Professional Marketing at the address below.

MARCEL DEKKER, INC.
270 Madison Avenue, New York, New York 10016
http://www.dekker.com

Printed and bound in India by Bhavish Graphics.

FOR SALE IN SOUTH ASIA ONLY

Preface

The objective of this book is to provide an up-to-date and critical evaluation of the application of biophysical tools and analysis for the determination of molecular transport across the skin. Both the nature of the passive permeability barrier and the impact of diverse penetration enhancement strategies are considered and discussed.

The rationale for such a text is based on the fact that, within the last two decades, there have been several quantum leaps of understanding in the physical principles underlying molecular diffusion across the stratum corneum. The major stimulus, of course, was the recognition that the lipid-filled, intercellular domains of this unique membrane were crucially important to barrier function. In turn, this led to detailed examination of the stratum corneum by the veritable arsenal of techniques available to the biophysicist. Suddenly, it was possible to discuss permeation mechanisms at the molecular level. Furthermore, realizing the opportunity presented, the pharmaceutical community could now revisit many unanswered questions about penetration enhancement and rethink the feasibility and optimization of transdermal drug delivery for both conventional substances and the more challenging species emerging from the biotechnology industry.

In planning the composition of this book, our first goal was to identify contributors with complete and "hands-on" knowledge of their fields. However, we did not limit ourselves exclusively to *éminences grises*—a conscious effort was made to invite representatives of the new generation of skin researchers, with a view towards presenting more novel and provocative ideas. Thus, the contributors to this text span the range of senior scientists, whose curricula vitae are bulging with pertinent publications, to the "new blood," whose theses are "hot off the press."

The result, we hope, is a comprehensive evaluation of what is known, a summary of what is happening now, and a perceptive look at what is to come in the area of mechanism and enhancement of molecular transport across the stratum corneum. The topics range from direct microscopic visualization, through "classic" scattering (x-ray, neutron) and spectroscopic (infrared, NMR, fluorescence, impedance) techniques, to modeling (mathematical, computer graphics) and structure–activity relationships (with and without enhancement). It is our intent that this menu will satisfy the seasoned gourmet in the field and that it will tempt others to take a place at the table. We believe that percutaneous absorption offers a challenging list of questions suitable for satisfying the most voracious of intellectual appetites.

Lastly, before inviting you to read on, a postscript of great sadness. In the final stages of the preparation of this work, the skin barrier function community lost one of its most remarkable contributors, Dr. Harry Boddé. Harry was a good friend, an outstanding colleague, and a scientist of the highest caliber. We dedicate this volume to this memory.

Russell O. Potts
Richard H. Guy

Contents

Contributors

William Abraham, Ph.D. Senior Manager, Advanced Materials, R&D, Cygnus, Inc., Redwood City, California

Myer Bloom, B.Sc., M.Dc., Ph.D. Emeritus Professor, Department of Physics, University of British Columbia, Vancouver, British Columbia, Canada

Joke A. Bouwstra, Ph.D. Associate Professor, Pharmaceutical Technology, Leiden-Amsterdam Center for Drug Research, University of Leiden, Leiden, The Netherlands

Ronald R. Burnette, Ph.D. Associate Professor of Pharmaceutical Sciences, School of Pharmacy, University of Wisconsin, Madison, Wisconsin

Sheree E. Cross, Ph.D. Senior Research Officer, Department of Medicine, University of Queensland, Brisbane, Queensland, Australia

John D. DeNuzzio, Ph.D. Senior Scientist, Becton Dickinson Research Center, Becton Dickinson and Company, Research Triangle Park, North Carolina

Gert S. Gooris Pharmaceutical Technology, Leiden-Amsterdam Center for Drug Research, University of Leiden, Leiden, The Netherlands

Richard H. Guy, Ph.D. Directeur Scientifique, Pharmapeptides, Centre Interuniversitaire de Recherche et d'Enseignement, Archamps, France

Jonathan Hadgraft The Welsh School of Pharmacy, University of Wales College of Cardiff, Cardiff, Wales

William I. Higuchi, Ph.D. Distinguished Professor, Department of Pharmaceutics and Pharmaceutical Chemistry, University of Utah, Salt Lake City, Utah

Neil Kitson, M.D., Ph.D., F.R.C.P.C.   Division of Dermatology, Faculty of Medicine, University of British Columbia, Vancouver, British Columbia, Canada

Pamela M. Lai   Department of Medicine, University of Queensland, Brisbane, Queensland, Australia

Aarti Naik, Ph.D., M.R.Pharm.S.   Department of Pharmaceutical and Biological Sciences, Aston University, Birmingham, England

Lourdes Nonato, B.S., Ph.D.   Graduate Group in Bioengineering, University of California—San Francisco, San Francisco, California

Louk A. R. M. Pechtold, M.Sc., Ph.D.   Pharmaceutical Technology, Leiden-Amsterdam Center for Drug Research, University of Leiden, Leiden, The Netherlands

Kendall D. Peck, Ph.D.   Research Scientist, Pharmaceutical and Analytical Research and Development, Abbott Laboratories, North Chicago, Illinois

Russell O. Potts, Ph.D.   Executive Director, Research, Cygnus, Inc., Redwood City, California

Randal W. Richards, Ph.D., D.Sc.   Interdisciplinary Research Centre for Polymer Science and Technology, University of Durham, Durham, England

Michael Stephen Roberts, B.Pharm., M.Sc., Ph.D., M.B.A., Dip. Tert. Ed. F.A.I.P.M.   Professor, Department of Medicine, University of Queensland, Brisbane, Queensland, Australia

Paul R. Street   The Welsh School of Pharmacy, University of Wales College of Cardiff, Cardiff, Wales

Jenifer L. Thewalt, Ph.D.*   University of British Columbia, Vancouver, British Columbia, Canada

Norris G. Turner, Pharm.D., Ph.D.   Department of Molecular Pharmacology, Stanford University School of Medicine, Stanford, California

---

Current affiliation: Assistant Professor, Department of Physics, Simon Fraser University, Burnaby, British Columbia, Canada

Adam C. Watkinson, B.Sc., Ph.D., M.R.S.C., C.Chem. Director, An-eX Analytical Services, Ltd., Cardiff, Wales

Stephen H. White, Ph.D. Professor, Department of Physiology and Biophysics, University of California—Irvine, Irvine, California

Nagahiro H. Yoshida Pharmacokinetics, Research Center Kyoto, Bayer Yakuhin Ltd., Kyoto, Japan

1
Visualization of Stratum Corneum and Transdermal Permeation Pathways

Norris G. Turner
Stanford University School of Medicine, Stanford, California

Lourdes B. Nonato
University of California—San Francisco, San Francisco, California

I. INTRODUCTION

The potential of using the skin as an alternative route for administering systemically active drugs has attracted considerable interest in recent years. However, the stratum corneum (SC), which is responsible for the skin's impermeability, is well known for its function as a protective barrier against the loss of physiologically essential substances and to the diffusion of potentially toxic chemicals from the external environment into the body. Generally, the SC is only permeable to small, lipophilic molecules. Thus, in order to expand the range of molecules available for transdermal drug delivery (TDD), it is necessary to employ enhancement technologies (i.e., chemical penetration enhancers, iontophoresis, sonophoresis) to controllably, reversibly, and safely reduce the resistance of the skin. Although there has been notable recent progress, the mechanisms of each of the different approaches used are far from being fully understood. A more fundamental understanding of the mechanism(s) of these novel drug delivery strategies is required to address the issues of feasibility and optimization.

This review chapter will focus on: (a) the microscopic techniques that

1

are currently used to visualize transport pathways across skin; and (b) recent mechanistic deductions and findings that have been generated using those techniques. Furthermore, the important aspects of transport pathway visualization that required additional study will be discussed.

II. BACKGROUND—VISUALIZATION TECHNIQUES

A. Light Microscopy

Advances in light microscopy have allowed the magnification of objects up to 1,000 times their original size and improved the resolution of the human eye from 0.1 mm to 0.2 µm (see Table 1 for a comparison of the different visualization techniques). With the aid of histochemical, fluorescence, and autoradiographic methods, in particular, the use of light microscopy in the biological sciences has revealed the substructure of tissues and dynamic processes within cells.

Table 1 Comparison of Direct and Indirect Visualization Methods

	Resolution	Advantages	Disadvantages
Direct visualization methods			
Transmission electron microscopy	~ 0.1 nm	Visualization of ultrastructure (intra- and intercellular SC)	Requires fixation/ sectioning Small areas studied Requires electron-dense compound Difficult to quantify
Light microscopy	~ 0.2 µm	Visualization of over-all morphology and appendages	Requires fixation and sectioning Requires radioactive or fluorescent compound
Indirect visualization methods			
Scanning electron microscopy	~ 1–100 nm	Visualization of 3-dimensional ultrastructure	Requires fixation/ sectioning
Freeze-fracture electron microscopy	~ 7–15 nm		

Table 1 Continued

	Resolution	Advantages	Disadvantages
Laser scanning confocal microscopy	~ 140 nm (lateral)	No fixation required	Cannot resolve intra- and intercellular distribution well
	~ 1 μm (axial)	Visualization of appendages Optical sectioning 3-Dimensional capabilities Quantifiable	Bleaching of sample Requires fluorescent compound with specific spectral properties
Deconvolution microscopy [with a charge-coupled device (CCD) camera]	90 nm (lateral) 400 nm (axial)	No fixation required Quantitative analysis on two- and three-dimensional images Extremely linear response to light intensity Light source provides illumination from UV to near-IR	Computationally very demanding Requires high capacity memory storage
Scanning electro-chemical micros-copy	~ 1 μm	Quantifiable Real-time measurement of ion flux	Limited to ion (electroactive) penetrants Measures only at skin surface
Vibrating probe electrode	~ 20 μm	No fixation Real-time measurement of direction and magnitude of ion flux	Difficult to correlate with specific ana-tomic structure Measures only at skin surface Technical challenges

B. Electron Microscopy

The invention of the electron microscope in the 1930s provided a thousandfold increase in magnification over the light microscope by taking advantage of the much shorter wavelength of the electron and enabling the visualization of the ultrastructure of tissues and cells. The two basic electron microscopes are the transmission electron microscope (TEM) and the scanning electron microscope (SEM). The TEM projects electrons through an ultrathin (i.e., 50-nm) sample and produces a two-dimensional image of the sample. The brightness of each region of the image is proportional to the number of electrons that are transmitted through it. The SEM directs a narrow beam (~2–3 nm) of electrons to the surface of a sample, producing secondary electrons that are detected by a sensor. Thus, the SEM appears to produce a three-dimensional image of the surface of the sample.

Specialized techniques have been developed in association with the electron and light microscopes that have enhanced and expanded their usefulness to the study of the skin. In autoradiography, radioactive isotopes are administered to the experimental subject, and tissue samples are collected after various times, then fixed and sectioned. A photographic emulsion (usually silver bromide) is placed in contact with the radioactive sample, which, in turn, produces a pattern in the emulsion based on the radiation energy emitted from the sample. The emulsion is developed by reducing the silver bromide to metallic silver. The autoradiograph, a picture of the tissue with the overlying metallic silver grains of the emulsion, is then viewed in the light or electron microscope. Autoradiography, in conjunction with microscopy, thus allows the visualization of transported radiolabeled compounds by following their penetration pathways into the sample tissue. In freeze-fracture electron microscopy (FFEM), replicas of fractured surfaces of frozen specimens are examined with the TEM. After samples are rapidly frozen and fractured, a replica of the surface is formed. It provides three-dimensional information about the general organization of tissues and cells and, in particular, about the lipid bilayers of cell and organelle membranes. In addition to morphological information, electron microscopy can be used to identify the chemical nature of components in samples by analysis of the types of energy emitted after the electron beam strikes the sample. In particular, x-ray microanalysis allows the identification and localization of a specific element in the specimen, based on the characteristic x-rays emitted by the element.

C. Laser Scanning Confocal Microscopy (LSCM)

LSCM is a powerful, relatively new tool for the examination of cellular structure and function, and it complements light and electron microscopy very well. The most attractive features of LSCM are its ability to optically section an intact, complex biological tissue and to rapidly produce high-resolution, two-dimensional images of the sample. Optical sectioning of a sample is achieved by the detection of fluorescence from a focal plane below the sample surface; out-of-focus light, however, is prevented from being detected due to the presence of a (user-controlled) physical aperture in front of the detector. This rejection of out-of-focus light results in a considerable improvement in both lateral resolution (improved by ~0.7 over conventional microscopy) and, more importantly, axial resolution. The focal plane can be changed by moving the microscope stage along the z-axis (either manually or with a step motor).

Although the use of fluorophores in LSCM applications is limited by the laser wavelengths available (for example, the krypton/argon laser, 488, 568, and 647 nm), this technique possesses numerous advantages over conventional imaging techniques (e.g., epifluorescence, electron microscopy). One of the most important advantages is that sample preparation for LSCM does not require tissue sectioning and fixation, which could modify both tissue structure and probe localization. Another key benefit of LSCM is that a series of optical sections collected at different focal planes (i.e., sample depths) may be digitally "stacked" to form either a three-dimensional reconstruction or a stereo image of the sample. In the fluorescence imaging mode, either the probe must be intrinsically fluorescent or a fluorescently labeled compound must be introduced into the tissue.

It is important to note that biological specimens imaged by LSCM should: (a) be sufficiently transparent to excitation light, (b) not strongly scatter light, and (c) possess low background fluorescence (i.e., autofluorescence) in the wavelength range of interest.

D. Scanning Electrochemical Microscopy (SECM)

Applications of this technique have ranged widely and have included the study of (a) electrochemical phenomena at electrode surfaces, (b) the properties of microporous membranes, and (c) the characteristics of biological samples. To date, Scott and co-workers [1–3] have uniquely adapted and applied SECM to the study of iontophoretic transport pathways across the skin.

SECM permits the real-time measurement of the local flux of an electroactive species across a porous membrane. Scott et al. [1,2,4] have adapted this technique to investigate the ion-conducting pathways across biological membranes under the conditions of an externally applied constant current. Thus, the SECM technique permits direct visualization and quantification of ion transport pathways of selective electroactive species across biological tissues, such as the skin (with a spatial resolution down to ~1 μm). The SECM technique is unique in that: (a) a high level of selectivity for electrochemically distinct species is offered; and (b) highly resolved two-dimensional maps of ion flux distribution over an area of the sample surface can be achieved. It is in this context that SECM permits the visualization and quantification of regions of high iontophoretic flux, which will be discussed later in this chapter.

Unlike LSCM, however, SECM cannot measure the ionic flux pathways *within* the skin. This technique offers information only about ionic fluxes at the surface of a sample; transport pathway information through the sample must be inferred.

E. Vibrating Probe Electrode (VPE) Technique

The main advantage of the VPE is that it provides a noninvasive means of detecting, in real time, the spatial distribution of extracellular ion flow across biological tissues. The VPE permits the detection of small, steady ionic currents from which one may obtain the magnitude and direction of the current vectors [5]. Use of this technique in conjunction with a microscope permits the investigator to correlate the current density vector with its corresponding anatomical region in the tissue [6]. Experimentally, the sample tissue is mounted in an Ussing chamber, constructed so that one side of the tissue is exposed for microscopic examination.

In contrast to SECM, the VPE cannot selectively distinguish a specific charge carrier from other charged species in the bathing electrolyte. The magnitude of the measured current is a composite of all transported ionic species. Thus, this technique permits one to identify the unique patterns of current distribution across the skin but not the chemical nature of the ions that produce these patterns of ion flow.

III. VISUALIZATION AND IDENTIFICATION OF TRANSDERMAL TRANSPORT PATHWAYS

A. Passive Diffusion Across the Stratum Corneum and Viable Epidermis

Light Microscopy

Histochemical studies of the skin in the 1940s and 1950s focused primarily on pathways of penetration of fats in vivo in humans [7,8] and rats [9]. The transport of topically applied substances (including olive oil, cod liver oil, and petrolatum) was followed by the addition of various dyes (Sudan IV [7,9] and Scarlet R [8]) to the solutions. Regardless of the dye or skin source used, the fats were found to penetrate "along the inside of the hairshaft" and into the sebaceous glands [7–9], with no penetration through the SC. In agreement with the above histochemical experiments, Witten and co-workers [10] reported that the application of radioactive mercury (0.5% aqueous Hg^{203}) in humans in vivo for 48 hours resulted in the localization of the mercury on the surface of the skin and within the viable epidermis and hair follicles.

Advances in autoradiography light microscopy have enabled a number of investigators [11–14] to demonstrate improved although limited mechanistic information about permeation pathways across the SC. To further increase its utility in drug delivery applications, this technique was adapted to allow visualization of the *generalized* distribution of radioactive materials in skin [14]. The modification involved storing the skin sample in a frozen state (postabsorption), thereby immobilizing the radioactive compound in the tissue. Currently, this visualization technique offers a means by which researchers can study the influence of the vehicle, dose, time of application, and other parameters on the macroscopic distribution of radiolabeled compounds across the layers of the skin (i.e., SC, viable epidermis, dermis, or pilosebaceous unit) following percutaneous absorption. However, light microscopy does not allow investigators to distinguish either between intercellular or transcellular pathways or among the more detailed structures of the pilosebaceous units.

In 1969, autoradiography was used to study the localization of a series of radioactive germicides, dissolved in soap and nonsoap detergents and shampoo, across guinea pig skin [14]. It was shown that for all of the germicides in each of the vehicles studied, radioactivity was concentrated predominantly in the SC. The time of application (i.e., 10 min) was not, however, varied in these experiments. Therefore, it was not possible for the authors to evaluate the manner in which the distribution of germicides along their permeation pathways changed, if at all, with time. Deposition of radioactivity in skin sites other than the SC (e.g., epidermis, dermis, hair follicles, and sebaceous glands) was variable. In a more recent study, Conte et al. [12] studied the skin distribution of a cream containing ^{14}C-flutrimazole, a topical antifungal, in normal and scarified (i.e.,abraded SC) mini-pig skin for varying time intervals (i.e., 2–24 hr). Autoradiography results, in contrast to the earlier work [14], revealed only minimal deposition of the lipophilic permeant was observed in the SC relative to the other epidermal layers. Permeation studies with ^{14}C-flutrimazole show its rapid absorption into the epidermis. The absence of localized SC deposits was therefore attributed to the high permeability of ^{14}C-flutrimazole across this layer. It should be mentioned that the shortest time of application in the latter study was 2 hours, compared to 10 minutes for germicide permeation in the earlier study. This disparity in application time makes it difficult to directly compare the distribution of germicides and ^{14}C-flutrimazole. Most certainly, the physicochemical properties of these permeants and their respective vehicles played a significant role as well.

Although follicular transport was not a major focus of the more recent study discussed above, distribution of ^{14}C-flutrimazole to hair follicles was observed to be significant in the few instances that these structures were visualized. As expected, penetration into scarified skin was greater than that into normal skin, presumably due to the damaged barrier function of the former skin. It was not possible, however, to evaluate differences in the distribution of ^{14}C-flutrimazole based on application time, due largely to the low resolution of the autoradiographic technique. Overall, the highest levels of radioactivity were observed in the basal layer of the epidermis close to the epidermal–dermal interface.

The limit of resolution for light microscopy (i.e., ~0.2–2.0 mm) in relation to its ability to visualize the regional deposition of radioactive substances (relative to the detailed anatomical features of the skin) does, indeed, have consequences that warrant further discussion. In the literature there exist several instances in which investigators have been unable to detect differences in the distribution characteristics of a radioactive compound when *certain* experimental conditions were varied. The group of Conte el al. [12], for example, had difficulty identifying qualitative changes in the distribution of ^{14}C-flutrimazole: (a) between normal and scarified skin; and (b) when the time of application was varied. In another study [11], higher doses of ^{3}H-estradiol applied to rat skin resulted in a masking of cellular and subcellular detail in the autoradiograms (see Fig. 1). Autoradiography was, however, able to distinguish qualitative differences in the distribution of ^{3}H-estradiol as the

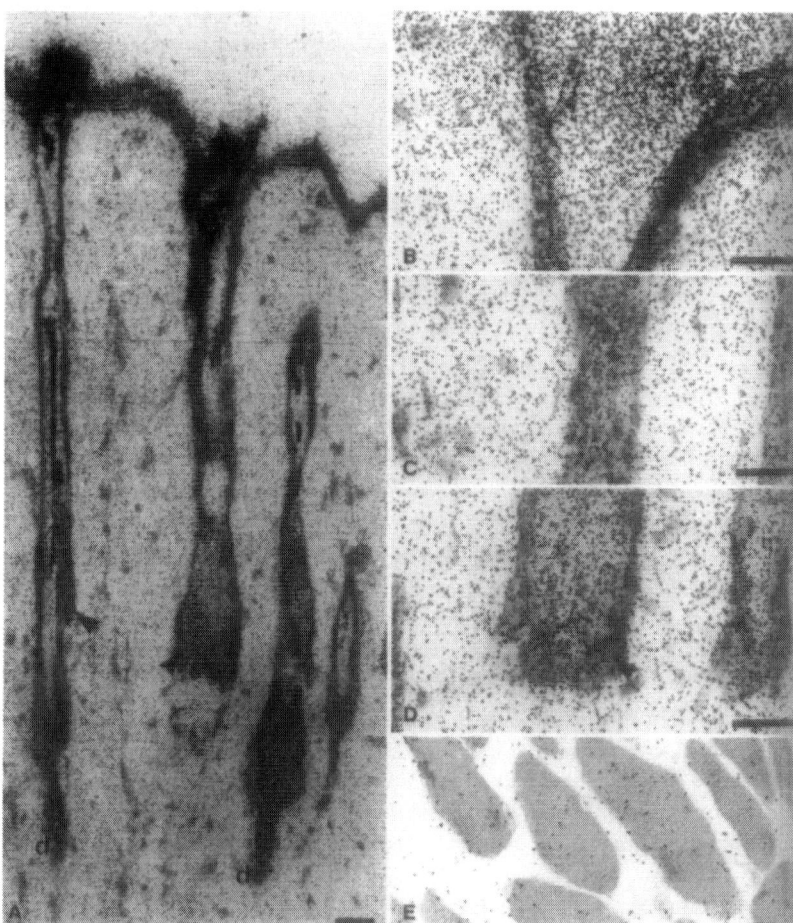

Figure 1 Autoradiogram of skin treated by the passive application of ^{3}H-estradiol, in dimethylsulfoxide, for 2 hours. The exposure time was 81 days. (A) A macroscopic view illustrating the regions of the epidermis, hair shafts, and sebaceous glands with the highest levels of radioactivity is shown. (The arrow points at a sebaceous gland.) Penetration gradients of radioactivity are apparent between the epidermis and dermis (B–C) and regions of hair shafts and the hypodermis (D–E). The scale bar is 25 μm. (Reprinted with permission from Ref. 11.)

vehicle was changed [i.e., dimethylsulfoxide (DMSO) vs. ethylene glycol]. Thus, depending on the extent to which the distribution of a radioactive substance changes when the experimental conditions are varied, autoradiography may or may not be able to resolve the differences.

Light microscopy has also been adapted to study the permeation characteristics of fluorescent compounds into the skin. Kao and co-workers employed fluorescence microscopy to investigate the influence of skin appendages on the in vitro percutaneous absorption of benzo[a]pyrene, an intrinsically fluorescent compound, across mouse skin [13]. To systematically study the influence of skin appendages on percutaneous absorption, an in-house mouse strain with three variants, phenotypically distinct only by hair density (i.e., high, medium, and low follicle density), was derived. However, because hair density was not quantified, it is difficult to know which mouse variant possesses a hair follicle density similar to that of humans. Photomicrographs revealed essentially no difference in the deposition of benzo[a]pyrene fluorescence along the SC and epidermal pathways between any of the three phenotypic variants. The extent of benzo[a]pyrene transport along the appendageal pathways, however, was different amongst the three phenotypic variants. Bright fluorescence was observed in the hair follicles, sebaceous glands, and deep dermal regions of the haired phenotype. Benzo[a]pyrene fluorescence was not observed, however, in the appendageal regions of the hairless mice; intermediate levels of fluorescence were observed in the fuzzy-haired mice. Overall, these studies suggest that the transappendageal penetration of this compound can contribute significantly to its total skin absorption.

In a parallel set of in vitro permeation studies, benzo[a]pyrene permeability was shown to be greater in animals with higher hair densities. These observations, together with the fluorescence microscopy results, further suggest that the follicular pathway of benzo[a]pyrene diffusion may represent a major route of passage. In contrast, testosterone, a compound well absorbed across the skin, showed a weak correlation between permeability and hair densitiy in vitro. Although it was not possible to visualize testosterone because of its lack of intrinsic flourescence, the authors deduced that this steroid, due to its high lipophilicity, rapidly diffuses through the intercellular pathways of the SC, with only minimal participation of the appendageal pathways. It may be hypothesized, then, that the follicular pathway may be more important for a compound such as benzo[a]pyrene that is less well absorbed into and across the SC.

In the development of topical drug delivery systems, it is important to understand the general distribution of a compound in skin *and* to know the precise ultrastructural localization of the permeant. It is, therefore, necessary to conduct both macroscopic (e.g., light microscopy) and ultrastructural (e.g., electron microscopy) measurements to fully and adequately evaluate the permeation pathways of substances across the skin.

Electron Microscopy

Initial transmission electron microscopy studies presented the SC as a composite of dead corneocytes separated by empty regions filled with debris or amorphous material [15–17]. Thus, the intercellular space of the SC appeared not to contribute to the barrier properties of the skin. Advances in fixation techniques [18], and evidence from other imaging techniques [19,20] and biophysical experiments [21–23], have indicated the complexity of the multilayered extracellular lipids of the SC and their importance in percutaneous transport. The problem of elucidating the functional role of each of the SC's components in the permeability barrier is further complicated by (a) the presence of appendages (i.e., hair follicles, sebaceous glands, and sweat glands) as alternate transport pathways, (b) the ongoing process of desquamation and desmosomal breakdown, and (c) the anisotropy of the SC, both within and between layers. Finally, differences in methodologies among investigators (e.g., source of skin, in vivo or in vitro studies, specific autoradiography and fixation protocols) makes a comparison of results difficult.

Studies using TEM and in situ precipitation to follow the pathway of topically applied compounds have focused on distinguishing between the intracellular and intercellular routes of transport of substances across the SC. In 1968, Silberberg [24] first used this technique to provide evidence that mercury, after topical application of 0.1% aqueous mercuric chloride, traverses across the SC in vitro via the intercellular spaces. But difficulties with fixation and processing prevented demonstration that the mercury aggregates were also present in the SC cells. Thus, the possibility that mercury may also have taken a transcellular route through the SC could not be excluded.

Using SEM and x-ray microanalysis, King and co-workers [25] followed the distribution of topically applied sulfur (10% precipitated sulfur in an aqueous cream base), lead (20% w/w, subacetate solution), zinc (calamine lotion), and fluorinated corticosteroids after topical application on the forearm of a human subject. It was found that the amount of sulfur, zinc, and lead were at higher concentrations in the deeper layers of the SC with increasing application time. The fluorinated corticosteroids were not detected within the skin. Information was not provided about the exact depth of penetration or the amount of each element found at different depths within the SC. It was, however, acknowledged that the combined SEM and x-ray microanalysis techniques are only able to resolve to depths of 1–3 μm and cannot determine whether the sulfur, zinc, or lead were localized inter- or intracellularly in the SC. Nonetheless, the data suggest that these elements did not penetrate via the hair follicles or sweat ducts.

Progress in characterizing the lipid composition of the SC suggested that the intercellular route may be important for the diffusion of lipophilic substances. Nemanic and Elias [26] overcame some of the initial problems associated with in situ precipitation and visualization, and presented quantitative evidence that n-butanol preferentially traversed human and neonatal mice SC via the intercellular domains (see Fig. 2). TEM studies revealed an extensive but irregular distribution of precipitate throughout the intercellular spaces of all layers of the SC, three times more than found in the corneocytes. Sharata and Burnette [27] exposed nude mouse skin to nickel II sulfate and mercuric chloride and localized the Ni^{2+} and Hg^{2+} tracers by immersion of the skin in aqueous ammonium sulfide. Confirming earlier observations, the tracers migrated primarily via the intercellular lipid route to the stratum granulosum/stratum corneum (SG/SC) interface. The tracers were also localized near the surface of corneocytes, possibly indicating an interaction of the metal with the cross-linked structure of the envelope.

More recently, Boddé and co-workers [28] used a similar in situ precipitation technique to investigate the transport pathway of mercury in the stratum corneum as a function of time. The diffusion of mercuric chloride (5% w/v in water) was followed in vitro in human skin for 0.25–48 hr. After exposure to mercuric chloride solution for 0.25 hr, the intercellular route predominated. But after 1 hr, apical corneocytes (closest to the SC surface) had taken up mercury intracellularly. In the lower SC, mercury remained in the intercellular space. At times longer than 10 hr, mercury was distributed uniformly throughout the apical corneocytes and was present in some of the medial cells, but was found only intercellularly in the lower SC. It was suggested that this "bimodal distribution" was related to a difference in properties of the cells of the upper and lower SC. It was postulated that apical corneocytes may provide more binding sites for the mercuric ion or that they may be more permeable. The sites of entrance of material into the upper cells of the SC was suggested to be partially degraded desmosomes. Thus, because mercury apparently preferentially entered the apical corneocytes and not the cells of the lower SC, transcellular transport may not contribute significantly to the diffusion of substances across the SC. Since mercury aggregates were present within the intercellular spaces at all levels of the SC at longer diffusion times, the intercellular pathway appeared to be the probable route of transport. Finally, the investigators further speculated that mercury and other small hydrophilic

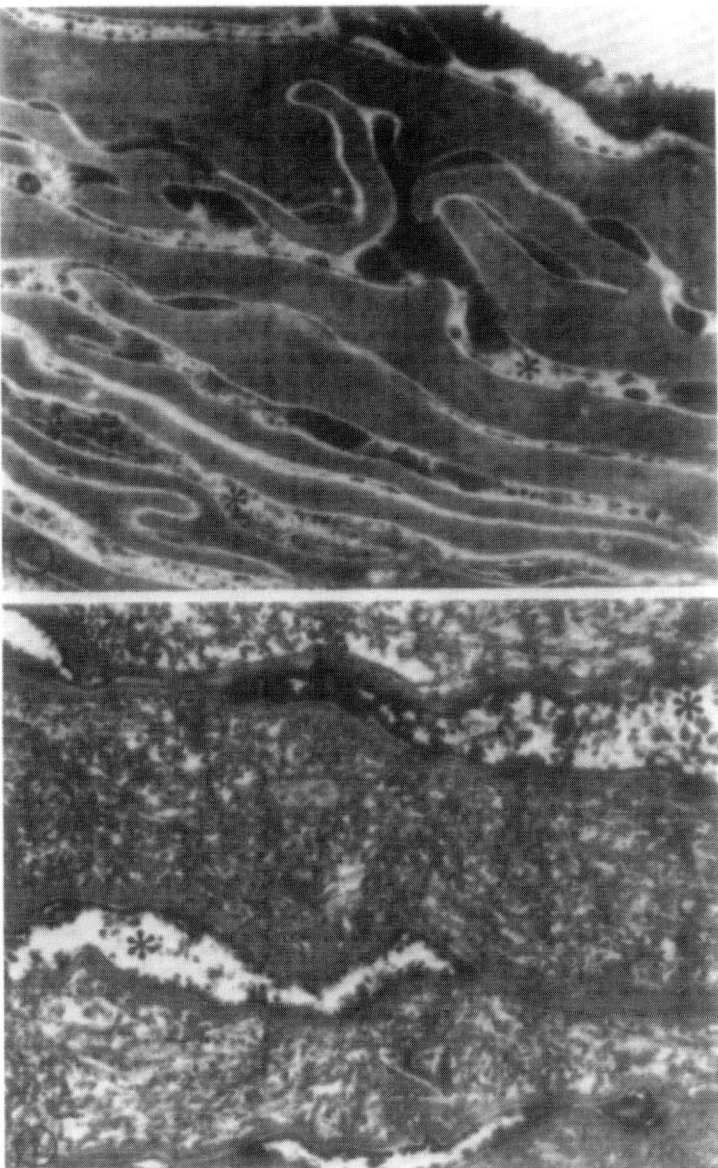

Figure 2 Electron micrograph of human stratum corneum after in situ precipitation of butanol (for 2 hr) following osmium vapor treatment. The authors found an irregular pattern of deposits throughout the intercellular spaces of the stratum corneum. The magnification is 45,600×. (Reproduced with permission from Ref. 26.)

species may travel through the intercellular spaces of the SC by surface diffusion along the polar headgroups of the lipids. In later work, the Leiden group [29] developed electron microscopy autoradiography and immunohisto-chemistry methods to examine the transport of topically applied estradiol and norethindrone across human SC in vivo. The results indicated that the steroids (24–48 hr application) also followed the "bimodal" distribution: the steroids were localized primarily in the intercellular space but were also found within apical corneocytes.

Since water regulation is a primary role of the skin, it is important to ask where the barrier to water and hydrophilic compounds resides within the stratum corneum. Hashimoto [30] attempted to localize the barrier by immer-sion of human skin samples (0.2 mm thick) in lanthanum nitrate for 3 days. Lanthanum was found in the intercellular spaces of all layers of the viable epidermis, with the exception of the junction between the stratum granulosum and the stratum corneum. Furthermore, lanthanum was not found between the corneocytes of the stratum corneum. Hashimoto suggested that the presence of tight junctions at the SG/SC interface may contribute to barrier function. Similar distributions of tracers were visualized by TEM of human skin incubated in ferritin for 24 hours [30] and in horseradish peroxidase for 1 hour [31], and of guinea pig skin immersed in lanthanum nitrate for 3 hours [17]. Squier and Hopps [31] suggested that the extruded contents of the lamellar bodies found within the stratum corneum intercellular space may be responsi-ble for the barrier to horseradish peroxidase transport. Major advances were made in a later set of experiments that more closely approximated the in vivo situation. These groundbreaking studies [20] used freeze-fracture electron microscopy (FFEM) to determine the pathway of water-soluble tracers through the skin in vivo and in vitro. Skin biopsies of neonatal mice were taken 30 minutes after either topical application or intradermal injection of horseradish peroxidase, thorium dioxide, or lanthanum nitrate. In vitro studies were performed by perfusing horseradish peroxidase or horse spleen ferritin from above and beneath epidermal sheets. The tracers applied topically to the skin were detectable only in the upper layers of the SC, although whether they were found intra- or intercellularly was not studied. Election microscopy of samples from intradermally injected mice revealed tracers in the dermis and viable epidermis but not in the stratum corneum. Transport appeared to be impeded at the SG/SC interface, at the sites of extrusion of the lamellar body contents. Micrographs of samples from the in vitro studies revealed that tracers were excluded from the cells and did not enter the intercellular spaces. After treatment with lipid solvents and surfactants, the water-soluble tracers pene-trated the SC via intercellular pathways. Thus, it was suggested that the intercellular lipids, arranged in lamellar sheets in the SC, are responsible for the barrier to transepidermal water loss.

Together with corroborating evidence from other nonmicroscopy techniques (infrared spectroscopy [32–34], differential scanning calorimetry [34,35], x-ray diffraction [23]) have also indicated that the intercellular lipid pathway provides the primary barrier to the passive diffusion of water- and lipid-soluble molecules across the SC.

Laser Scanning Confocal Microscopy

Only a few laser scanning confocal microscopy (LSCM) studies have examined the *passive* permeation pathways of molecules across the skin. Cullander and Guy [36] showed that calcein, a multiply charged fluorophore, penetrates minimally into the SC of hairless mouse skin (HMS). Similar studies by Turner et al. [37a] have confirmed this observation. Indeed, it is the hydrophilic, charged nature of calcein that prevents its facile partitioning into the lipophilic intercellular spaces of the SC. Although some penetration of calcein into the SC intercellular domains, and into the pilary canal of the hair follicles, is observed, the total *passive* epidermal transport of calcein was negligible.

Nile red (NR) is a highly lipophilic compound that has been used as a fluorescent probe [36–38] to trace epidermal permeation pathways under various experimental conditions. Nile red readily and extensively partitions into the intercellular lipid regions of the SC; it diffuses significantly through the intercellular pathways of the stratum granulosum and stratum spinosum and, to a lesser extent, in the cytoplasmic spaces of those two layers. Veiro and Cummins [38] studied the distribution of NR in human and pig skin. Nile red penetrated poorly into the basal layer of the skin samples, whether the application time was 30 seconds or 15 minutes. Recently, Turner et al. [37b] have followed NR diffusion across HMS for 4 hours and have found results consistent with the earlier study. There were two inconsistencies, however: (a) NR was localized in relatively high concentrations around the perimeter of the hair follicle in the basal layer, whereas the earlier study reported negligible distribution into this area; and (b) a high affinity of NR for the hair shaft was observed, a finding that had not been previously reported. These discrepancies may be attributed to the different times of permeation.

The use of LSCM to identify the preferred permeation pathways of chemicals as a function of their physicochemical properties offers some clear advantages. Percutaneous absorption experiments, using molecules of varying physicochemical properties, followed by visualization of the transport, should allow general trends to be observed. For example, the hydrophilic, charged nature of calcein prevents it from penetrating significantly into the intercellular spaces of the SC, an essentially lipophilic milieu. On the other hand, NR, a lipophilic dye, diffuses extensively in the lipidlike intercellular spaces of the SC. Although morphological details of skin structure are not always clearly resolved by LSCM, valuable information about the site-specific localization of fluorescent probes in skin may be obtained (see Fig. 3). Thus, similar to light microscopy autoradiography, LSCM allows visualization of the *generalized* distribution of compounds in skin. The greatest advantage of LSCM, though, is that the lateral and axial resolutions are better than those of the light microscope. This advantage permits permeation pathways to be monitored as a function of depth in the skin. The weakness of LSCM, however, is the requirement that the permeant be fluorescent and that its fluorescence be excitable by the available laser light wavelengths used in LSCM. These criteria severely constrain the number and, more importantly, the physicochemical diversity of the compounds available for investigation.

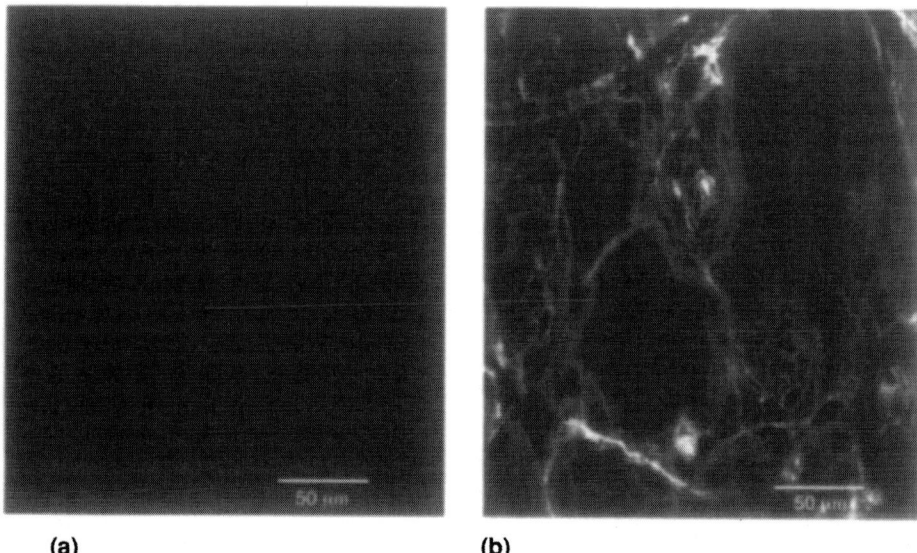

(a)   **(b)**

Figure 3   Confocal fluorescence images obtained following: (A) passive diffusion of calcein for 4 hr, and (B) passive diffusion of Nile red for 4 hr. The optical section was obtained nominally at 10 μm below the skin surface. Magnification is 40×.

B. Diffusion Routes Across the Stratum Corneum in the Presence of Penetration Enhancers

Percutaneous penetration enhancement techniques fall primarily into two categories: physical and chemical. Physical penetration enhancement involves an externally applied force to augment the delivery of the target agent across the skin. Examples are iontophoresis (the use of a small electric current), sonophoresis (the use of ultrasound), and electropermeabilization (the use of short-duration, high-voltage electric pulses). Further discussion of these subjects is presented later in this chapter and in other parts of the book. Aprotic solvents [dimethylsulfoxide (DMSO), dimethylformamide (DMF), and dimethylacetamide (DMA)], which were used to accelerate the permeation of diverse drugs; however, problems with irritancy, toxicity, and odor have limited their use [39]. Recent research suggests that other chemical penetration enhancers, such as oleic acid, azone, and sodium lauryl sulfate, exert their major effect on the intercellular spaces of the SC [40–42].

Light Microscopy

Different light microscopy techniques, such as autoradiography and quantitative fluorescence microscopy (QFM), have been used to examine the influence of penetration enhancers on percutaneous absorption.

Given the resolution of light microscopy (i.e., autoradiography, fluorescence microscopy), the *general* position of either radioactive or fluorescent chemicals after penetration into the skin can be determined. However, it is not possible to resolve the presence of these substances within the intercellular spaces of the SC, an obviously important site of action for penetration enhancers. In 1959, the penetration of the anionic surfactants sodium laurate and sodium dodecyl sulfate (SDS) into human skin was studied [43]. Although the SC remained *intact* during the diffusion experiments, subsequently (just prior to autoradiography) the SC was *removed entirely* for sodium laurate and only *partially* for SDS experiments by tape stripping. Autoradiograms showed that sodium laurate penetrated significantly into the epidermis and upper dermis, although overall resolution of the skin structure was poor. On the other hand, very little SDS was detected in the epidermal or dermal layers. Based on these observations, the authors were unable to draw unambiguous conclusions as to why both of these agents elicit skin irritation, given that only the sodium laurate appeared to penetrate into the deeper layers of the skin. In fact, the premise upon which the interpretation was based may have been flawed: in the paper, it was claimed that if a substance penetrated *only* into the SC, simple dryness might result, but severe skin irritation would occur *only* if the agent penetrated into the viable cells of the epidermis. This explains why the SC was removed in the study design. Little, if any, significance was attributed to the potential role of the SC in mediating skin irritation. As demonstrated more recently [44], however, when an agent exerts a severe enough effect on the SC lipids such that barrier function is impaired, a series of biochemical changed can be initiated that ultimately may result in skin irritation.

Lieb et al. [45] employed a QFM technique to study the influence of liposomes (and other "enhancing" vehicles) on the delivery of a fluorophore into the pilosebaceous units of the hamster ear. This model was used specifically to study targeting to the pilosebaceous unit. The long-term aim of this work was to develop liposomal formulations that can effectively treat follicular diseases such as alopecia and acne. The hair follicle density of the male Syrian hamster ear is ~1000 follicles/cm^2, which is similar to that of the human scalp (~800 follicles/cm^2) and face (~770 follicles/cm^3) skin. The QFM-detected deposition of carboxyfluorescein (CF) into pilosebaceous units was greatest ($p < 0.05$) when delivered from a multilamellar liposomal vehicle as compared to the other formulations tested (i.e., HEPES buffer, propylene glycol, ethanol, sodium lauryl sulfate, and a control lipid mixture). However, an important limitation of this visualization technique is that resolution of skin structures (including pilosebaceous units) was poor in the presence of deposited CF. Nevertheless, results from independent measurements using the same study design correlated very well with the QFM data.

Electron Microscopy

The in situ precipitation technique and transmission electron microscopy have been used to investigate the effect of DMSO on percutaneous absorption in the mouse barrier [27] and human SC [46]. Sharata and Burnette examined ultrastructural changes in mouse stratum corneum by determining the distribution of sulfide precipitates of topically applied, water-soluble tracers (Hg^{2+} and Ni^{2+}) after application of enhancer [27]. For skin pretreated with DMSO, mercury and nickel precipitates were found within swollen basal stratum corneum cells as well as intercellularly and associated with the cell envelopes, but not below the stratum corneum–stratum granulosum interface. It was concluded that treatment with DMSO, as well as with other dipolar aprotic solvents such as DMF and DMA, alters the passive intercellular diffusion pathway by expanding the size of the basal stratum corneum cells, resulting in an increased free volume for tracer diffusion.

Boddé and co-workers [46] studied the effect of DMSO and propylene glycol pretreatment (24 hours) on the route of penetration of mercuric chloride in human skin in vitro as a function of time (see Fig. 4). DMSO-induced effects allowed the diffusion of mercury past the SG/SC interface (as compared with PBS-treated controls) to the stratum spinosum, but did not alter the "bimodal" distribution of tracer that they had previously observed in untreated skin. This is in contrast with the earlier investigation [27], in which DMSO was shown to alter the basal corneocytes and thus to enhance intracellular transport. Boddé and co-workers also found that propylene glycol pretreatment did not alter the localization or extent of tracer diffusion as compared with controls. Thus, the two studies revealed different effects of DMSO and other enhancers on the penetration profile of mercury, possibly because of differences in skin source and study design. Differential scanning calorimetry experiments suggest that DMSO may interact with the lipid polar head groups and thus affect lipid packing [47]. However, it has also been proposed that DMSO may amplify the intracellular pathway and thereby decrease the intercellular lipid diffusional resistance [40].

Azones (azacycloheptan-2-ones) have been found to enhance the transdermal transport of antibiotics [48], peptides [49], and glucocorticosteroids [48]. The effect of azones on the stratum corneum or on the route of

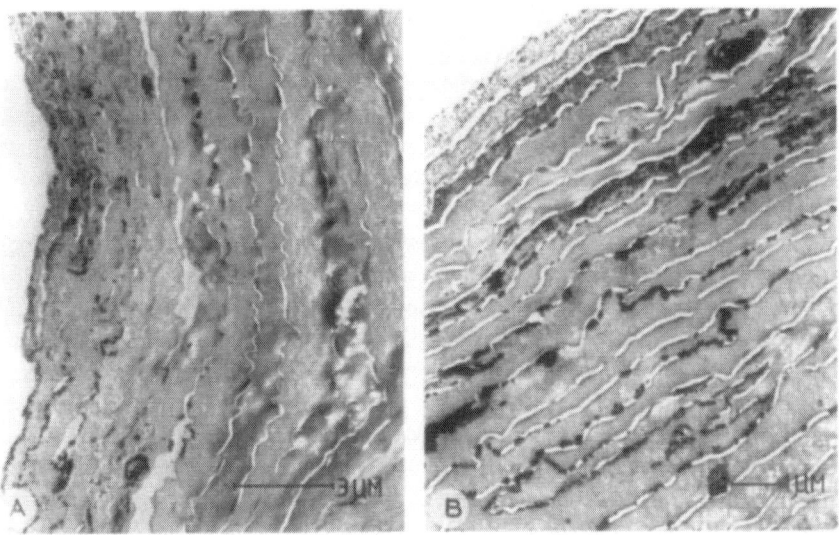

Figure 4   Electron micrograph of DMSO-pretreated human stratum corneum in vitro. Boddé and co-workers propose that DMSO increases mercury penetration but does not affect the "bimodal" distribution visualized in untreated skin. (Reproduced with permission from Ref. 46.)

penetration of various compounds has been studied by various microscopy techniques: in situ precipitation with transmission electron microscopy [46], freeze-fracture electron microscopy [50], and scanning electron microscopy [51]. Using transmission electron microscopy, Boddé and co-workers studied the effect of skin pretreatment with hexadecyl azone (10% v/v propylene glycol) on the diffusion of mercuric chloride in human skin in vitro for 24 hours. They found a comparable pattern of mercury distribution to that found in untreated skin: mercury tracers were localized within the apical corneocytes and in some of the medial cells, but were found only intercellularly in the lower SC; hexyl azone (10% v/v propylene glycol) enhanced this bimodal distribution, similar to the effect of DMSO [46]. Interestingly, dodecyl azone (10% v/v propylene glycol) enhanced only the intercellular, and not the intracellular, distribution of mercury. Hoogstraate and co-workers utilized freeze-fracture electron microscopy (FFEM) to visualize human skin after 24-hr azone pretreatment and percutaneous application of a peptide (desglycinamide arginine vasopressin) [50]. Although dodecyl azone (0.15 M propylene glycol) enhanced peptide transport 3.5-fold, it did not alter the SC lipid lamellar pattern. Most recently, scanning electronic microscopy (SEM) of hairless rat skin pretreated with dodecyl azone (55% ethanol) revealed an increase in the distance between the corneocytes [51]. But it is difficult to compare or determine transport pathways using FFEM or SEM, which provide different levels of structural detail and do not allow direct visualization of the stratum corneum. Again, conflicting results from various investigators may result from the use of skin from different sources (human [46,50], rat [51], or mouse [52]) and from the use of different vehicles (propylene glycol [46,50] or ethanol [51]).

Ogiso and co-workers [53] investigated the effect of n-octyl-b-D-thioglucoside (OTG) on the transdermal penetration of fluorescein isothiocyanate–labeled (FITC) dextrans (4400, 9600, and 69,000 Da) through hairless rat skin. In their work, it had been shown that OTG enhanced the penetration of peptides such as eel calcitonin [54] and ebiratide [53,54]. Scanning electron microscopy revealed that OTG treatment caused the dissociation of corneocyte cell membranes, an effect that increased with increasing treatment time. It was postulated that OTG acted by forming new "pores" produced by the exfoliation of cell membranes; however, it was unclear whether this implied that the disruption of the corneocyte membrane provided a pathway through the corneocyte or whether it resulted in disorganization of the intercellular lipid lamellae.

In recent years, liposomes have been used to increase skin permeability, but conflicting theories have been presented for their mechanism of action. Hofland and co-workers [55], using freeze-fracture electron microscopy (FFEM), investigated three commercially available liposomal formulations (NAT 50, NAT 89, and NAT 106, from Nattermann phospholipid GmbH) on human abdominal stratum corneum in vitro. The three formulations differed primarily in their phosphatidylcholine (PC) content (NAT 89; 10% PC; NAT 50: 28% PC, and NAT 106: 85% PC). NAT 50 and NAT 89 were adsorbed at the suspension–stratum corneum interface. NAT 50 did not appear to alter the stratum corneum beneath the interface, whereas NAT 89 caused the formation of irregular structures with a rough fracture surface down to 2 μm into the stratum corneum. This suggests that this formulation may have caused a structural alteration of the intercellular lipid bilayers and that the liposomes may have penetrated at least partially into the stratum corneum. NAT 106, the formulation containing the highest amount of phosphatidylcholine, appeared to induce the greatest changes in the ultrastructure of the stratum corneum. FFEM observations demonstrated flattened, spherical structures throughout the lipid bilayers, which may be explained by a mixing of the NAT 106 lipids with the stratum corneum lipids and the consequent formation of new lipid structures, which may then provide a new pathway for drug transport. NAT 106 also caused corneocyte swelling. It should be noted that, although NAT 106 provoked the greatest morphological changes in the SC, all three liposomal formulations were able to enhance greatly the topical delivery of betamethasone. Clearly, further studies of the effect of liposomes on SC structure are required.

Scanning Electrochemical Microscopy (SECM)

As previously discussed, electron, light, and confocal microscopy techniques may be used to visualize the position of electron-dense precipitates, radioactive substances, and fluorescent probes, respectively, in the sample tissue. However, none of these techniques possess the capability both to visualize *and* to selectively measure the flux of a molecule across the skin. SECM, however, permits the measurement and subsequent imaging of the local flux of an electroactive species across biological membranes. Scott et al. [3] used SECM to investigate the effect of pretreatment of the penetration enhancer sodium dodecyl sulfate (SDS), on the ion transport rate and transport pathways of $Fe(CN)_6^{-4}$ across hairless mouse skin. Increasing the time of SDS exposure from 10 min to 30 min increased the overall (porous and nonporous) transport of $Fe(CN)_6^{-4}$ by 17-fold. More specifically, the SDS-induced increase in $Fe(CN)_6^{-4}$ transport was found to be associated with nonporous (i.e., intercellular) transport routes, while transport via porous routes was significantly reduced. The fraction of $Fe(CN)_6^{-4}$ transport through pores, as measured by

SECM, was decreased by 8%, 23%, and 65% (from pretreated iontophoretic flux values) for 10-, 20-, and 30-minute pretreatment with SDS, respectively. It was concluded that the penetration enhancement effect of SDS alters the nonporous structures of the skin (i.e., keratin-filled corneocytes, intercellular lipid matrix).

Laser Scanning Confocal Microscopy

Simonetti and co-workers [56] visualized the transport pathways of Nile red (NR) through human skin in vitro using laser scanning confocal microscopy (LSCM). Nile red was formulated in three different solvents, each of which is considered to have penetration-enhancing ability: polyethylene glycol (PEG400), propylene glycol (PG), and dimethylsulfoxide (DMSO), LSCM showed that NR in DMSO distributed predominantly through the intercellular spaces of the SC and into the cytoplasmic spaces of the viable epidermis. Unlike absorption from DMSO, its penetration of NR from PEG400 and PG was negligible.

C. Iontophoretic Transport Pathways Across the Stratum Corneum and Epidermis

When an electric potential is imposed across the skin, as in iontophoresis, ions will move along the pathways of lowest electrical resistance. Although the exact anatomical location of these low-resistance shunt pathways has not been well characterized, recent microscopy studies have shed mechanistic insight on the problem. Experimental variables of particular importance that have been shown to strongly influence the preferred iontophoretic transport pathways include: (a) the physicochemical nature of the penetrant; and (b) the penetrant's affinity for the different environments available (e.g., hair follicle, sweat duct, intercellular lipids). These unresolved and, in some cases, controversial issues will be discussed in the context of both classical and recent microscopy investigations.

Light Microscopy

In two different series of investigations, (a) discrete sites of high ionic flux have been stained during the iontophoresis of charged dyes, and (b) microelectrodes have been used to measure spatially the electric potential gradient during current passage. Abramson in 1942 [57] and later Grimnes in 1984 [58] concluded that the sweat duct openings at the surface of human skin were most frequently associated with the highest iontophoretic flux. This conclusion was based on (a) the detection of oxidized sites on a metal electrode plate that was placed in contact with the skin, and (b) visualization of methylene blue deposition. In the latter study, the use of a wide-angle dissecting microscope to examine the surface of the skin confirmed the presence of methylene blue at the entrance to the sweat glands, with little or no dye in the hair follicles. It should be pointed out, parenthetically, that two current, practical applications of iontophoretic transport support a role for the sweat gland: (a) the cystic fibrosis test involves iontophoresis of pilocarpine to *induce* sweating (so that a measurement of Cl^- is possible), suggesting delivery of the drug into the sweat gland apparatus; and (b) iontophoresis of tap water is used to treat hyperhidrosis (i.e., excessive sweating), again implying at least some level of "targeting" to the eccrine ducts.

The animal species selected for use in either in vivo or in vitro iontophoretic experiments (whether human, pig, hairless rat, or hairless mouse) will, indeed, influence the distribution of a molecule along its transport pathways. Accordingly, the interpretations of results must take certain critical factors into consideration, such as: (a) the hair follicle density of the animal model; and (b) the existence or inexistence of an eccrine sweat duct. In pig skin, for example, although eccrine sweat glands are not present, their hair follicle density ($11/cm^2$) is purportedly similar to that found in human skin [59]. Monteiro-Riviere et al. [60] used light microscopy to examine the mechanism of iontophoretic transport. Mercuric chloride (7.4%) was iontophoresed into pig skin in vivo for 1 hr (current density: 200 $\mu A/cm^2$), at the end of which biopsies were taken and exposed to ammonium sulfide vapor to precipitate and localize the mercury. Light microscopy revealed significant distribution of the precipitate into the intercellular domains of the SC and localization into the upper portion (~100 μm) of the hair follicle (see Fig. 5). The density of the precipitate in the skin was directly proportional to the time of exposure to ammonium sulfide vapor. Based on the collective results, it was concluded that iontophoretic transport of mercuric chloride occurred predominantly via the intercellular pathway, less so along the follicular route.

To visualize the iontophoretic transport pathways of fluorescein across mammalian skin, Burnette and Ongpipattanakul [61] positioned an optical microscope on the receiver (dermal) side of excised human skin and iontophoresed the fluorophore. Discrete, localized sites of fluorescein transport were visualized (see Fig. 6). A set of microelectrodes were then rastered across the visualized pathways and the corresponding voltage gradient was measured. For each of the resistance measurements, the maximum potential difference detected was directly over the center of the visualized pathways, verifying that the discrete sites of fluorescein transport did, indeed, correspond to sites of

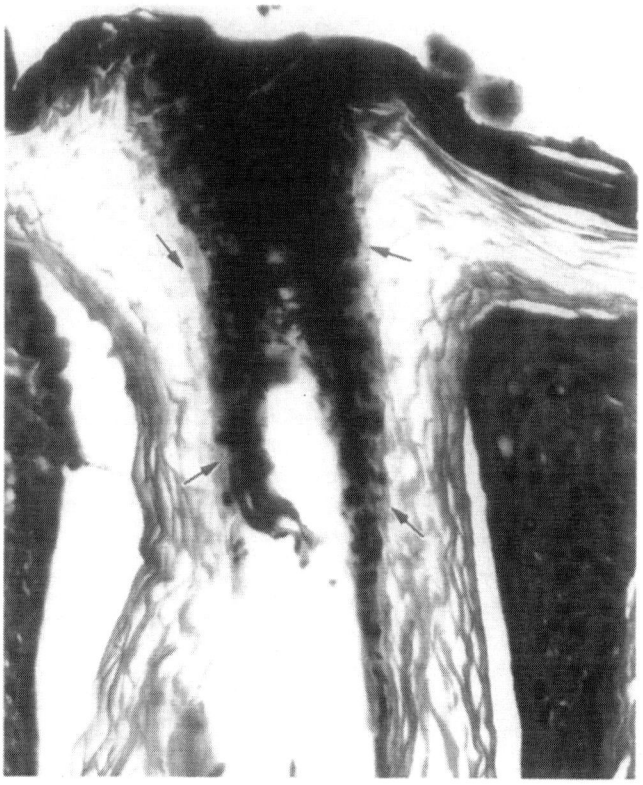

Figure 5 Light micrograph of mercuric sulfide. Mercuric chloride was applied to pig skin in vivo under the influence of a 200-μA/cm^2 current density for 1 hr. The time of ammonium sulfide development was 15 minutes (hair follicle). Magnification 625×. (Reproduced with permission from Ref. 60.)

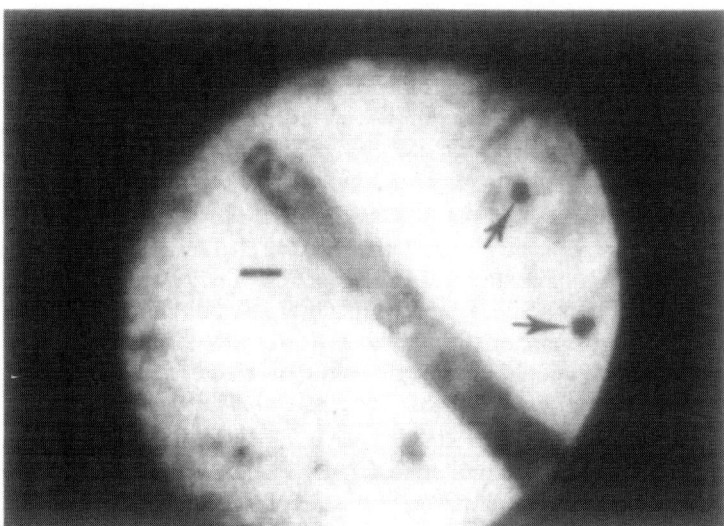

Figure 6 Light micrograph of the transport of fluorescein dye across full-thickness female human breast skin. Constant current was applied for 10 min at a current density of ~0.16 mA/cm^2. Arrows point to discrete localized sites of fluorescein dye deposition. The central gray bar passing through the image field is a shadow of the Ag/AgCl electrode. The scale bar is 1 mm. (Reproduced with permission from Ref. 27.)

high current flow. Thus, it was concluded that the iontophoretic transport pathway of fluorescein occurred at least in part through low-resistance shunt routes across the SC barrier (e.g., via hair follicles, sweat ducts, or imperfections in the skin).

Another set of variables that have been shown to influence the preferred iontophoretic transport pathways taken are the physicochemical properties of the penetrant. Jadoul et al. [62] employed light microscopy autoradiography, together with tape stripping and tissue sectioning, to directly visualize the iontophoretic transport pathways of two model compounds across hairless rat skin in vivo: (a) fentanyl, a lipophilic species; and (b) the more polar thyrotropin releasing hormone (TRH). Constant current iontophoresis was performed for 1, 4, and 6 hours at a current density of 0.33 mA/cm^2. Under both passive and iontophoretic conditions, the accumulation of fentanyl in the SC was high and permeation to the underlying epidermis was limited. The iontophoretic delivery of fentanyl into follicular structures was low relative to its accumulation in the bulk SC. TRH, on the other hand, penetrated the SC to a greater extent following iontophoresis. Significant levels of TRH were also noted in the hair follicle after current passage (relative to passive diffusion). Thus, the physicochemical properties of the permeant molecule can influence, to a large extent, the preferred iontophoretic transport pathways taken. Perhaps not surprisingly, it has been found that lipophilic species, even with the application of an iontophoretic current, prefer the lipid-rich intercellular regions of the SC, while more polar (charged) species appear to seek out the appendageal structures. Recently, a similarly designed study was conducted by Turner et al. [37b] in which confocal microscopy was used to examine the differential distribution of Nile red and calcein across hairless mouse skin under both passive and ionophoretic conditions. The results corroborated those of the earlier autoradiographic study. In short, it was observed that the hydrophilic molecule showed a greater tendency, under the influence of current, to be localized in the hair follicle, whereas the lipophilic molecule was more likely to be localized in high concentrations in the SC. Moreover, the distribution profile of the lipophilic molecule was not significantly affected whether current was passed or not.

Electron Microscopy

To date, Monteiro-Riviere and co-workers [60] have published the only studies using electron microscopy to examine the mechanism of iontophoretic transport. They applied mercuric chloride (7.4%) in vivo in pigs for 1 hr (current density: 200 μA/cm^2) and subsequently exposed the biopsies to ammonium sulfide vapor to precipitate and localize the mercury, similar to earlier passive transport studies [28]. The micrographs revealed that mercuric chloride traverses intracellularly through the first few layers and intercellularly through the remainder of the stratum corneum. The authors concluded that the intercellular pathway is the predominant route for passive and iontophoretic drug delivery systems. However, it is difficult to eliminate follicular transport as a possible pathway, since only small areas can be examined at a time (~1 mm^2) and the low density of hair follicles (11/cm^2) makes it difficult to study them with the electron microscope.

Vibrating Probe Electrode (VPE)

Distinct from the previous methods employed, the vibrating probe electrode (VPE) allows determination of the magnitude *and* direction of current flow, in real time [63]. The magnitude of the measured current is, of course, a sum over all transported ionic species. Thus, this technique permits the unique patterns of current distribution across the skin to be identified, but not, however, the chemical nature of the ions that are responsible. Cullander and Guy [5,36] used the VPE to study iontophoretic current flow under relevant conditions of pH, ionic strength, and applied current density. The results were largely consistent with those from other visualization studies and showed site-specific ionic flow during current passage across HMS. Iontophoretic transport was primarily appendageal, with certain structures (e.g., small hair follicles) apparently carrying most of the current. Of special note, though, was the detection of current flow at sites not yet identified with specific structures of the skin. Unfortunately, technical challenges (such as positioning the probe at a constant height above the skin surface) have prevented realization of the full potential of this technique.

Scanning Electrochemical Microscopy (SECM)

The scanning electrochemical microscope permits the real-time measurement of the local flux of ionic species across a porous membrane [64]. Scott et al. [1,4,65] have adapted this technique to investigate, mechanistically, the ion-conducting pathways across the skin under externally applied constant current. The SECM technique permits visualization (with a spatial resolution down to ~1 μm) and quantification of iontophoretic transport pathways of selective electroactive species. The SECM technique is unique from other visualization techniques in that: (a) a high level of selectivity for electrochemically distinct species (i.e., $Fe(CN)_6^{4-}$, Fe^{3+}) is possible; and (b) well-resolved two-dimensional maps of ion flux distribution over an area of the sample surface can be achieved. It is in this context that SECM permits the visualization and quantification of regions of high iontophoretic flux (see Fig. 7). To complement the SECM method, counterdirectional iontopohoretic transport of two different iron salts resulted in the formation of an easily identifiable precipitate (Prussian blue (PB) [66]), thereby selectively staining the skin at sites of high iontophoretic flux. Video microscopy was used to monitor the appearance of these high-ionic-conductance pathways (see Fig. 8). Counterdirectional iontophoresis was conducted across HMS for up to 2 hours, at current densities in the range 10–200 μA/cm² [65]. The number of PB "spots" observed by video microscopy increased dramatically with increasing time of current application. Moreover, the total skin resistance was inversely proportional to the number of PB deposits on the epidermal skin surface. When current was applied for 2 hours at the maximum current density (200 μA/cm²), the average density of "pores" (874 ± 138/cm²), as determined by SECM, was not significantly different from the average density of hair follicles (760 ± 150/cm²) assessed by optical microscopy. This suggests, therefore, that the

A)

B)

Figure 7 SECM image (A) and optical image (B) acquired over the same 1-mm^2 region of hairless mouse skin visualize the *real-time* iontophoretic deposition of $Fe(CN)^{-4}$ at a current density of 40 $\mu A/cm^2$. The bright spot in A corresponds to high $Fe(CN)^{-4}$ flux above a "pore." The dark spot in B corresponds to the site of Prussian blue deposition at the "pore" opening. (Reproduced with permission from Ref. 65.)

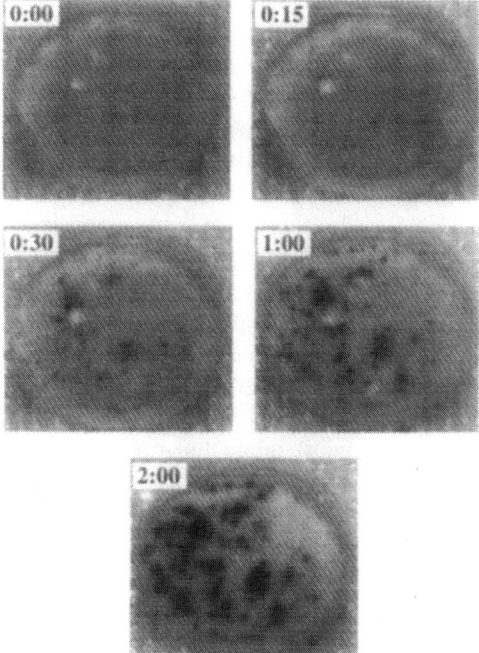

Figure 8 Video images of the appearance of high-ionic-conductance pathways during iontophoresis of $Fe(CN)^{-4}$ and Fe^{+3}. Counterdirectional iontophoresis was conducted across HMS for up to 2 hours at a current density of 40 $\mu A/cm^2$. The dark spots are localized deposits of Prussian blue dye at "pore" openings. (Reproduced with permission from Ref. 65.)

anatomical correlate of these discrete pathways of high ionic conductance ("pores") may, in fact, be the hair follicles.

Taken together with the other work described above, the SECM results emphasize the importance of appendageal pathways in iontophoresis. However, it is clear that both the SECM and the VPE show that *non*appendageal routes exist as well, and that neither technique can visualize or quantify the pathways of ion flow *within* the skin. Further mechanistic work addressing these gaps in our knowledge is therefore warranted.

Laser Scanning Confocal Microscopy

In the early 1990s, laser scanning confocal microscopy (LSCM) was employed [36] to directly visualize the iontophoretic transport pathways of fluorescent species across the skin. In this study, three fluorescent probes were examined: (a) calcein (a charged hydrophilic species), (b) NBD-diethanolamine (an uncharged polar molecule), and (c) Nile red (an uncharged lipophilic moiety). Constant-current iontophoresis across hairless mouse skin (HMS) in vitro was carried out at 0.4 mA/cm^2 for 20 minutes. For both calcein and NBD-diethanolamine, the confocal images revealed penetration into the intercellular and follicular pathways to approximately the same extent. In the SC, distribution of the two probes along intercellular pathways was also observed. In the viable epidermis, the fluorophores were found predominantly in the hair follicles. Nile red, however, was observed primarily in the intercellular lipids of the SC and in both inter- and intracellular regions of the viable epidermis. The extent to which these initial findings can be generalized to other permeants and to different experimental conditions is yet to be determined.

While this earlier research strongly suggests, in a mostly qualitative fashion, that appendageal and (to some extent) intercellular pathways are important in iontophoresis, this deduction is not quantitative and is based primarily upon measurements recorded at inner or exterior surfaces of the skin. To expand on the earlier investigations, studies were recently conducted to visualize *and* quantify with LSCM the penetration of (a) calcein and (b) a series of FITC-labeled cationic poly-L-lysines (of molecular weights 4 kDa, 7 kDa, and 26 kDa) along the iontophoretic transport pathways *within* the skin. In addition, quantification of transported fluorescent material along the penetration pathways (e.g., intercellular vs. follicular) was conducted [37c].

Constant-current iontophoresis of calcein, at 0.5 mA/cm^2, was conducted across HMS for 1, 2, 4, and 8 hr. For each experiment, the corresponding passive control was performed under identical conditions, except that no current was passed. All LSCM images showed that the passive permeation of calcein into the skin was minimal, regardless of the duration of calcein exposure. With iontophoresis, however, significantly increased penetration of calcein into HMS was observed, at each of the sampled skin depths, for 1-, 2-, 4-, and 8-hr transport. Also notable was that, at increasing skin depths, iontophoresis localized progressively higher concentrations of fluorescence in the hair follicles (relative to the intercellular regions). Penetration of calcein into the intercellular regions was highest in the more superficial skin layers (i.e., < 10 μm below the surface), becoming progressively less significant in the deeper layers (i.e., > 20 μm) [37a].

To augment the visualization of electrotransport, it was a key objective to quantify the regionally distributed fluorescence in the digitized confocal images. A method was therefore developed to assess the relative contribution of iontophoretic transport pathways [i.e., follicular (F) versus nonfollicular

(NF)] for calcein across the skin. The quantitative transport data from confocal images were expressed as: (a) *absolute transport #*—the fraction of the total transported fluorescence along a designated transport route (i.e., either F or NF); and (2) *normalized transport #*—the fraction of the total transported fluorescence *per unit area* along a designated transport route (i.e., either F or NF). It was found that the F route was a more efficiently targeted (by ~4-fold) iontophoretic transport pathway (per unit surface area) than the NF route. However, in absolute terms the NF pathway still apparently accounted for a much greater overall fraction of calcein transport than the F pathway (by ~4-fold). This is explained by the large surface area difference between F (~3–7%) and NF (~93–97%) regions. Although the extent of iontophoretic delivery of calcein was not visually remarkable via NF pathways through the skin, the accumulated amount over such a large surface area (relative to F regions) was significant. Nonetheless, F iontophoretic transport pathways do serve as important shunt routes through the SC barrier, especially given their significant contribution to transport, relative to the small fractional surface area occupied [37a].

An important goal of iontophoresis is to enhance the delivery of high molecular weight (MW) therapeutic agents across the skin. Using three fluorescently labeled poly-L-lysines (FITC-PLL) (of MWs 4 kDa, 7 kDa, 26 kDa), the extent and distribution of iontophoretic skin penetration was investigated as a function of MW using LSCM. It was found that, relative to the passive controls, iontophoresis greatly enhanced the penetration of the 4-kDa FITC-PLL, slightly elevated the delivery of the 7-kDa FITC-PLL, but had no effect on the transport of the larger, 26-kDa FITC-PLL (compared to the passive controls). Quantitative analyses of LSCM images revealed that iontophoresis increased transport via F pathways *only slightly* more than that through NF pathways for the 4-kDa and 7-kDa FITC-PLL molecules. Thus, it is *visually* apparent (by comparison of calcein and FITC-PLL transport study results) that the iontophoretic transport pathways taken are importantly determined by the physicochemical properties (including size and charge) of the penetrant [37c].

D. Transport Routes Across the Stratum Corneum for Ultrasonically Enhanced Drug Delivery

Sonophoresis (or phonophoresis) is a technique to enhance percutaneous penetration via the application of ultrasonic energy. Review of the sonophoresis literature, however, shows that the effects of ultrasound have been variable. For example, largely unsuccessful earlier studies with various common drugs used ultrasound frequencies of 1–3 MHz at 1–3 W/cm^2 [67,68], whereas a more recent study demonstrated the successful enhancement of salicylic acid delivery at higher frequencies (10 and 16 MHz) and lower power [69]. Even more dramatic, however, are results published within the last year [70] indicating that ultrasound at a much lower frequency (20 KHz) (100 pulses/sec at intensities of 12.5–225 mW/cm^2) can promote the transdermal delivery of quite large species, including insulin (~6 kDa), interferon-γ (~17 kDa), and erythropoeitin (~48 kDa). Another earlier study with insulin had reported similar data [71]. Despite the excitement provoked by these observations, however, the feasibility of this approach for drug delivery in a practical sense is yet to be established.

Electron Microscopy

To determine sonophoretic transport route(s) at the ultrastructural level, Bommannan and co-workers [72] visualized guinea pig skin with transmission electron microscopy (TEM) after the application of colloidal lanthanum hydroxide (an electron dense tracer) and treatment in vivo with 10- or 16-MHz ultrasound (0.2 W/cm^2). In control samples, the tracer did not appear to penetrate into the stratum corneum. But in samples exposed to sonophoresis, the tracer was found in localized areas of the intercellular space, which may correspond to the "lacunae" (polar head-group domains) described by Hou and co-workers [73] as polar or head-group domains. In addition, sonophoresis for 5 minutes (at both 10 and 16 MHz) did not appear to alter the morphology of the epidermal cells, whereas damage to cells was observed after 20 minutes of treatment (16 MHz). Thus, sonophoresis appears to cause the permeation of the tracers via the intercellular route within the stratum corneum.

In 1994, Menon and co-workers [74] similarly used TEM to visualize tracers in the stratum corneum after sonophoresis treatment. They applied colloidal lanthanum and fluorescein-conjugated dextran (MW 40,000) to hairless mouse skin and treated the site with 15 MHz (0.1 W/cm^2) for 5 minutes. As before, the tracers were observed in intercellular "lacunae" at different levels of the stratum corneum (see Fig. 9). Electron microscopy of horizontal sections further revealed that the tracers were found within interconnected lacunae. It was suggested that sonophoresis may cause lipid-phase separation, thereby forming continuous channels that divide the lipid bilayers and amplify an intercellular transport pathway.

Laser Scanning Confocal Microscopy

In a more recent examination of sonophoretic delivery, Mitragotri et al. [75] employed confocal microscopy to characterize the ultrasound-enhanced trans-

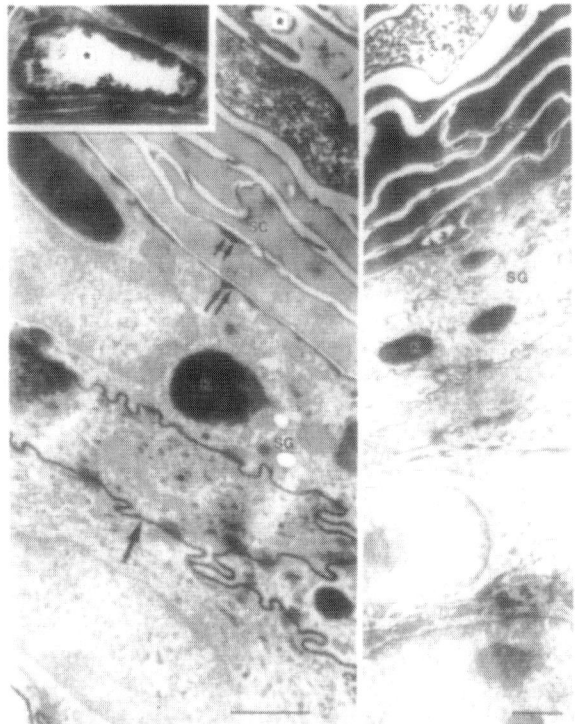

Figure 9 Electron micrograph demonstrating tracer penetration within the stratum corneum intercellular spaces (★) and at the SC–SG interface (→) following sonophoresis. The scale bar is 1 μm. (Reproduced with permission from Ref. 74.)

port of fluorescein. They hypothesized that ultrasound-induced cavitational effects produce increased oscillations of SC lipids, which, in turn, leads to increased structural disorder of SC lipids (and, thereby, to increased permeability). To test this hypothesis, a confocal assay was developed to evaluate the hydrogen peroxide–induced oxidation of fluorescein by measuring photobleaching of compound in the SC. Confocal microscopy was used to monitor the diminishing fluorescein concentration (fluorescence intensity) in the SC as a function of ultrasound exposure (see Fig. 10). It was concluded that loss of fluorescence is suggestive of cavitation as the dominant mechanism for sonophoretic enhancement. However, much more work is necessary to test this proposal.

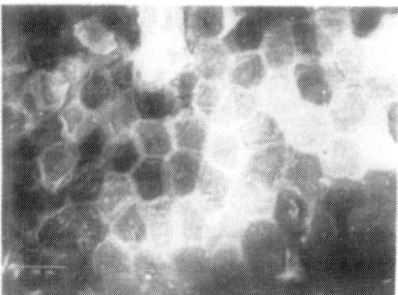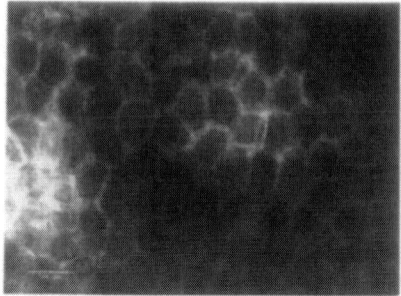

Figure 10 Confocal micrographs that show the diminishing fluorescein concentration (fluorescence intensity) in the SC as a function of ultrasound exposure. *Left—*heat-stripped human cadaver skin loaded with fluorescein. *Right—*skin exposed to ultrasound for 30 min. (Reproduced from Ref. 75.)

IV. SUMMARY

Visualization techniques have provided significant insights into the mechanism of passive and enhanced transdermal drug delivery. Studies utilizing light microscopy of radiolabeled and fluorescent compounds have contributed important information about the general distribution of topically applied substances throughout the structures of the epidermis and dermis. Light microscopy investigations have also been useful in indicating the role of skin appendages (i.e., hair follicles, sebaceous glands) in passive and electrically enhanced drug delivery, although limited resolution makes it difficult to distinguish intra- and intercellular environments.

Transmission, freeze-fracture, and scanning electron microscopy have contributed ultrastructural information about passive transport, particularly *within* the stratum corneum. Advances in fixation protocols for transmission electron microscopy have preserved the intercellular bilayers of the SC and have corrobrated their role in both passive and enhanced drug delivery. Scanning and freeze-fracture electron microscopy have supplemented transmission electron microscopy by supplying three-dimensional representations of the transport pathways within the SC.

Confocal and scanning electrochemical microscopy of fluorescent and electroactive species, respectively, have provided complementary information to that from the other microscopy techniques. Both these newer methods have the advantage of using the skin without fixation, thus avoiding possible artifacts associated with its chemical preservation. Confocal microscopy has improved our ability to localize fluorophores in the appendages, while scanning electrochemical microscopy has allowed simultaneously the measurement of flux and the visualization of ionic substances in real time. These methods have significantly increased our knowledge of the role of hair follicles and sebaceous glands in chemically and electrically enhanced drug delivery.

Ongoing optimization of visualization techniques will undoubtedly further elucidate the routes of molecular transport across the skin under varying conditions. Certainly, more research is required into the effects of the various enhancement methodologies on the structure of the skin, on the skin of subjects from varying age groups, and, most importantly, in humans in vivo. In conclusion, to advance our understanding of the mechanism of transport of substances in both passive and enhanced drug delivery, visualization studies are necessary for intelligently addressing the feasibility and optimization of current and future transdermal drug delivery methods.

ACKNOWLEDGMENTS

Financial support for L.B.N. was provided by a National Science Foundation Fellowship, and support for N.G.T. was provided by the U.S. National Institutes of Health (GM15585-03). Grant support was provided to both L.B.N. and N.G.T. on HD-27839 and DA-09292. We also owe a great debt of gratitude to Richard H. Guy and Yogeshvar N. Kalia for their critical and very helpful comments and suggestions about the manuscript.

REFERENCES

1. Scott, E. R., White, H. S. and Phipps, J. B. Direct imaging of ionic pathways in stratum corneum using scanning electrochemical microscopy. *Solid State Ionics 53–56*:176–183, 1992.
2. Scott, E. R., White, H. S. and Phipps, J. B. Iontophoretic transport through porous membranes using scanning electrochemical microscopy: Application to in vitro studies of ion fluxes through skin. *Anal. Chem. 65*:1537–1545, 1993.
3. Scott, E. R., Phipps, J. B. and White, H. S. Direct imaging of molecular transport through skin. *J. Invest. Dermatol. 104*:142–145, 1995.
4. Scott, E. R., White, H. S. and Phipps, J. B. Scanning electrochemical microscopy of a porous membrane. *J. Mem. Sci. 58*:71–87, 1991.
5. Cullander, C. and Guy, R. H. Sites of iontophoretic current flow into the skin: Identification and characterization with the vibrating probe electrode. *J. Invest. Derm. 97*:55–64, 1991.

6. Foskett, J. K. and Scheffey, C. Scanning electrode localization of transport pathways in epithelial tissues. In: *Methods in Enzymology.* New York, Academic Press, 1989, vol. 171, p. 792.

7. Strakosch, E. Studies on ointments. I. Penetration of various ointment bases. *J. Pharmacol. Exper. Ther. 78*:65–71, 1943.

8. Harry, R. Skin penetration. *Br. J. Derm. Syphilis. 53*:65–82, 1941.

9. Eller, J. and Wolff, S. Permeability and absorptivity of the skin. *Arch. Derm. Syphilology 40*:900–923, 1939.

10. Witten, V., Grayson, L. and Birnbaum, V. Studies of the mechanism of allergic eczematous contact dermatitis. I. Findings on human skin with radioactive bichloride of mercury. *J. Investigative Derm. 28*:339–346, 1957.

11. Bidmon, H. J., Pitts, J. D., Solomon, H. F., Bondi, J. V. and Stumpf, W. E. Estradiol distribution and penetration in rat skin after topical application, studies by high resolution autoradiography. *Histochem. 95*:43–54, 1990.

12. Conte, L., Ramis, J., Mis, R. et al. Percutaneous absorption and skin distribution of [14C]flutrimzaole in mini-pigs. *Arzneimittelforschung 42*(6):847–853, 1992.

13. Kao, J., Hall, J. and Helman, G. In vitro percutaneous absorption in mouse skin: Influence of skin appendages. *Tox. & App. Pharm. 94*:93–103, 1988.

14. Rutherford, T. and Black, J. G. The use of autoradiography to study the localization of germicides in skin. *Br. J. Derm. 81*(Suppl. 4):75–87, 1969.

15. Brody, I. Intercellular space in normal human stratum corneum. *Nature 209*:472–476, 1966.

16. Snell, R. Intercellular debris in the stratum corneum of the human epidermis. *J. Invest. Derm. 47*:698–702, 1966.

17. Wolff, K. and Schreiner, E. An electron microscopic study on the extraneous coat of keratinocytes and the intercellular space of the epidermis. *J. Invest. Derm. 51*:418–430, 1968.

18. Madison, K., Swartzendruber, D., Wertz, P. and Downing, D. Presence of intact intercellular lipid lamellae in the upper layers of the stratum corneum. *J. Invest. Derm. 88*:714–718, 1987.

19. Landmann, L. Epidermal permeability barrier: Transformation of lamellar granule-disks into intercellular sheets by a membrane-fusion process, a freeze-fracture study. *J. Invest. Derm. 87*:202–209, 1986.

20. Elias, P. and Friend, D. The permeability barrier in mammalian epidermis. *J. Cell. Bio. 65*:180–191, 1975.

21. Golden, G., Guzek, D., Harris, R., McKie, J. and Potts, R. Lipid thermotropic transitions in human stratum corneum. *J. Invest. Derm. 86*:255–259, 1986.

22. Friberg, S., Osborne, D. and Tombridge, T. X-ray diffraction of human stratum corneum. *J. Soc. Cosmet. Chem. 36*:349–354, 1985.

23. Bouwstra, J., Gooris, G., van der Spek, J. and Bras, J. Structural investigations of human stratum corneum by small angle x-ray scattering. *J. Invest. Derm. 97*:1005–1012, 1991.

24. Silberberg, I. Percutaneous absorption of mercury in man. *J. Invest. Derm.* 50:323–331, 1968.

25. King, C., Moore, N., Marks, R., and Nicholls, S. Preliminary studies into percorneal penetration and elemental content of the stratum corneum using x-ray microanalysis. *Arch. Derm. Res.* 263:257–265, 1978.

26. Nemanic, M. K., and Elias, P. M. In situ precipitation: A novel cytochemical technique for visualization of permeability pathways in mammalian stratum corneum. *J. Hist. & Cytochem.* 28(6):573–578, 1980.

27. Sharata, H. and Burnette, R. Effect of dipolar aprotic permeability enhancers on the basal stratum corneum. *J. Pharm. Sci.* 77:27–32, 1988.

28. Boddé, H. E., van der Brink, I., Koerten, H. K. and de Haan, F. H. N. Visualization of in vitro percutaneous penetration of mercuric chloride; transport through intercellular space versus cellular uptake through desmosomes. *J. Contr. Rel.* 15:227–236, 1991.

29. Neelissen, J., de Haan, F., Junginger, H. and Boddé, H. Microscopical visualization of transport routes of estradiol and norethindrone (acetate) across human stratum corneum in vitro. In *Prediction of Percutaneous Penetration.* Montpelier, 1993.

30. Nordquist, R., Olson, R. and Everett, M. The transport, uptake, and storage of ferritin in human epidermis. *Arch. Derm.* 94:482–490, 1966.

31. Squier, C. and Hopps, R. A study of the permeability barrier in epidermis and oral epithelium using horseradish peroxidase as a tracer in vitro. *Br. J. Derm.* 95:123–129, 1976.

32. Ongpipattanakul, B., Burnette, R., Potts, R. and Francoeur, R. Evidence that oleic acid exists in a separate phase within stratum corneum lipids. *Pharm. Res.* 8:350–354, 1991.

33. Potts, R. and Francoeur, M. Lipid biophysics of water loss through the skin. *Proc. Nat. Acad. Sci. U.S.A.* 87:3871–3873, 1990.

34. Golden, G. M., McKie, J. E. and Potts, R. O. Role of stratum corneum lipid fluidity in transdermal drug flux. *J. Pharm. Sci.* 76(1):25–28, 1987.

35. Potts, R. and Francoeur, M. The influence of stratum corneum morphology on water permeability. *J. Invest. Derm.* 96:495–499, 1991.

36. Cullander, C. and Guy, R. Visualization of iontophoretic pathways with confocal microscopy and the vibrating probe electrode. *Solid State Ionics 53–56*:197–206, 1992.

37a. Turner, N. G. and Guy, R. H. Confocal visualization and quantification of iontophoretic current pathways across mammalian skin, submitted.

37b. Turner, N. G. and Guy, R. H. Dependence of iontophoretic transport upon penetrant physicochemical properties, submitted.

37c. Turner, N. G., Ferry, L., Cullander, C. and Guy, R. H. Iontophoresis of poly-L-lysines: transport as a function of molecular weight measured by confocal microscopy, submitted.

38. Veiro, J. A. and Cummins, P. G. Imaging of skin epidermis from various origins using confocal laser scanning microscopy. *Derm. 189*:16–22, 1994.

39. Barry, B. Optimizing percutaneous absorption. In: B. Maibach, ed. *Percutaneous Absorption* 1989, pp. 531–554.

40. Barry, B. W. Mode of action of penetration enhancers in human skin. *J. Contr. Rel. 6*:85–97, 1987.

41. Sato, K., Timm, D. E., Sato, F. et al. Generation and transit pathway of H^+ is critical for inhibition of palmar sweating by iontophoresis in water. *J. Appl. Physiol. 75*(5):2258–2264, 1993.

42. Clemessy, M., Couarraze, G., Bevan, B. and Puisieux, F. Mechanisms involved in iontophoretic transport of angiotensin. *Pharm. Res. 12*(7):998–1002, 1995.

43. Su, M. H., Srinivasan, V., Ghanem, A. H. and Higuchi, W. I. Quantitative in vivo iontophoretic studies. *J. Pharm. Sci. 83*(1):12-7, 1994.

44. Wilhelm, K. P., Cua, A. B., Wolff, H. H. and Maibach, H. I. Surfactant-induced stratum corneum hydration in vivo: Prediction of the irritation potential of anionic surfactants. *J. Invest. Dermatol. 101*(3):310–315, 1993.

45. Lieb, L. M., Ramachandran, C., Egbaria, K. and Weiner, N. Topical delivery enhancement with multilamellar liposomes into pilosebaceous units: I. In vitro evaluation using fluorescent techniques with the hamster ear model. *J. Invest. Dermatol. 99*(1):108–113, 1992.

46. Boddé, H. E., Kruithof, M. A. M., Brussee, J. and Koerten H. K. Visualization of normal and enhanced $HgCl_2$ transport through human skin in vitro. *Int. J. Pharm. 53*:13–24, 1989.

47. Bouwstra, J., Pesschier, L., Brussee, J. and Boddé, H. Effect of *N*-alkyl-azoheptan-2-ones including azone on the thermal behavior of human stratum corneum. *Int. J. Pharmaceut. 52*:47–54, 1989.

48. Stoughton, R. Enhanced percutaneous penetration with 1-dodecylazocycloheptan-2-one. *Arch. Dermatol. 118*:474–477, 1982.

49. Bannerjee, P. and Ritschel, W. Transdermal permeation of vasopressin, II. Influence of azone on in vitro and in vivo permeation. *Int. J. Pharmaceut. 49*:199–204, 1989.

50. Hoogstraate, A., Verhoef, J., Burssee, J., IJzerman, A., Spies, F. and Boddé, H. Kinetics, ultrastructural aspects and molecular modelling of transdermal peptide flux enhancement by *N*-alkylazacycloheptanones. *Int. J. Pharmaceut. 76*:37–47, 1991.

51. Ogiso, T., Iwaki, M., Bechako, K. and Tsutsum, Y. Enhancement of percutaneous absorption by laurocapram. *J. Pharmaceut. Sci. 81*:762–767, 1992.

52. Lambert, W., Higuchi, W., Knutson, K. and Krill, S. Dose-dependent enhancement effects of azone on skin permeability. *Pharmaceut. Res. 6*:798–803, 1989.

53. Ogiso, T., Paku, T., Masahiro, I. and Tanino, T. Mechanism of the enhancement effect of *n*-octyl-β-D-thioglucoside on the transdermal penetration of fluorescein isothiocyanate-labeled dextrans and the molecular weight dependence of water-

soluble penetrants through stripped skin. *J. Pharmaceut. Sci. 83*:1676–1681, 1994.

54. Ogiso, T., Iwaki, M., Yoneda, I., Horinouchi, M. and Yamashita, K. Percutaneous absorption of elcatonin and hypocalcemic effect in rat. *Chem. Pharm. Bull. 39*:449–453, 1991.

55. Hofland, H. E., Bouwstra, J. A., Boddé, H. E., Spies, F. and Junginger, H. E. Interactions between liposomes and human stratum corneum in vitro: Freeze fracture electron microscopical visualization and small angle x-ray scattering studies. *Br. J. Dermatol. 132*(6):853–866, 1995.

56. Simonetti, O., Hoogstraate, A. J., Bialik, W., et al. Visualization of diffusion pathways across the stratum corneum of native and in-vitro-reconstructed epidermis by confocal laser scanning microscopy. *Arch. Dermatol. Res. 287*(5):465–473, 1995.

57. Abramson, H. and Engel, M. Skin Reactions. XII. Patterns produced in the skin by electrophoresis of dyes. *Arch. Dermatol. Syphilology 44*:190–200, 1942.

58. Grimnes, S. Pathways of ionic flow through human skin in vivo. *Acta Derm. Ven. (Stockh.) 64*:93–98, 1984.

59. Bronaugh, R. L., Stewart, R. F. and Congdon, E. R. Methods for in vitro percutaneous absorption studies. II. Animal models for human skin. *Toxicol. Appl. Pharmacol. 62*(3):481–488, 1982.

60. Monteiro-Riviere, N., Inman, A. and Riviere, J. Identification of the pathway of iontophoretic drug delivery: Light and ultrastructural studies using mercuric chloride in pigs. *Pharmaceut. Res. 11*:251–256, 1994.

61. Burnette, R. R. and Ongpipattanakul, B. Characterization of the pore transport properties and tissue alteration of excised human skin during iontophoresis. *J. Pharm. Sci. 77*(2):132–137, 1988.

62. Jadoul, A., Hanchard, D., Thysman, S. and Préat, V. Quantification and localization of fentanyl and TRH delivered by iontophoresis in the skin. *Int. J. Pharm. 120*:221–228, 1995.

63. Jaffe, L. F. and Nuccitelli, R. An ultrasensitive vibrating probe for measuring steady extracellular currents. *J. Cell. Bio. 63*:614–628, 1974.

64. Lee, C., Kwak, J. and Bard, A. J. Application of scanning electrochemical microscopy to biological samples. *Proc. Natl. Acad. Sci. 87*:1740–1743, 1990.

65. Scott, E. R., Laplaza, A. I., White, H. S. and Phipps, J. B. Transport of ionic species in skin: Contribution of pores to the overall skin conductance. *Pharm. Res. 10*(12):1699–1709, 1993.

66. Gadsby, P. D. Visualization of the barrier layer through iontophoresis of ferric ions. *Medical Instrumentation. 13*(5):281–283, 1979.

67. Benson, H., McElnay, J. and Harland, R. Use of ultrasound to enhance percutaneous penetration of benzydamine. *Phys. Ther. 69*:113–118, 1989.

68. McElnay, J., Matthews, M., Harland, R., and McCafferty, D. The effect of ultrasound on the percutaneous absorption of lignocaine. *Br. J. Clin. Pharmacol. 20*:421–424, 1985.

69. Bommannan, D., Okuyama, H., Stauffer, P. and Guy R. H. Sonophoresis. I. The use of high-frequency ultrasound to enhance transdermal drug delivery. *Pharm. Res.* 9(4):559–564, 1992.

70. Mitragotri, S., Blankschtein, D. and Langer, R. Ultrasound-mediated transdermal protein delivery. *Science* 269:850–853, 1995.

71. Tachibana, K. Transdermal delivery of insulin to alloxan-diabetic rabbits by ultrasound exposure. *Pharm. Res.* 9(7):952–954, 1992.

72. Bommannan, D., Menon, G. K., Okuyama, H., Elias, P. M. and Guy, R. H. Sonophoresis. II. Examination of the mechanism(s) of ultrasound-enhanced transdermal drug delivery. *Pharm. Res.* 9(8):1043–1047, 1992.

73. Hou, S., Mitra, A., White, S., Menon, G., Ghadially, R. and Elias, P. Membrane structure in normal and essential fatty acid-deficient stratum corneum: Characterization by ruthenium tetroxide staining and x-ray diffration. *J. Invest. Derm.* 86:215–223, 1991.

74. Menon, G. K., Bommannan, D. B. and Elias, P. M. High-frequency sonophoresis: Permeation pathways and structural basis for enhanced permeability. *Skin Pharmacol.* 7:130–139, 1994.

75. Mitragotri, S., Edwards, D. A., Blankschtein, D. and Langer, R. A mechanistic study of ultrasonically enhanced transdermal drug delivery. *J. Pharm. Sci.* 84(6):697–706, 1995.

2

X-Ray Analysis of the Stratum Corneum and Its Lipids

Joke A. Bouwstra and Gert S. Gooris
University of Leiden, Leiden, The Netherlands

Stephen H. White
University of California—Irvine, Irvine, California

I. INTRODUCTION

The rate-limiting step for the diffusion of most drugs through the skin occurs in the stratum corneum that forms the outermost layer of the skin. Although the corneocytes of the stratum corneum must play a role in limiting diffusion processes, the primary diffusion barrier is the intercellular lipid domains located between the corneocytes. Knowledge of the physical properties and molecular structure of these domains and of the corneocytes is essential for the development of strategies for the transdermal delivery of drugs. The most direct method for obtaining structural information about those lipids and proteins that are arranged in regular (repeating) arrays is by means of small- and wide-angle x-ray diffraction measurements. Small angle x-ray diffraction (SAXD) provides information about structural features with large repeat distances on the order of 50–150 Å (1 Å = 0.1 nanometer [nm]); wide-angle x-ray diffraction (WAXD) reports information from features with small repeat distances (typically 3–10 Å). SAXD and WAXD measurements have been used extensively for determining the structures and phase behavior of lipid and lipid–peptide mixtures and for obtaining structural information from biological membranes (Franks and Levine, 1981; Blaurock and Worthington, 1966). The primary structural element of biological membranes is the lipid bilayer, comprised principally of phospholipids (e.g., phosphatidylcholine) and cholesterol. Mixtures of these lipids dispersed in water or deposited from organic solvents on glass substrates commonly form multilamellar arrays of bilayers that are particularly suitable for diffraction studies. Figure 1 shows a schematic representation of the type of diffraction pattern obtained from multilayers comprised of bilayers with fluid alkyl chains oriented on a glass surface. SAXD measurements yield information about the structure in a direction normal to the bilayer plane, whereas WAXD provides information about the lateral packing of the lipids parallel to the bilayer plane. Unlike cell membranes, which consist of a single bilayer, the lipids of the stratum corneum are arranged naturally as multilamellar arrays that are quite amenable to diffraction studies. In further contrast to cell membranes, the major lipid components of the stratum corneum are ceramides, free fatty acids, cholesterol, and triglycerides (Wertz, et al., 1992; Lampe et al., 1983); phospholipids are virtually absent.

The first x-ray studies of the horny layer (stratum corneum, SC) of the skin were carried out by Swanbeck in 1959 (Swanbeck and Thyresson, 1962; Swanbeck and Thyresson, 1961; Swanbeck, 1959) using tissue obtained from the sole of the human foot and from patients suffering from ichthyoses and psoriasis. In 1973, Wilkes et al. (1973) examined the structure of human and neonatal rat stratum corneum using WAXD and thermal analysis. Although these pioneering studies clearly demonstrated the feasibility of obtaining important structural information using diffraction methods, no further work was reported until Friberg and Osborne (1985) published a brief account of SAXD studies of human stratum corneum and White et al. (1988) described a detailed SAXD and WAXD investigation of intact SC, extracted lipids, and isolated "couplets" (corneocyte envelopes plus intercellular domains) from hairless mice. Very recently, human stratum corneum has been investigated by two groups (Bouwstra et al., 1992b; Bouwstra et al., 1991; Garson et al., 1991) using a synchrotron radiation source that improves the quality of the diffraction patterns. Mouse stratum corneum has been reinvestigated by Bouwstra et al. (1994), who also reported the first studies of the lipid structure of pig stratum corneum (Bouwstra et al., 1995a).

The primary goal of this chapter is to review comprehensively the x-ray diffraction literature concerned with normal, diseased, and penetration-enhancer-treated skin. Because diffraction methods have not been widely utilized in SC structural studies until rather recently, we begin the chapter with a review of the basic principles of diffraction not only as an aid to the reader but also to encourage others to consider the possibility of using x-ray diffraction as means of studying the stratum corneum and its lipids.

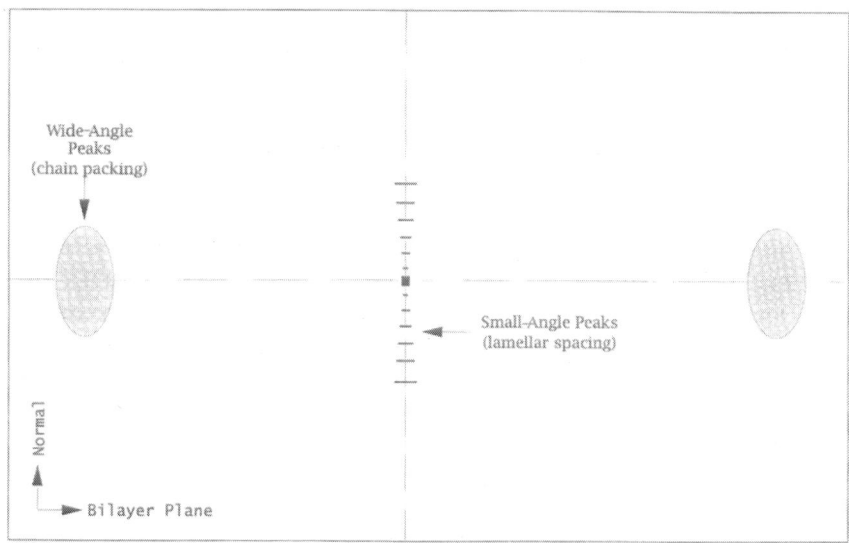

Figure 1 Schematic representation of a "typical" diffraction pattern from an oriented lamellar lipid structure. The x-ray beam producing the pattern is normal to the page, with the lamellae roughly parallel to the beam and the horizontal (equator) so that the lipid alkyl chains are vertical (meridian). The position of the beam is marked by the small square in the center of the pattern, which represents the beam stopper that absorbs the direct beam to prevent overexposure of the x-ray film. Repeating structures with small spacings produce diffraction spots at large angles (far from the beam), while those with large spacings produce spots at small angles (close to the beam) because of Bragg's Law. The centerlines of the lipid alkyl chains are typically 4–5 Å apart and diffract at large angles. Because fluid chains are disordered (variable spacing), the diffraction spots are broad and "fuzzy." Because the chains are oriented roughly normal to the equator, the diffraction lies along the equator. The spacings between the horizontal lamellae are typically 50–100 Å and yield diffraction spots (lines) at equal intervals along the meridian described by Bragg's Law because of constructive interference due to the regular lattice. The six lines on either side of the beam are assigned integer values beginning with 1 that correspond to the Bragg order n (Eq. 3) of the diffraction peak. Note that the small-angle lines become progressively wider as n increases. This is due to the so-called orientational disorder arising from fluctuations of the lamellae around the horizontal plane (see Fig. 3). If the lamellae are perfectly horizontal, all spots are circular because they are images of the incident beam. The type of experimental arrangement that produces the diffraction pattern is shown in Fig. 4.

II. GENERAL PRINCIPLES OF STRUCTURE DETERMINATION BY X-RAY DIFFRACTION

The general principles of x-ray diffraction are described well in a number of standard texts (Rhodes, 1993; Woolfson, 1970; Warren, 1969). We focus here on the essential ideas necessary for understanding diffraction from the stratum corneum. The x-rays incident on a sample interact with the electron clouds of the sample's molecules and are scattered onto a detector, such as photographic film, that records the positions and intensities of the scattered x-rays. The recorded x-ray diffraction pattern is determined by molecular geometry and electron density of the sample. The maximum possible amplitudes of the scattered x-rays are directly proportional to the electron densities of the scattering centers of the structure. However, the intensity of the x-rays observed at a particular position on the detector is determined by constructive and destructive interference of x-rays scattered from different parts of the sample's "unit cell." (The unit cell is the basic three-dimensional pattern of molecules that can be used to reproduce the entire lattice comprising the sample by repetitive translations along the x-, y-, and z-coordinates.) These interference effects arise directly from phase differences of the scattered x-rays caused by the differences in spatial position of the atoms in the unit cell. X-ray measurements take place over a time period that is large compared to the time scale of molecular motions, so the diffraction pattern can only provide information about the time-averaged electron density distribution of the sample.

The diffraction pattern of the scattered x-rays, including intensities, can be calculated from the electron density distribution of the sample by means of Fourier transforms. Equation 1 shows the calculation of the structure factors $F(hkl)$ for an orthorhombic unit cell of dimensions $a \times b \times c$ from the electron density $\rho(x,y,z)$ and the exponential phase-factor term. The integers h, k, and l specify the order of the diffraction peaks and are related to the Miller indices that specify the reflecting planes within the crystal producing the diffraction spots (vide infra). An observed intensity I is calculated from $I = F(hkl)F(hkl)* = |F(hkl)|^2$, where

$$F(hkl) = \iiint \rho(x,y,z)e^{\,2\pi i\,(hx/a + ky/b + lz/c)}\,dV \tag{1}$$

The sample's structure (i.e., electron density distribution) can be calculated by inverse Fourier transformation using the amplitudes [i.e., the $F(hkl)$] and phase factors (the exponential term) of the scattered x-rays using Eq. 2:

$$\rho(x,y,z) = \frac{1}{V} \sum_{h=-\infty}^{\infty} \sum_{k=-\infty}^{\infty} \sum_{l=-\infty}^{\infty} F(hkl)e^{-2\pi i\,(hx/a + ky/b + lz/c)} \tag{2}$$

Unfortunately, the measured intensities of the scattered x-rays are devoid of the phase information that is essential for calculating the structure. This is the so-called "phase problem," whose solution generally requires special methods. It is simplified when the molecular geometry of the sample (the unit cell) is centrosymmetric [i.e., $\rho(x,y,z) = \rho(-x,-y,-z)$] because then the phase angles, which in general range from 0 to 2π radians, are restricted to 0 or π, so the $F(hkl)$ have phases of $+1$ or -1. Fortunately, most bilayer structures are centrosymmetric, so the phase problem is greatly simplified.

The determination of a molecular structure in crystalline form involves measuring the intensities of the scattered x-rays, determining phases, and iteratively constructing model structures whose calculated intensities agree within experimental error to the observed intensities. The calculated intensities converge to the measured ones as the models converge to the correct structure. A primary requirement for this method is knowledge of the composition of the unit cell, including the atomic compositions of the constitutent molecules. This approach has been used successfully for determining the structures of phospholipids in a crystalline state (Pascher et al. 1992). However, most natural lipid systems do not satisfy all of the requirements for crystallographic refinement.

A major problem with cell membranes is that they naturally exist only as a single bilayer rather than as ordered arrays. Although one can in principle determine the structure of a specimen only one unit cell thick, this is generally impractical. Fortunately, some membrane systems, such as nerve myelin (Franks et al. 1982; Franks and Levine, 1981; Blaurock, 1982) and the intercellular lipid domains of SC (Bouwstra et al. 1991; White et al. 1988), naturally form multilamellar arrays that can be treated as one-dimensional "crystals." The structure in the plane of the layer cannot be generally determined because the lipids may be in disordered fluid state or, if in a crystalline or gel state, have no preferred orientation relative to the layer normal. In such cases "the structure" consists of the projection of the electron densities of the constituent molecules onto an axis normal to the plane of the layers. Such a structure is referred to as an *electron density profile*. Under certain circumstances, one can carry out a crystallographic-type refinement procedure for simple fluid bilayer systems that leads to the time-averaged transbilayer distribution of the principal lipid structural groups that make up the profile (Wiener and White, 1991a; Wiener and White, 1991b).

An additional major problem with natural membrane systems is that the composition of the one-dimensional unit cell may be unknown because of the presence of proteins of unknown structure and composition. Nevertheless, it is possible to model the electron density profile of a multilamellar system to arrive at a crude model for the distribution of lipids and proteins. The models improve considerably if the lipid composition and lipid structures are known. In any case, the basic crystallographic structural method is used: The model is refined on the basis of comparisons between the calculated and the experimentally determined intensities through an iterative process.

III. ORIGIN AND CHARACTERISTICS OF THE DIFFRACTION PATTERN

As an example, consider a specimen with atoms arranged in a regular pattern to form a lattice as shown in Fig. 2. Some of the incident x-rays that pass through this lattice scatter from the atoms as spherical waves. These waves have a fixed phase relationship, so in certain directions in space they add constructively while in others they add destructively. This causes the diffracted x-rays to be observed in only certain directions. Although the mathematical description of the spatial distribution of these diffracted intensities can be quite complex in general (Warren, 1969), the basic principle is easily understood for the simple situation depicted in Fig. 2. It is important to recognize that two coordinate systems are present: One of is that of the laboratory defined by the axis of the x-ray beam, and the other is the coordinate system of the sample defined by its crystal lattice. The lattice in Fig. 2 consists of atoms separated by a distance a along the x-axis and a distance b along the y-axis. This two-dimensional lattice represents the layout of the atoms on the xy-plane passed through an orthorhombic crystal, with atoms separated along the z-axis (normal to the plane of the page) with a spacing c. We associate with the x-, y-, and z-axes integers h, k, and l specifying the diffraction orders and Miller indices associated with those directions. A plane encompassing any three atoms defines a lattice plane that is one member of a family of parallel planes separated from one another by a fixed distance d determined by the lattice parameters a, b, and c. Constructive interference will be observed when the chosen lattice planes make an angle θ (with respect to the x-ray beam) defined by Bragg's law

$$2d \sin \theta = n\lambda \tag{3}$$

where d is the separation between the planes, λ is wavelength of the x-rays (typically 1.54 Å), and n is an integer specifying the "order" of the diffraction peak. Because so many different families of planes exist, constructive interference will be observed in many different (but not arbitrary) directions as the crystal is rotated with respect to the incident beam. Indeed, the diffraction experiment involves the systematic rotation of the crystal in the x-ray beam to produce as many diffraction peaks as possible. Bragg's law (Eq. 3) is illustrated in Fig. 2, where two sets of planes (normal to page) have been constructed. The set shown in Fig. 2A passes through each layer of atoms in the direction of the x-axis and are thus separated by the distance $d = b$. The other set of planes, shown in Fig. 2B, pass through atoms offset from one another by one lattice constant in the x- and y-directions. One can easily show that in this case the separation of the planes is $d = ab/\sqrt{a^2 + b^2}$.

For constructive interference to occur from the set of planes in Fig. 2A, the difference in the path length $2s = 2d \sin \theta$ between x-rays scattered from the atom marked A and the atom marked B must be an integral multiple of the wavelength λ as given by Eq. 3. Thus, a diffraction peak will be observed when the lattice plane makes an angle defined by $\theta_1 = \arcsin (\lambda/2b)$. This is the so-called first-order diffraction peak, because $n = k = 1$. The second-order peak ($n = k = 2$) will be observed when $\theta_2 = \arcsin (2\lambda/2b)$, as shown by the dashed rays in Fig. 2A. Because the x-ray beam is fixed in space, this second peak can be observed only by rotating the crystal relative to the beam. An alternate way of expressing θ_2 is as $\arcsin [\lambda/2(b/2)]$, which would be equivalent to a first-order diffraction from planes with a spacing of $b/2$. We may in general think of the nth-order diffraction peak as arising from hypothetical planes separated by a distance d/n, where d is the true separation of the physical planes in the crystal. The hypothetical planes are described formally by Miller indices $(h/n,k/n,l/n)$, and the plane under discussion has Miller indices (010), so $k/n = 1$. The hkl indices are usually used in the definition of the spacing between planes so that here we have been discussing the distances $d(0k0)$ between the (010) planes.

Three additional concepts may be introduced by means of Fig. 2A. First, all measurements of the diffracted beams are made relative to the incident x-ray beam so that the diffracted beam leaves the crystal at an angle 2θ, as illustrated. Thus, while the diffraction condition is determined by the angle between the incident and diffracted beams relative to a lattice plane, the *measured* position of the diffracted beam is determined relative to the incident beam. Second, there is a *reciprocal* relation between the spacing between lattice planes and the positions of the diffraction spots; small lattice spacings give diffraction spots with large values of 2θ. This leads to two types of "space." The crystal coordinate system is in "real space," whereas the diffrac-

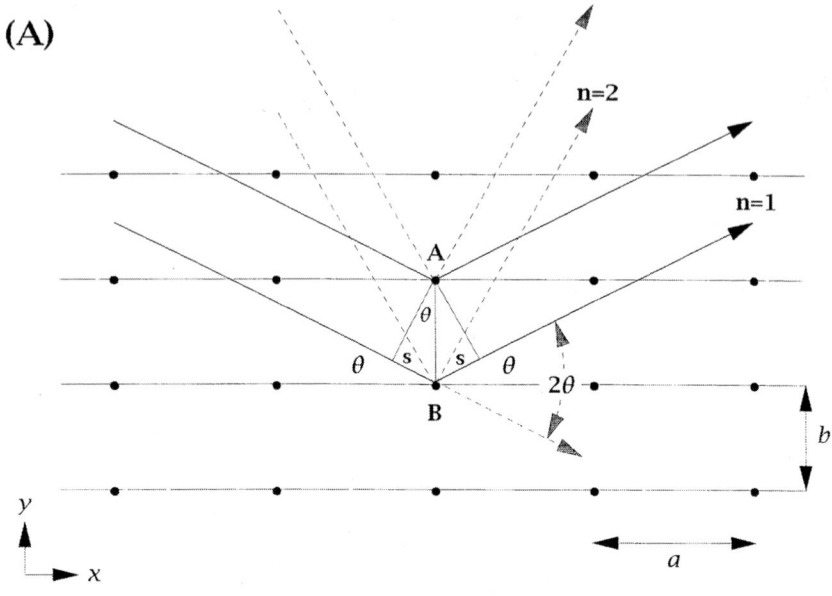

(A)

(B)

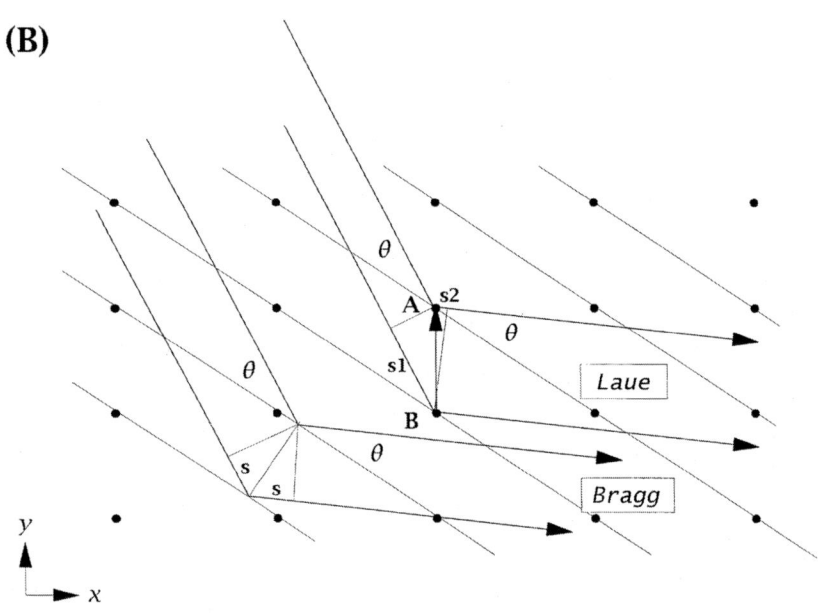

Figure 2 Principles of the diffraction x-rays from a crystal lattice. The dots represent atoms arranged on a rectangular lattice with unit cell dimensions $a \times b$. (A) Illustration

tion pattern seen in the laboratory coordinate system is in "reciprocal space." The measured intensities may be plotted as a function of angle (θ), but it is more common to plot them as a function of the magnitude of the reciprocal lattice vector $S = (2 \sin \theta)/\lambda$ [equal to $1/d(hkl)$ at the diffraction maxima] or the magnitude of the wave vector $Q = 2\pi S = (4\pi \sin \theta)/\lambda$ [equal to $2\pi/d(hkl)$ at the diffraction maxima]. Third, diffraction occurs because of intereference between x-rays scattered from atoms. Note, however, that the diffraction geometry shown applies anywhere along the lattice planes, so the mathematics are unchanged by translating the geometrical arrangement to any arbitrary position along the lattice planes that does not include any atoms.

In the Bragg formulation of diffraction we thus refer to reflections from lattice planes and can ignore the positions of the atoms. The Laue formulation of diffraction, on the other hand, considers only diffraction from atoms but can be shown to be equivalent to the Bragg formulation. The two formulations are compared in Fig. 2B for planes with Miller indices (110). What is important in diffraction is the difference in path length between x-rays scattered from two atoms. The distance $s1 + s2$ in the Laue formulation is the same as the distance $2s$ shown for the Bragg formulation. The Laue approach is by far the more useful one for complicated problems and leads to the concept of the *reciprocal lattice* (Blaurock, 1982; Warren, 1969) and the reciprocal lattice vector $\vec{S} = \vec{Q}/4\pi$ that makes it possible to create a representation of the crystal lattice in reciprocal space.

The structure factors used in the determination of a model structure and the unit cell dimensions and space group are derived from diffraction patterns

---

of Bragg's law in which the layers of atoms are viewed as diffracting planes arranged so that the planes form an angle θ with the incident and reflected beams. The beams reflected from successive layers are out of phase by an amount $2s$, so constructive interference is obtained for values of θ for which $2s = \lambda$ (the wavelength of the x-rays; typically 1.54 Å). For the arrangement shown, $s = b \sin \theta$, so $2b \sin \theta = \lambda$ (Bragg's law). Constructive interference occurs whenever the sample is oriented relative to the beam such that $2s = n\lambda$ ($n = 1$, 2, 3, etc.). Thus, Bragg's law becomes $2b \sin \theta = n\lambda$. For bilayer diffraction with $b \approx 50$ Å, $\theta \approx 1°$, so $\sin \theta \approx \theta$. This results in Bragg's law's being satisfied at integral multiples of θ and results in the regular spacing of diffraction lines shown in Fig. 1 (B). Illustration of Laue's more realistic and versatile view of the diffraction condition in which diffraction occurs by scattering of x-rays from individual atoms rather than hypothetical planes. In this case, constructive interference occurs when $s1 + s2 = n\lambda$. A different set of diffraction planes has been chosen here to illustrate that the Bragg condition can be satisfied by any set of parallel planes that can be constructed from the atoms on the lattice.

recorded on film or some other detector. The structure factor amplitudes are obtained from the square root of the intensities after they are corrected for geometrical effects (Blaurock, 1982) and the unit cell information from the symmetries and spacings of the patterns.

In addition to this information, however, the diffraction pattern also provides information on the quality of the crystal lattice and the thermal motion of the atoms in the unit cell. Figure 3 shows examples of the diffraction patterns that would be observed under various circumstances for the lattice shown in Fig. 2. The examples assume diffraction from the (010) and (100) planes of the lattice that are, respectively, planes parallel to the xz-plane (Fig. 2A) and yz-plane (not shown). A diffraction pattern for a crystalline sample is recorded by rotating a crystal in the x-ray beam to record systematically the reflections from the various lattice planes. To see the diffracted intensities for the example under consideration, the crystal would be mounted with its z-axis parallel to the x-ray beam and then rotated about the x-axis to obtain reflections from the (010) planes with spacings of $d(0k0)$ and about the y-axis to obtain reflections from the (100) planes with spacings of $d(h00)$. All of the reflections are recorded on a single "frame" of a two-dimensional detector or a single piece of photographic film.

The diffraction pattern obtained for a "perfect" crystal shown in Fig. 3A can be interpreted as follows. First, the arrays of spots are orthogonal because the crystal is orthorhombic. Second, the spots tend to be evenly spaced for small angles because $\sin\theta \approx \theta = n\lambda/d$. Third, the spots themselves are images of the x-ray beam deflected from the z-axis according to Bragg's law and, ignoring details such as sample size, will all have the same spatial distribution on the detector surface if the crystal is perfect. Perfection is rarely achieved in crystals and in some cases is even undesirable (Warren, 1969). Most crystals are in reality made up of a mosaic of many small crystals that are slightly disoriented with respect to one another. That is, their x-, y-, and z-axes are not perfectly parallel, so each small crystal in the mosaic diffracts slightly off-axis. As a result, the diffraction pattern can be smeared slightly into circular arcs, as shown in Fig. 3B. An extreme case is shown in Fig. 3C. Here the sample is composed of a crystal that has been shattered into a powder, causing all orientations to be present. This example is inaccurate, however, because only the (010) and (100) reflections are shown. If all orientations are present in the beam, then one would also see reflections from other lattice planes as well. Note in Fig. 3A, B, and C that the widths of the diffraction peaks along the x- and y-axes remain narrow and are the same for all the spots. This means that although the crystal

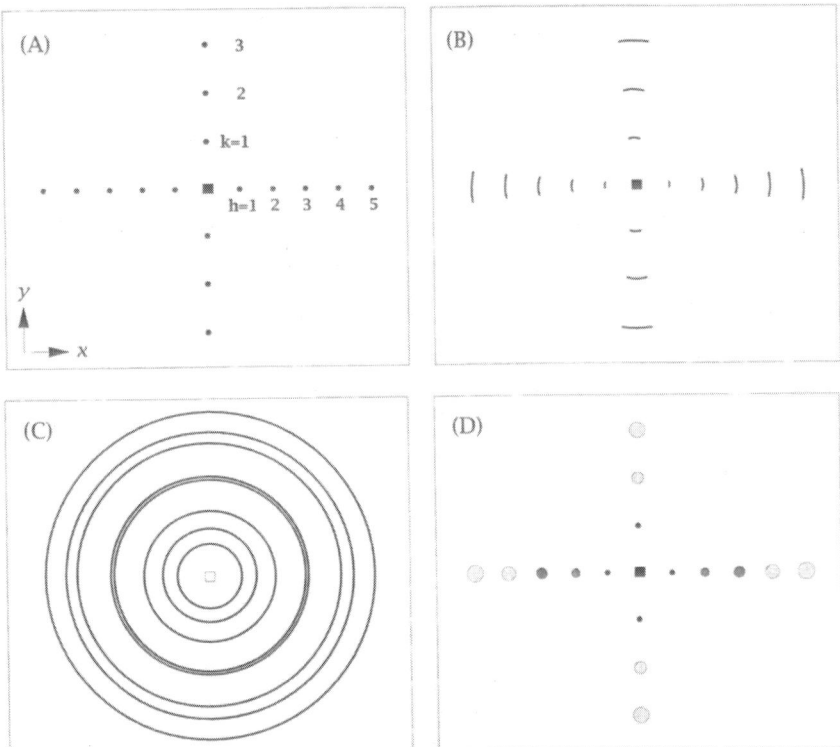

Figure 3 Schematic representations of diffraction patterns from samples with various characteristics. (A) Diffraction from a perfect lattice corresponding to the rectangular arrangement of atoms shown in Fig. 2. The x-ray beam is normal to the plane of the paper. Diffraction orders $k = 1, 2, 3, \ldots$ are obtained by rotating the crystal around the x-axis and orders $h = 1, 2, 3, \ldots$ by rotating the crystal around the y-axis. (B) Most real crystals actually consist of a "mosaic" of smaller crystals that are slightly disoriented relative to one another. This results in a smearing of the spots into arcs. This is an example of orientational disorder. (C) The extreme case of orientational disorder in which the crystal is broken up into many small fragments that are randomly disordered over a 360° range so that the arcs in B become full circles. This situation occurs in powdered crystals and is therefore called a *powder diffraction pattern*. (D) In this case, the spacing between points on the lattice is irregular, so Bragg's law is satisfied over a range of angles. This results in a progressive broadening of the lines as the diffraction order increases.

is a mosaic, the small crystals comprising it are nearly perfect in terms of the quality of the lattice.

Poor crystals have imperfect lattices that are basically attributable to variations in the composition of the unit cell, which cause the $d(hkl)$ spacings to vary throughout the crystal. These variations destroy long-range order in the crystal and lead to a broadening of the diffraction peaks as a function of the order of diffraction, as illustrated in Fig. 3D. A simple way of understanding this effect is to imagine that each small crystal of the mosaic had slightly different lattice spacings. This would cause the diffraction spots from each to have slightly different spacings along the x- and y-axes so that the observed patterns are an amalgamation of these different spacings. If one of these hypothetical small crystals has a first-order peak at θ while another one has a first-order peak at $\theta + \Delta\theta$, the differences in spacing progressively increase by $n \cdot \Delta\theta$ as n increases. Therefore, as shown in Fig. 3C, the spots will progressively increase in size with n. An important consequence of this is that the intensity is spread over an increasingly large area, and for sufficiently large n eventually disappears into the background noise. The higher-order diffraction peaks will be lost. Because they are essential for an accurate structural model, the resulting structures will be underresolved and therefore inaccurate.

Another effect that can be observed in the diffraction patterns is disorder due to the thermal motion of the atoms in the unit cell. This disorder is independent of lattice defects and arises from the thermal fluctuations of the atoms around their mean positions and is an inherent feature of the molecules under investigation. The effect on the diffraction pattern is a steady decrease in amplitude with increasing diffraction order without any changes in the widths of the spots along the x- and y-axes. This effect is best understood by means of a simple example.

Consider an atom at some position in the unit cell. Its electron density projected onto one of the axes, say, the x-axis, will have the shape of a Gaussian curve:

$$\rho(x) = \frac{b}{A\sqrt{\pi}} \exp\left\{ -\left[\frac{(x - X_1)}{A} \right]^2 \right\} \tag{4}$$

where b is the scattering length related to the number of electrons, X_1 is the mean position of the atom, and A is the $1/e$ half-width of the distribution that describes the time-averaged fluctuation of the atom around its mean position. The structure factors from this atom can be calculated by Fourier transforming Eq. 4:

$$F(h) = 2b \exp\left[-\left(\frac{\pi A h}{d}\right)^2\right] \cos\left(\frac{2\pi X_1 h}{d}\right) \tag{5}$$

The structure factor, whose square gives the intensity of the diffraction peak, is composed of three terms. The first is the scattering length (i.e., electron density) and the third is the cosine term that is the magnitude of the Fourier component. The second term in the equation is a negative exponential that dampens the magnitude of the structure factor due to the thermal motion described here by the $1/e$ half-width, A. If A is small, then the exponential term is close to 1 and there will be little damping. As A increases, however, the damping term becomes rapidly smaller, causing the structure factor to decrease in size. As an example, if $A = 1$ Å (approximately the radius of an atom), then one can expect to observe about 25–30 orders of diffraction in a typical experiment. If $A = 3$ Å, then only 8–10 orders of diffraction can be observed, as discussed in detail by Wiener and White (1991a). This exponential term is the so-called thermal factor and the exponent $(\pi A h/d)^2$ is referred to as the "B factor" because the thermal factor is usually written $\exp(-B)$.

Although the effects of thermal motion might be considered undesirable in crystallography, they provide, in fact, important information about the properties of the molecules under study (see, for example, Finzel et al., 1984). In terms of refining a crystal structure, the structure factors calculated assuming the atoms to be rigidly fixed on the lattice will be too large compared to the observed structure factors. The thermal factors for each atom reduce the sizes of the calculated structure factors by an amount appropriate for the thermal motion present.

This discussion has shown that the diffraction pattern can reveal three types of disorder, as discussed fully by several authors (Wiener and White, 1991a; Blaurock, 1982; Hosemann and Bagchi, 1962). Thermal disorder is generally referred to as *disorder of the first kind* and lattice disorder as *disorder of the second kind*. The disorder due to the mosaic nature of the sample is referred to as *orientational disorder*. Thermal disorder and small amounts of orientational disorder are not particularly troublesome in the diffraction experiment. Lattice disorder, on the other hand, can be extremely problematic because one can never achieve a fully resolved image of the structure since there are too few structure factors available to obtain a faithful model. Thermal disorder simply means that the position of the atoms are "smeared" in some fashion, determined by the equation of state of the molecules. If the lattice is excellent so that all of the structure factors observable within the limits of the thermal motion are obtained experimentally, the resulting model will be a faithful representation of the molecules, *including* their thermal motion.

IV. DIFFRACTION MEASUREMENTS ON BILAYER SYSTEMS

A. Diffraction from Bilayers

The stratum corneum, nerve myelin, collagen, and keratin are examples of partially ordered systems that lack long-range order in all three dimensions that is necessary for standard crystallographic analysis. Alpha-keratin, for example, is composed, in part, of bundles of α-helices arranged as coiled coils (Fraser and MacRae, 1973), much like a rope. The problems are that the coiled coils are frequently interrupted by nonhelical regions, the patterns of amino acids along the lengths of the polypeptide sequences are not uniformly repetitious, and the amino acid repeating units in the individual chains are not in register with one another. There is sufficient order and repetition to obtain diffraction patterns, but it is insufficient for obtaining the level of detail we have come to expect in protein crystallography. Highly specialized and technically demanding methods are required to extract useful structural information from fiber systems and have been useful for examining the structure of hard keratins (Fraser and MacRae, 1973). Lipid bilayer and cell membrane systems are a class of partially ordered systems that is particularly relevant to studies of the stratum corneum intercellular lipid domains. These systems form multilamellar arrays that produce good diffraction patterns (Fig. 1) in at least one dimension (normal to the lamellae) that can be analyzed in a relatively straightforward manner to obtain electron density profiles of the individual bilayers.

Bilayer systems in vitro are generally examined either as bulk dispersions in water, in which case powder diffraction patterns are obtained (Fig. 3C), or as oriented multilamellar arrays. The methods of analysis are similar in both cases, but oriented systems are preferred because one has a better chance of seeing the highest-order diffraction peaks since the diffracted intensity is concentrated into a smaller area on the detector. The disadvantage of oriented systems is that they are easiest to work with at low hydration, although excellent (but technically demanding) methods exist for studying them in excess water (Smith et al., 1990). The classic bilayer diffraction experiment using oriented multilamellar arrays of fluid phospholipids that produces diffraction patterns like that shown in Fig. 1 is illustrated in Fig. 4 and serves as the basic paradigm. The closely spaced sharp lines along the meridian in Fig. 1 are due to the small angle diffraction normal to the bilayer

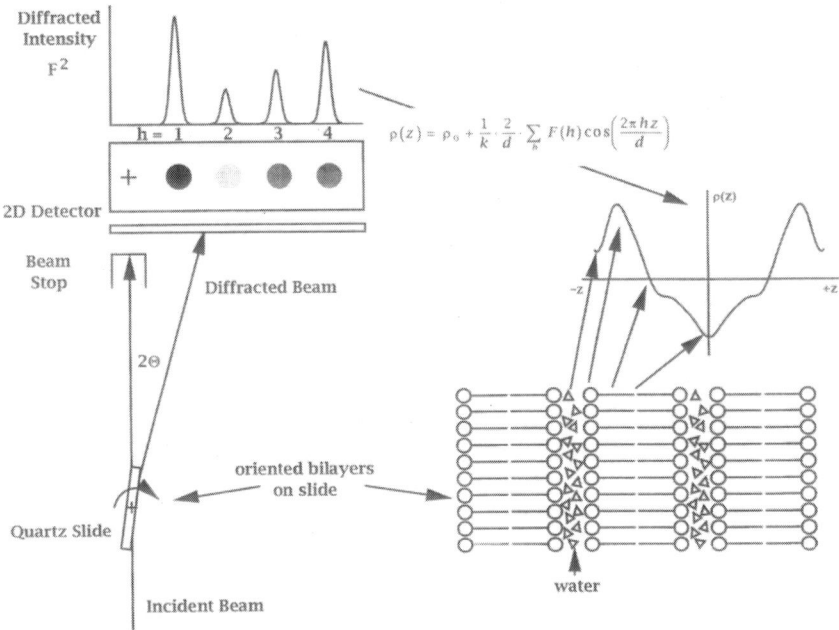

$$p(z) = p_0 + \frac{1}{k} \cdot \frac{2}{d} \cdot \sum_h F(h) \cos\left(\frac{2\pi h z}{d}\right)$$

Figure 4 Summary of the method for obtaining the structure of a bilayer from an oriented multilamellar sample. The diffraction pattern (shaded circles) is that expected from a multibilayer sample oriented perfectly parallel to the glass slide that is rotated in the x-ray beam. The intensities of the spots are proportional to square of the structure factors $F(h)$, which causes the phases (+1 or −1 in this case; see text) to be lost. If the phases can be determined, then the electron density profile $p(z)$ can be determined by Fourier transformation, as shown. The correlations of the peaks and valleys of $p(z)$ with the features of the bilayer are illustrated. This figure is based upon Fig. 1 of an article by White et al. (1986).

plane and typically correspond to a repeat period of about 50 Å. The broad, diffuse peaks along the equator are due to the highly disordered fluid alkyl chains and are centered at spacings corresponding to 4.5–4.6 Å. The fact that the wide-angle and small-angle patterns lie along perpendicular lines demonstrates the existence of the bilayer with acyl chains normal to the plane of the bilayer. If the bilayer is in a gel state, these diffuse peaks are replaced by single sharp lines corresponding to a spacing of 4.2 Å arising from a more orderly hexagonal packing arrangement of the alkyl chains. The chains may also assume a number of different crystalline packing arrangements that form characteristic rectangular or oblique subcells. The different subcells and the packing arrangements of the alkyl chains have been described in detail by Abrahamsson et al. (1978) and Small (1986).

An electron density profile for a bilayer system can be obtained from the diffracted intensities by Fourier transformation (Eq. 1), as illustrated in Fig. 4. Fluid bilayers have a great deal of thermal motion, so the resulting profiles (Fig. 4) have smooth, broad peaks. Although thermal motion precludes the possibility of atomic level resolution, basic information on the location of headgroups and water is easily obtained. More detailed images of bilayers that describe the transbilayer distributions of the principal structural groups of the lipids can be obtained using neutron diffraction (Büldt et al., 1979; Zaccai et al., 1979) or a combination of x-ray and neutron diffraction (Wiener and White, 1992). Neutron diffraction is useful because of the large difference in the scattering strength of hydrogen and deuterium (Schoenborn, 1975) that permits specific atoms or groups of atoms to be identified through specific deuteration.

B. The Relationship Between Electron Density and Diffraction Pattern

The most important goal of the membrane or bilayer diffraction experiment is to obtain the electron density profile of the membrane. Although one most often uses multilamellar arrays of membranes, one can in some cases obtain diffraction patterns for single bilayers prepared as unilamellar vesicles (Lewis and Engelman, 1983; Wilkins et al., 1971). It is important to understand the relationship between diffraction patterns obtained from single bilayers and from bilayers in stacks because the pattern can be strongly affected if the number N of repeating units is small ($N < 10$). The intercellular lipid domains of the SC frequently have a small number of repeating units (Hou et al., 1991). The small-angle diffraction pattern for a single bilayer consists of a continuous scattering curve rather than a series of discrete diffraction spots. That is, the observed intensity I is a continuous function of the scattering angle θ. Recalling that $Q = 2\pi S = 2\pi \cdot 2 \sin \theta / \lambda$, $I(Q)$ may be calculated from the electron density $\rho(x)$ of a single membrane from

$$F_m(Q) = \int_0^d \rho(x) e^{iQx}\, dx \qquad (6)$$

where d is the thickness of the bilayer and $F_m(Q)$ is the continuous Fourier transform (structure factor) of the electron density. The intensity observed in the scattering experiment is obtained from

$$I(Q) = F_m(Q) \cdot F_m(Q)* = |F_m(Q)|^2 \qquad (7)$$

where $F_m(Q)*$ is the complex conjugate. The process of squaring the continuous Fourier transform removes the phase information that is necessary for reconstructing the electron density from the intensity (vide infra). In principle, however, it is possible to obtain the electron density profile unambiguously from the continuous scattering curve of a single membrane under some circumstances (Franks and Levine, 1981; Blaurock, 1982).

A membrane diffraction pattern with discrete rather than continuous intensities results when the membranes are stacked together to form a multi-lamellar array. The electron density of the array can be described by the function

$$\rho(x + nd) = \rho(x), \quad n = 1, 2, \ldots N - 1 \qquad (8)$$

for $0 \leq x \leq d$, where d is the thickness of a single bilayer. The structure factor function for the array is the sum of the $F_m(Q)$ for each membrane in the array and may be written as (Franks and Levine, 1981)

$$F(Q) = \left\{ \sum_{n=0}^{N-1} e^{iQnd} \right\} F_m(Q) \qquad (9)$$

The term in brackets is referred to as the *interference function* and may be written (Franks and Levine, 1981)

$$G(Q) = e^{\frac{iQ \cdot (N-1)d}{2}} \left[\frac{\sin(NQd/2)}{\sin(Qd/2)} \right] \qquad (10)$$

This function will have maxima when all terms in the series have a value of $+1$, which occurs only when $Qnd/2\pi = m$, with $m = 0, \pm 1, \pm 2$, etc. Because both n and m are integers, this equation will be satisfied for all n if $Qd/2\pi$ is also an integer:

$$\frac{Qd}{2\pi} = h, \quad h = 0, \pm 1, \pm 2, \ldots \qquad (11)$$

This is simply a restatement of Bragg's law, since $(Q/2\pi)d = Sd = 2s \sin \theta / \lambda$. The interference function for a stack of membranes will thus consist of a series of sharp peaks located at points $S = \pm h/d$ in reciprocal space. One can show that the peaks of the interference function will have widths on the order of $1/Nd$ and amplitudes N. Therefore, if the number of membranes in the stack is large, the peaks are very narrow, so the interference function samples the continuous Fourier transform of the membrane electron density function at intervals of $1/d$. That is, the standard lamellar diffraction pattern is obtained but is now interpreted as sampling at intervals $1/d$ of the continuous Fourier transform of a single bilayer.

C. Problems Peculiar to the Stratum Corneum

The bottom line for the preceding analysis is that the observed diffraction pattern is the product of two fucntions: a shape function related to the electron density of a single membrane, and an interference function related to the lattice of the stack of membranes. The sharpness of the observed peaks is related inversely to the number of membranes in the stack, a fact that makes it possible to estimate the number of repeating units in the lattice (Blaurock, 1982). As N decreases, the multilamellar diffraction peaks broaden, so the diffraction pattern approaches the continuous transform as $N \rightarrow 1$. As a rule of thumb for bilayer systems, the multilamellar diffraction patterns begins to be significantly affected only for $N < 10$ (Lesslauer and Blasie, 1972). Electron micrographs suggest that values of N less than 10 are likely to be encountered in most lipid regions of the SC (Swartzendruber et al., 1995). An additional complication is that the micrographs suggest wide variations in N throughout the SC. Finally, we do not know how good the lattice may be in any given location of the SC, nor do we know if the composition of the unit cells is uniform throughout the SC.

D. The Phase Problem

The electron density of the unit cell (Eq. 1) is obtained from the structure factor amplitudes $|F(hkl)|$ and phase factors $\exp[-2\pi i(hkl)]$ by means of Eq. 1, but the diffraction experiment yields only the amplitudes, since $I = |F(hkl)|^2$. Because $|F(hkl)|^2 = F(hkl)F(hkl)*$, the phase information is lost. This makes the inverse procedure of calculating an electron density profile from the experimental intensities a nontrivial exercise. This is the phase problem. As noted earlier, the phase problem is greatly simplified for centrosymmetric unit cells because the imaginary part of the Fourier transform vanishes, causing the phases to be limited to 0 (phase factor $= +1$) or π (phase factor $= -1$). The problem reduces to simply determining the signs of the structure factors. In general, however, the Fourier transform consists of a real and an imaginary part because the phases can adopt all values between 0 and 2π. Several methods (Blaurock, 1982) are available for solving the phase problem. For centrosymmetric multilamellar bilayer systems, the solution of the phase problem (choosing signs for the structure factors) is relatively straightforward if the Bragg spacing of the system can be changed by varying the hydration and if the electron density profile of a single bilayer is relatively unaffected by hydration (Franks and Levine, 1981). The earlier discussion indicated that for multilamellar systems with a large number of bilayers in the stack, the structure factors represent a sampling of the continuous Fourier transform of the electron density at intervals $1/d$, so if d is varied the sampling moves along the continuous transform and one can infer the phases by relatively simple procedures (Franks and Levine, 1981). Unfortunately, this "swelling method" cannot be applied to the SC because the intercellular lipid domains do not swell or shrink as hydration is changed. Heavy-atom labeling (Franks et al., 1978) is a possibility that has not yet been explored, but the labeling must not change the structure (i.e., the labeled structure must be isomorphous with the unlabeled structure).

V. X-RAY DIFFRACTION STUDIES THE STRATUM CORNEUM

Diffraction work relevant to the skin can be divided broadly into two groups: keratin structure and SC structure. Studies of the structure of keratin began in the 1930s and holds an honorable and distinguished position in the history of protein crystallography and structure. As will be discussed later, diffraction from keratin is not always seen in diffraction studies aimed at the intercellular lipid domains. Nevertheless, it is useful to summarize briefly x-ray diffraction characteristics of keratins before focusing on lipid-oriented studies. Questions about the lipid of the stratum corneum first emerged in the studies of Swanbeck (1959) and Swanbeck and Thyresson (1962, 1961) that were directed primarily toward understanding the organization of keratin in human skin. After the brief discussion of diffraction from keratins, we summarize diffraction studies on the stratum corneum of several different species, including humans. Although the earliest diffraction work involving lipids was performed by Swanbeck (1959) on human SC and by Wilkes et al. (1973) on neonatal rat SC, we begin the discussion with studies (White et al., 1988) on adult mouse SC, because those were the first comprehensive studies that could usefully serve as a paradigm for SC diffraction experiments.

A. X-Ray Diffraction Studies of Keratins

There are several thorough reviews of the structures of keratins that the interested reader should consult (Steinert and Cantieri, 1983; Baden and Kubilus, 1983; Fraser and MacRae, 1973). Here, our intention is to focus on the diffraction patterns obtained from different types of keratin so that diffraction from keratin can be distinguished from diffraction originating from other SC structures.

Keratins are roughly classified according to their sulfur content and mechanical properties and are broadly divided into hard keratins (nails, feathers, etc.) and soft keratin (primarily skin). They can also be classified according to the type of x-ray diffraction pattern they produce: α-keratin, β-keratin, feather keratin, and soft ("amorphous") keratin (Fraser and MacRae, 1973). Our classification of protein secondary structure as α-helix and β-sheet originated from the classification scheme for keratins. Unstretched porcupine quills produce the classic α-keratin pattern that consists of diffuse equatorial spots with a 9.8-Å spacing and meridional lines with a 5.15-Å spacing. The meridional spacing expected for an α-helix is $3.6 \times 1.5 = 5.4$ Å, but the helices form coiled coils that cause this length to be foreshortened to 5.15 Å. The 9.8-Å spots result from the center-to-center spacing of the parallel α-helices. That is, an α-helix has a diameter of about 9.8 Å. Upon stretching, porcupine quills produce strong equatorial reflections at 9.7 and 4.7 Å and relfections along the period, with the dominant one being at 3.3 Å, corresponding the amino acid repeat of a fully extended polypeptide chain. This is the pattern of β-keratin. Feather keratins produce highly oriented and richly detailed diffraction patterns.

In contrast to the other keratins, which produce diffraction patterns with high orientation and detail, soft keratin produces unoriented (i.e., powder) diffraction patterns with diffuse rings that have spacings of about 4.5 and 9.5 Å. Soft keratin, the type found in the skin, is believed to have little secondary structure. The pattern observed in a particular case undoubtedly depends upon species and preparation conditions.

B. Mouse Stratum Corneum

The earliest studies on mouse stratum corneum were carried out by Elias et al. (1983) by means of WAXD, using intact stratum corneum, membrane couplets (isolated corneocyte envelopes with adherent intercellular lipid domains), and extracted lipid. Two reflections at 3.75 and 4.16 Å were observed in both intact SC and isolated couplets that were attributed to the packing of the lipid chains into a crystalline arrangement. In a similar but more complex study, White et al. (1988) examined the structures in excess water of hairless mouse SC and its isolated couplets and lipids over a wide range of temperatures, using both WAXD and SAXD. Diffraction attributable to soft keratin was not observed. Unlike SC scale, fresh full-thickness mouse SC tissue seems generally not to produce soft-keratin patterns (S. H. White, unpublished observation). The SAXD pattern of SC at 25°C revealed four strong lamellar spacings ($h = 2, 3, 4, 5$) that corresponded to a repeat distance of 131 Å (Fig. 5, top). The wide-angle pattern revealed two strong sharp reflections, at 3.75 and 4.16 Å, and a diffuse one at 4.6 Å (Fig. 5, bottom). All three lines disappeared in delipidated SC and couplets and could therefore be attributed unequivocally to lipid alkyl chains. Two additional sharp lines that resisted delipidation were observed for SC and couplets at 4.6 Å and 9.4 Å (Fig. 5, bottom). Because these lines were also observed in couplets that were keratin-free, they were attributed to the corneocyte envelope. However, the 4.6-Å line was somewhat weakened in delipidated SC and couplets, and it is probable that there was a sharp lipid diffraction line at the same position. Assuming this to be the case,

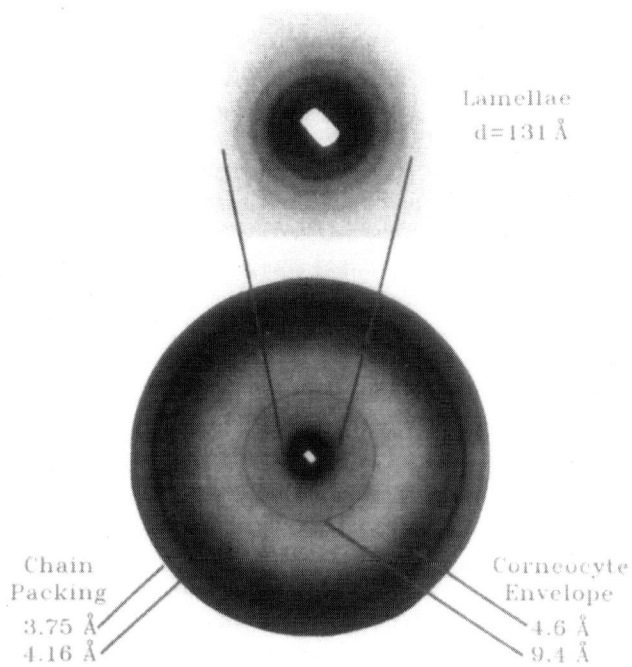

Figure 5 Murine stratum corneum: normal full thickness. Powder diffraction patterns obtained from mouse SC at 25°C. The upper figure shows the small-angle lamellar pattern produced by the intercellular lipid domains, with a repeat period of 131 ± 2 Å. The lower figure shows the wide-angle pattern produced by the lipid alkyl chains and the corneocyte envelope. See text. (Data from White et al., 1988.)

the line spacings are close to the values of 4.61, 4.12, and 3.75 Å observed for triglycerides with orthorhombic alkyl-chain packing (Small, 1986).

In addition to the 4.6-Å and 9.4-Å lines, delipidated membrane couplets also produced a weak reflection at 3.9 Å (White et al., 1988). None of the reflections were temperature dependent, consistent with a nonlipid origin. It was suggested that these reflections originated from their corneocyte envelope, although they could also have originated from protein in the intercellular spaces. In any case, the spacings corresponded quite well to those observed from crystals of β-polyglutamate salts that form antiparallel β-sheets (Keith et al., 1969). Interestingly, the corneocyte envelope originates from soluble precursor proteins comprised of multiple repeats of the sequence QEEEQGQL that become highly cross-linked by transglutaminases to produce ε-(γ-gluta-myl)lysine bonds (Peterson et al., 1983; Goldsmith, 1983).

At 45°C, the SAXD lamellar pattern became somewhat diffuse, while the wide-angle 3.75-Å and 4.16-Å lines were replaced by a single sharp reflection at 4.12 Å. These wide-angle changes indicate that the lipids' alkyl chains undergo a phase transition that is most likely an orthorhombic to hexagonal lattice. A similar change has been observed in a more recent study in human stratum corneum (vide infra). When the temperature was raised to 70°C, the 4.12-Å line was replaced by a diffuse band at 4.6 Å, indicating that all of the lipid was in a fluid state. No SAXD lamellar diffraction was apparent at this temperature. When the SC was returned to 25°C, all of the diffraction peaks originally observed returned, including those assumed to be from proteins, indicating that the changes were reversible. The wide-angle diffraction peaks observed in intact SC and couplets at various temperatures were also observed in the extracted lipids. Interestingly, however, the extracted lipids did not form lamellar phases, but rather phases characterized by rectangular or oblique lattices. All of these phases had unit cell parameters that were considerably smaller than the repeat period of 131 Å for the SC lamellar phase. This observation led to the conclusion that another component must be present in the intercellular lipid domains in situ to organize them into a lamellar phase. The fact that the lamellar diffraction of the SC was recovered when the temperature was returned to 25°C from 70°C is consistent with this conclusion. Had there not been an "organizing" component present, diffraction patterns similar to those observed from the extracted lipids would have been expected. The SC lamellar repeat is too large to be a single bilayer, so White et al. (1988) concluded that the basic repeat unit must be a two-bilayer structure. Further, because of the presence of both even and odd lines in the lamellar pattern, it was concluded that the individual bilayer substructures had to be highly asymmetric, as was demonstrated by simple electron density models. White et al. (1988) proposed that the asymmetry resulted from a putative protein component that organizes the lipids into a lamellar phase. However, there are other possibilities for the missing component. For example, the lipid extraction might not have extracted all of the lipid components evenly that are not linked to the corneocyte envelope, so that either a critical lipid was missing or the detailed composition of the extracted mixture differed from the in situ mixture.

In another study of mouse SC, performed by Bouwstra et al. (1994) using a synchrotron x-ray source, a second lamellar structure with an apparent Bragg spacing of 60 Å was observed. In addition, the first-order peak for a 134-Å lamellar repeat was seen clearly. However, after heating to 120°C and then cooling down to room temperature, only a 135-Å lamellar structure was observed. This behavior was also found in human stratum corneum (Bouwstra et al., 1991). Reheating resulted in the disappearance of the lamellar pattern at 60°C, which is much higher than before recrystallization from 120°C. Despite the similarity in repeat distance, severe differences apparently exist between the structures present before and after recrystallization. These changes are most likely due to protein denaturation and/or irreversible changes in the lipid mixing.

Bouwstra et al. (1991) also reported a sharp reflection from mouse SC corresponding to a repeat distance of 33.5 Å that is often characteristic of crystalline cholesterol. S. H. White (unpublished) has observed multiple lines in fatty-acid–deficient mice characteristic of monohydrated cholesterol. The exact pattern seen, however, varies greatly among specimens. Bouwstra et al. (1992b) also did not observe the very obvious 4.6- and 9.4-Å lines seen by White et al. (1988) and suggested this was due to variations between donors, which is quite likely. Consistent with this conclusion, these two lines are frequently, but not always, absent in studies of human SC (Bouwstra et al., 1992b).

C. Neonatal-Rat Stratum Corneum

One of the earliest diffraction studies was that of Wilkes et al. (1973) on neonatal-rat stratum corneum carried out using WAXD combined with differential thermal analysis. They also investigated the dependence of the diffraction pattern on the orientation of the sample. With the x-ray beam normal and perpendicular to the surface of the SC, two strong reflections, corresponding to repeat distances of 4.2 and 3.7 Å, were observed that were assigned to crystalline lipids. In addition, two halos were observed, at 9.8 and 4.6 Å, that were attributed to protein. Because they could not find a 5.15-Å reflection that is often seen in α-keratin from hard tissues (Fraser and MacRae, 1973), they concluded that the protein was not keratin. However, it seems clear in retrospect that these lines probably originated from soft keratin. In any case, from the orientation of the lipid and protein reflections, the erroneous conclusion was reached that the lipids were associated with the proteins according to the lipid-protein structure proposed in the late '50s by Swanbeck (1959) for human stratum corneum. In this model it was assumed that the lipids were coated as a sheet around the keratin proteins. In the early '70s it was shown that the lipids were organized in lamellar sheets in the intercellular regions (Breathnach et al., 1973).

Extraction of the lipids with organic solvents resulted in the disappearance of the 4.2- and 3.7-Å reflections, confirming that these reflections were from lipids. The 3.7-Å reflection disappeared at 40°C, and the 4.2-Å reflection disappeared at approximately 70°C, corresponding to thermal transitions detected calorimetrically at similar temperatures. The two protein reflections were not affected by temperature. Recrystallization of the lipids in the stratum corneum result in the same wide-angle diffraction pattern as untreated stratum corneum. The recrystallization was not affected by the water content in the stratum corneum.

D. Human Stratum Corneum

The first x-ray studies on SC were performed on human stratum corneum in the late 1950s by Swanbeck (1959). The specimens consisted of 0.5-mm-thick flakes of horny layer from the sole of the foot. The following reflections were observed: Two wide-angle relfections were observed corresponding to spacings of 3.7 and 4.2 Å (attributed to SC lipids), a diffuse 10-Å band, two small-angle peaks corresponding to spacings of 95- and 145-Å, a broad, diffuse 40–60-Å peak, and a very weak peak at 30 Å. The orientation and the positions of the wide- and small-angle peaks and a comparison of the observed patterns with theoretical scattering curves based on cylinders led Swanbeck to conclude that the patterns arose from proteins arranged in cylinders that were covered by a lipid layer. This model was also used by Wilkes et al. (1973) to interpret their diffraction data (vide ultra). Subsequent studies on keratin-free samples are not consistent with this interpretation, and it is unlikely that the lipid-coated protein filament model is correct (White et al., 1988). Recent x-ray studies (Hou et al., 1991) and electron microscopic observations (Madison et al., 1987) clearly show that the intercellular domains are organized as lamellae.

In addition to the 3.7- and 4.2-Å lipid lines reported by Swanbeck (1959), Wilkes et al. (1973) also reported a 4.6-Å lipid reflection. They also performed measurements at elevated temperatures, and, as for rat stratum corneum, they observed a lipid transition at 40°C that was accompanied by the disappearance of the 3.7-Å reflection. The 4.2- and 4.6-Å reflections were observed to disappear at 70°C, but the disappearance of the 4.6-Å reflection has not been confirmed by other studies (see below). Wilkes et al. (1973) did not observe reflections characteristic for α-keratin, which was not in agreement with the findings of Goldsmith and Baden (1970) and Baden et al. (1980, 1973). Baden et al. (1973) found the α-keratin reflection, but performed their experiments either on material isolated by cutting thin sheets from the palm, probably callus, or on keratin isolated from hair and stratum corneum (Baden et al., 1980). The α-keratin reflection was also found in callus in a recent study by Garson et al. (1991), who present a thorough discussion of variations in keratin diffraction patterns attributable to sample preparation and anatomical region.

Garson et al. (1991) have reported a comprehensive synchrotron x-ray study of SC structure on intact stratum corneum, its membrane couplets, and callus performed at ambient temperature and humidity. Importantly, they were able to examine their specimens carefully at different orientations relative to the x-ray beam and thereby confirm electron microscopic observations that most of the lamellar structures are aligned parallel to the surface of the skin (Hou et al., 1991; Swartzendruber et al., 1989; Wertz et al., 1989). In perpendicular orientation, diffuse bands at approximately 4.5 and 9.5 Å were detected, indicating the presence of amorphous keratin. The 9.5-Å reflection became anisotropic in the parallel configuration (see Fig. 6), so 9.6-Å meridional and 9.3-Å equatorial reflections were observed. They concluded that the reflections originated from deformed β-keratin with the chain axis aligned perpendicular to the surface of the stratum corneum.

Although Garson et al. (1991) reported many reflections attributed to lipid, only a few of them were interpreted. Peaks were observed at 65, 33.5, 45, 22.5, and 14 Å, which were attributed to two lipid domains with spacings of 65 and 45 Å. Surprisingly, Garson et al. (1991) suggested that these spacings corresponded to the narrow and wide intercellular lipid bands frequently observed in RuO_4-stained SC (Swartzendruber et al., 1989). This is quite unlikely, since reflections correspond to entire repeating units in a structure and not to single lipid bands within the repeating unit. Garson et al. (1990,1991) also suggested that the 33.5-Å repeat lamellar pattern that produced reflections at 33.5, 16.8, 8.2, and 4.1 Å was due to crystalline cholesterol. However, this assignment seems uncertain based upon either the triclinic crystal structure of cholesterol monohydrate (Craven, 1976) that should produce $d(00l)$ reflections for $l = 1$–5 at 33.95, 16.98, 11.32, 8.49, and 6.79 Å or the triclinic crystal

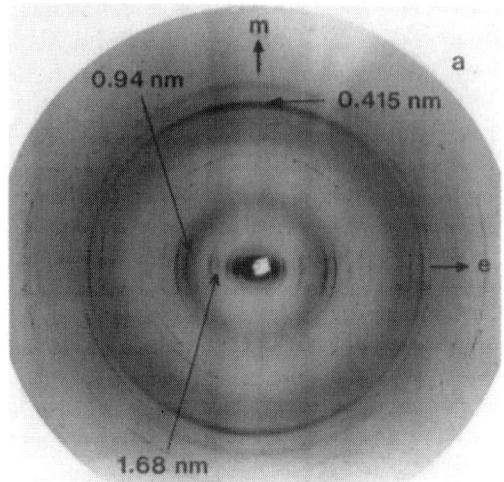

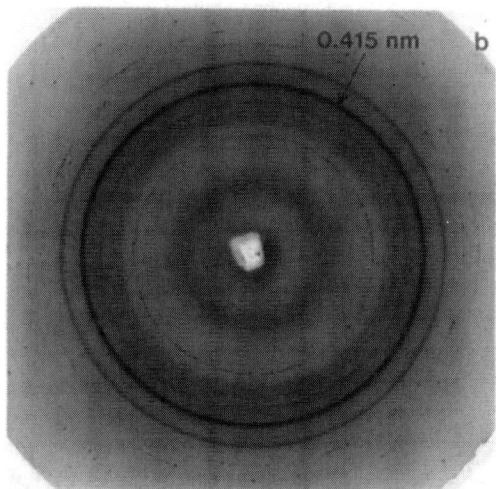

Figure 6 Wide-angle diffraction pattern from human SC oriented (a) parallel and (b) perpendicular to the plane of the SC. (From Garson et al., 1991.)

structure of anhydrous cholesterol (Shieh et al., 1977), which produces strong reflections at 33.6, 16.8, 6.24, 5.74, 5.23, 5.09, and 4.90 Å. Although the reflections observed by Garson et al. (1990) at 33.5 and 16.8 Å are consistent with anhydrous cholesterol, the 8.2- and 4.1-Å reflections are not. The origin of the latter pair is thus uncertain. Various dotted rings and spots in the diffraction patterns were also reported in various specimens but showed large variations in appearance. The origin of the reflections are uncertain but were also reported in later studies (Bouwstra et al., 1992b). Finally, Garson et al. (1991) reported the presence of an unidentified component with reflections at 9.4, 9.4/2 = 4.7, and 9.4/3 = 3.1 Å. These reflections were claimed to be similar to those reported by White et al. (1988) for the murine corneocyte envelope that appeared at 9.4, 4.6, and 3.9 Å. The latter, however, cannot be indexed as a family of layer lines. For this reason and because Garson et al. (1991) reported the disappearance of these reflections in human SC couplets, it is not clear that the patterns originate from the same structure.

Bouwstra et al. (1991) have also examined human SC by WAXD and SAXD using a synchrotron source. They, however, looked closely at the lipid structure of the SC as function of temperature, water content, and lipid recrystallization procedures. Unlike Garson et al. (1991), who used standard x-ray film, Bouwstra and her colleagues used an electronic quadrant detector that has the advantages of high dynamic range for the detection of weak diffraction peaks against the high background scattering signals of human SC and high resolution at small angles. The disadvantage of the quadrant detector is that information on orientation is difficult to obtain. As shown in Fig. 7, Bouwstra et al. observed two doublet peaks in the small-angle region, a weak and a strong, each consisting of a main position and a shoulder at a slightly higher Q (i.e., scattering angle). The main position of the strong diffraction peak and the shoulder of the weak diffraction peak were interpreted as the first- and second-order peaks of a lamellar phase, with a repeat distance of 64 Å, in agreement with some of the patterns observed by Garson et al. (1990, 1991). Recrystallization of specimens after heating to 120°C produced sharp lamellar diffraction peaks ($l = 2, 3, 4, 5, 6$) and a shoulder ($l = 1$) that correspond to a Bragg spacing of 134 Å (120°C curve, Fig. 8). Comparison of this curve with the scattering curve obtained from untreated stratum corneum (25°C curve in Fig. 8, 20% curve in Fig. 7a) led to the conclusion that the shoulder of the strong doublet and the main peak of the weak doublet corresponded to orders 3 and 4 of a 134-Å lamellar structure. This interpretation thus suggested that in the untreated specimen, two lamellar structures are present. A complication in the interpretations is that one of the reflections of polycrystalline cholesterol is located at the position of the fourth-order diffraction peak of the 134-Å

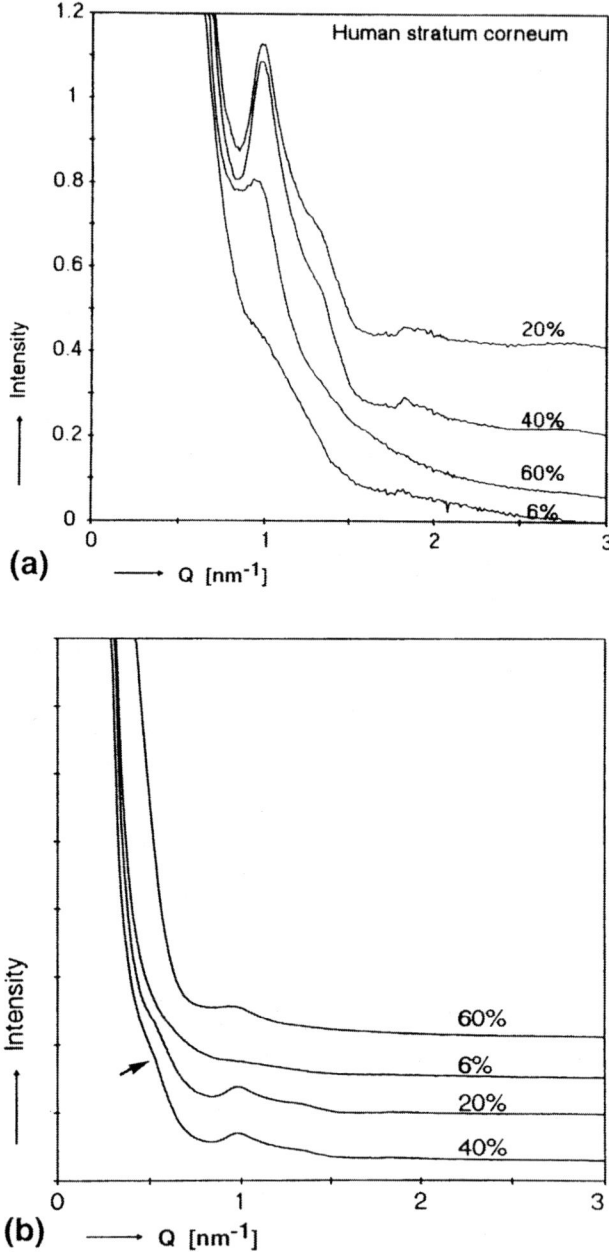

Figure 7 X-ray scattering curves from human SC hydrated to different extents. (a) Scattering curves hydrated to levels from 6% (w/w) to 60% (w/w). The shoulder on the

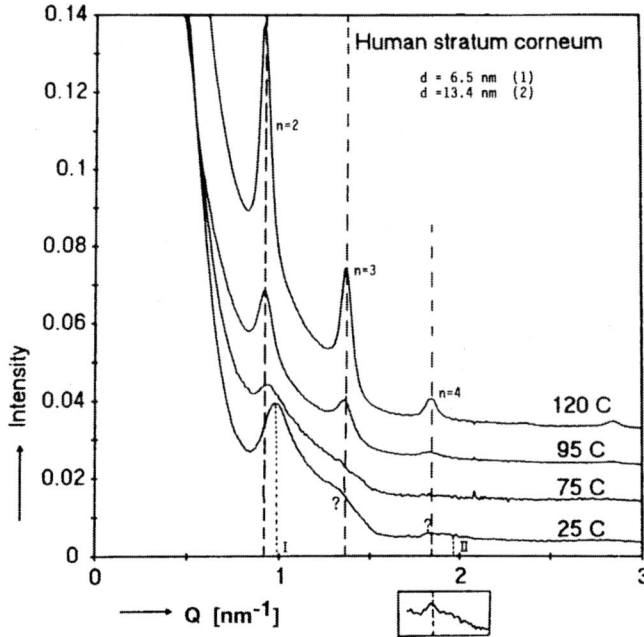

Figure 8 Scattering curve from human SC after heating to various temperatures followed by cooling to room temperature. The temperatures to which the SC was heated are indicated. $n = 1$, 2, etc. refer to the orders of diffraction peaks from a lamellar structure with a Bragg spacing of 134 Å. $n = $ I, II refer to peaks corresponding to a lamellar structure with Bragg spacing of 64 Å. (Data from Bouwstra et al., 1991.)

lamellar structure. However, wide-angle measurements of untreated SC produce diffraction peaks that can be indexed as orders 5 through 10 of a 134-Å lamellar structure and as order 2 of the 64-Å lamellar structure (Bouwstra et al., 1992b).

Between 60 and 75°C, a disordering of the lamellar structure appears to occur that coincides roughly with a thermal transition (Bouwstra et al., 1989; Golden et al., 1986; van Duzee, 1975). The scattering curve measured at 75°C, shown in Fig. 9, shows only a shoulder on the descending scattering curve,

main peak disappears at 60%. (b) Scattering curves for conditions in part (a) plotted on a different scale to show the first-order peak (shoulder on the descending curve; arrow) corresponding to a Bragg spacing of 134 Å. (Data from Bouwstra et al., 1991.)

Bouwstra et al.

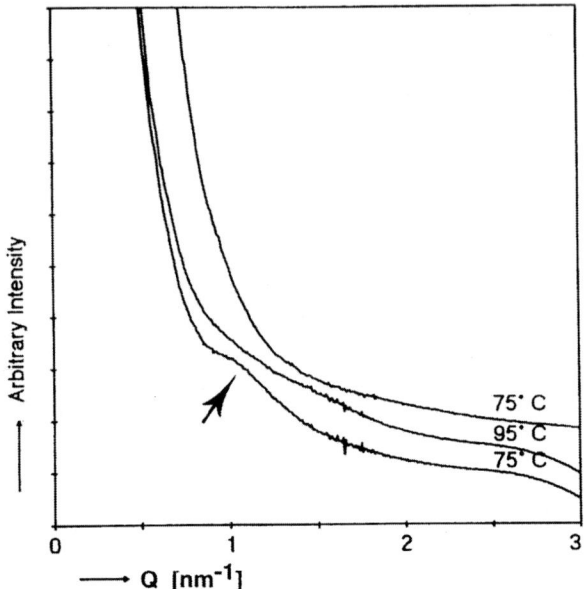

Figure 9 Scattering curves from human SC at 75 and 95°C. On both curves a small shoulder appears (arrow) that disappears after heating to 120°C followed by recrystallization at room temperature and then reheating to 75°C.

while at 95° C (above the third thermal transition) only a shift of the shoulder on the scattering curve was observed, which disappeared upon heating to 120°C. Recrystallization from 120°C resulted in the disappearance of the shoulder at 75°C. This is in agreement with thermal analysis: Heating to 120°C, cooling down, and reheating results in a shift of the thermal transition from 87°C to around 70°C (Bouwstra et al., 1989; Golden et al., 1986), which is that temperature at which the second thermal transition takes place.

Regarding the lateral packing of the lipids, Bouwstra et al. (1992b) observed reflections at 3.78 and 4.17 Å at room temperature that are likely due to an orthorhombic arrangement. However, the authors indicate that the 4.17-Å reflection might be obscured by the one at 4.12 Å, so it is also possible that some lipid is present in a hexagonal arrangements. It is even possible that lipids in a fluid phase are present but obscured by the diffuse keratin ring at 4.6 Å. At approximately 40°C, a change in lateral packing from crystalline to hexagonal appears to take place, because the 3.78-Å line could not be observed at 45°C. A similar transition was also found in mouse stratum corneum (White et al., 1988). Another interesting and related phenomenon is the behavior of the gel-to-fluid transition determined by wide-angle x-ray scattering (Bouwstra et al., 1992b). In the first heating run to 120°C, the hexagonal lateral packing disappeared between 75 and 95°C, while after recrystallization from 120°C the hexagonal lateral packing disappeared between 60 and 75°C (see Fig. 10). The third thermal transition seems to be related to a change from hexagonal to fluid packing of the lipids and to the fact that this transition is influenced by the denaturation of proteins that occur between 90 and 120°C. The influence of protein denaturation on the phase transition observed between 75 and 95°C was inferred from other studies (Bouwstra et al., 1989; Golden et al., 1986).

Bouwstra et al. (1991) also performed SAXD and WAXD measurements at hydration levels ranging from 6 to 60% (w/w). No swelling of the lamellae could be observed. But there did sometimes appear to be a disordering of the 134-Å lamellar system at water contents of 60% w/w. Hydration had no apparent effect on the lateral packing of the lipids. No swelling was observed in mouse SC by Hou et al. (1991) either, and it therefore is clear that almost no water is present in the lamellar phases. However, the presence of a few water molecules per lipid cannot be excluded. In fact, the presence of water is indicated by a decrease in lipid transition temperatures (Golden et al., 1986) and an increase in lipid disordering (Alonso et al., 1995) at increasing water content in SC. In two recent papers (Shah et al., 1995a, 1995b), studies of the physical properties of nonhydroxy and α-hydroxy ceramides demonstrated swelling of the lamellae at increasing water content. However, the ceramides were prepared either by modification of bovine brain ceramides or by synthesizing the ceramides from sphingosine, but it is not known whether the physical properties of these ceramides are similar to those found in SC. That only small amounts of water are present in the lamellar phases is consistent with the known structure of ceramindes, fatty acids, and cholesterol that have small lipid headgroups and probably form tight hydrogen-bond networks (Löffgren and Pascher, 1977; Swartzendruber et al., 1989). Extensive swelling of bilayers in the presence of water is a feature characteristic of phospholipids with large headgroups with ample space for free water. Such lipids are not present in SC. Nevertheless, water is a very potent penetration enhancer, and stratum corneum can take up enormous amounts of it. This leads one to believe that water absorption must occur in the corneocytes and, in some fashion, in the intercellular domains. Water has, in fact, been recently observed in the SC intercellular regions in separate domains by freeze-fracture electron microscopy (van Hal et al., 1996).

The strong reflections found in the powder pattern of anhydrous crystalline cholesterol (see above) have also been found in the pattern of human

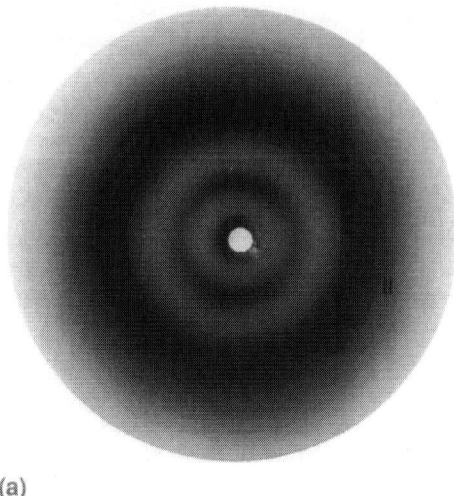

(a)

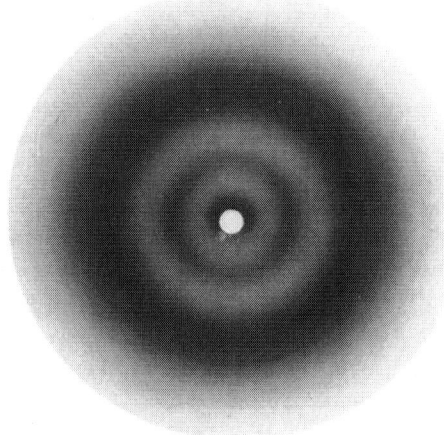

(b)

Figure 10 Wide-angle diffraction patterns from human SC oriented parallel to the incident beam at a temperature of 75°C. (a) A 4.17-Å reflection due to hexagonal lipid packing is seen (labeled I) along with reflections at 3.6, 4.6, and 7.16 Å. The ring marked II has not been observed in any other donor. (b) Diffraction pattern obtained after recrystallization of the lipids from 120°C. The 4.17-Å reflection has disappeared. (Data from Bouwstra et al., 1992b.)

stratum corneum (Bouwstra et al., 1992b). Often, the intensities of the choles-terol reflections were not uniform in the plane of the film but showed a preferential orientation as a function of the azimuthal angle oriented parallel to the SC. Cholesterol crystals may possibly be intercalated in the lipid bilayers to cause the preferred orientation. The disappearance of the choles-terol reflections occurred between 60 and 95°C and probably depends on the size of the crystals.

Besides the unidentified compound with spacings of 3.1, 4.7, and 9.4 Å reported by Garson et al. (1991), Bouwstra et al. (1992b) also found two other reflections, at 3.6 and 7.17 Å, that could not be identified. The reflections were arc shaped and did not change upon heating between 20 and 120°C and are therefore most probably due to thermostable proteins because they were also observed in chloroform/methanol-extracted SC.

E. Pig Stratum Corneum

The lamellar and lateral packing of intercellular domains of pig stratum corneum differs from both human and mouse SC (Bouwstra et al., 1995a). SAXD scattering curves indicate the existence of at least two lamellar struc-tures, with repeat periods of 60 and 132 Å. As for mouse and human SC, the lamellar repeats were largely unaffected by the hydration level. The most striking difference is the existence of only the hexagonal lateral packing of the lipids, as evidenced by a single wide-angle line of 4.15 Å at room temperature. No reflections could be observed that are indicative for a crystalline packing of the lipids (see Fig. 11). Recrystallization from 120°C resulted in a single lamellar structure, with a repeat distance of 132 Å.

VI. X-RAY DIFFRACTION STUDIES OF LIPIDS EXTRACTED FROM STRATUM CORNEUM

White et al. (1988) studied the phase behavior of whole-lipid extracts from mouse stratum corneum to excess water using the same temperature range as for the intact tissue. The wide-angle pattrns were exactly the same as those of the intact stratum corneum at all corresponding temperatures. Thus, the lateral packing of the chains in the extracted lipids seem to be identical to that of the intact SC. However, the small-angle patterns of the extracts differed dramati-cally from the intact case. The most important observation was that no lamellar phase was observed. The small-angle peaks at 25°C and 45°C seemd to correspond to two-dimensional oblique and rectangular lattices, respectively,

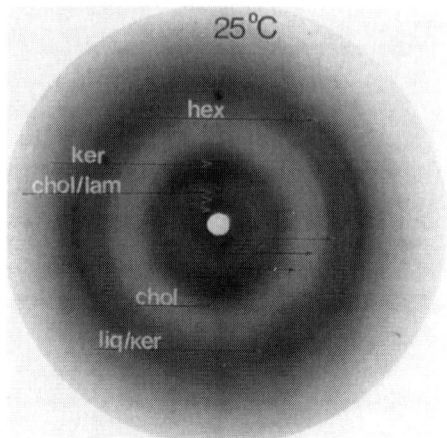

Figure 11   Diffraction pattern from pig SC at 25°C. Only diffraction from hexagonal (hex) lipid-chain packing is seen, together with the cholesterol (chol), keratin (ker), and the higher-order lamellar (lam) reflections. (Data from Bouwstra et al., 1995a.)

and none of the cell dimensions approached the 131-Å lamellar repeat observed in intact SC. At 70°C, the lipids formed a reversed hexagonal phase that has also been observed when skin lipid liposomes are heated to 70°C (Abraham, 1991) (J. A. Bouwstra, M. A. de Vries, and G. S. Gooris, unpublished). Very recently, however, large Bragg spacings have been obtained from lipid mixtures in excess water (pH = 5, the same as intact SC) comprised of varying mole ratios of cholesterol and ceramides isolated from pig stratum corneum (McIntosh et al., 1996; Bouwstra et al., 1995b; Bouwstra et al., 1996b). The ceramides alone form crystalline structures, but upon the addition of cholesterol two lamellar phases were observed in the lipid mixtures with cholesterol/ceramide molar ratios between 0.4 and 2 (Bouwstra et al., 1996b). The phases had periodicities of 52 and 122 Å. Hexagonal lateral packing, typical of intact pig SC, was also observed. McIntosh et al. (1996) observed that in the absence of ceramide 1, the long periodicity phase was not present. In addition, Bouwstra et al. (1996a) reported that by using only ceramide 1, ceramide 2, and cholesterol, two lamellar phases, with repeat periods of 52 and 120 Å, were formed, similar to the phase behavior of mixtures prepared from total pig SC ceramide fraction and cholesterol.

The above results show that while total lipid extracts do not necessarily form the same lamellar arrangement observed in intact stratum corneum, it is possible with lipids alone (i.e., ceramides and cholesterol in certain ratios) to obtain diffraction patterns similar to those obtained from SC. Abraham et al. (1987) studied the effect of Ca^{2+} ions on the fusion of vesicles consisting of extracted pig SC ceramides, free fatty acids, cholesterol, and cholesterol sulfate. Interestingly, it appeared that skin lipid liposomes were transformed from unilamellar to multilamellar and finally to lamellar sheets after addition of Ca^{2+} to the suspension. This occurred, however, only when free fatty acids were intercalated to the liposomes. This is consistent with the hypothesis of Landmann (1984) that the formation of broad interrupted layers in the intercellular space occurred by fusion of the membranes originating from the membrane-coated granular disks, indicating that Ca^{2+} may be important for the formation of lamellae in vivo.

VII. MODEL CALCULATIONS

Although a means for solving the phase problem for the SC does not yet exist, model calculations based upon intensities provide useful information. White et al. (1988) noted two features of the small-angle patterns that were important. First, a Bragg spacing of about 130 Å cannot be easily reconciled with a single bilayer structure; the basic repeat is most likely the result of two bilayers. Second, there was no odd–even effect in the observed patterns. Diffraction patterns for myelin membranes show very weak odd orders and strong even orders of diffraction (Worthington and Blaurock, 1969), and the simplest models demonstrate that this is expected if the two bilayers of the unit cell have very similar structures with only slight asymmetries. The lack of the odd–even effect for the SC indicates that the bilayers of the unit cell must be highly asymmetric, and White et al. (1988) attributed the asymmetry to a protein component.

Bouwstra et al. (1991) carried out more detailed calculations using the five orders of diffraction data obtained from SC with lipids recrystallized from 120°C. They used an iterative procedure that involved varying the bilayer electron density profile until the intensities calculated from the three-parameter model agreed with the observed intensities. In the case of mouse stratum corneum, the peaks are clearly resolved in untreated stratum corneum (Bouwstra et al., 1994; White et al., 1988), but in human SC the calculations can be carried out only after recrystallization of the lipids, because the peaks are unresolved in untreated skin. The results of their calculations are shown in Fig. 12. The electron density strip model shows three high and three low

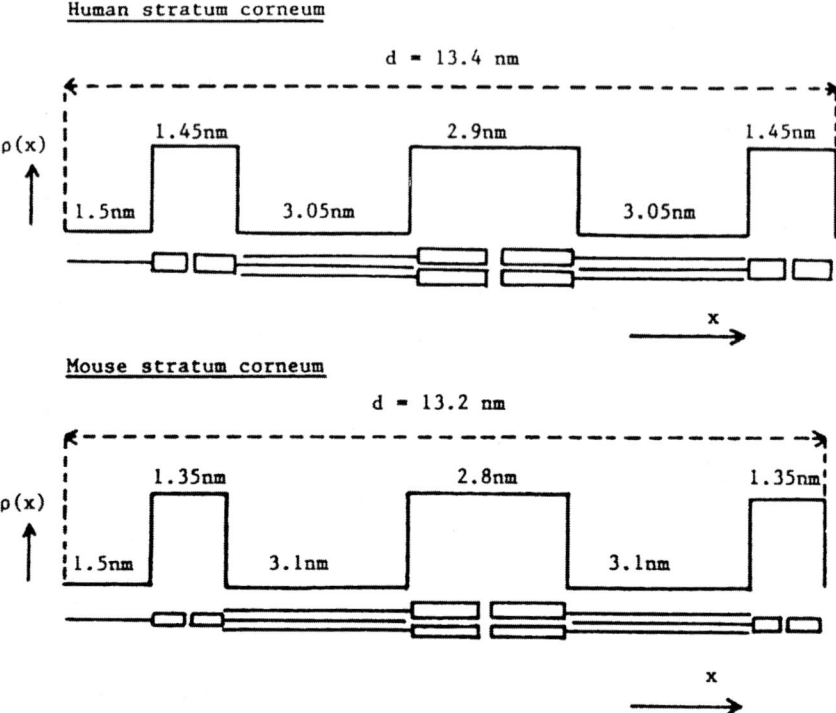

Figure 12 Models for electron density profiles of human and mouse stratum corneum intercellular lipid domains. Fourier transformation of the profiles produce diffracted intensities consistent with the observed ones. The unit cell spacings of the human and mouse SC are 134 Å and 132 Å, respectively.

electron density regions. The low electron density regions probably correspond with alkyl chains, while the high electron density regions correspond with the headgroup regions of the lipids. However, the width of the headgroup regions cannot be explained by lipids alone, which have only diminutive headgroups. Further, because the diffraction patterns are not affected by hydration, the width of the regions cannot be explained by the presence of water either. The most likely explanation is that protein or some other substance is present in these regions. The low-electron-density alkyl-chain regions are characterized by a broad–broad–narrow pattern, in reasonable agreement with results obtained by transmission electron microscopy using RuO_4 staining (Swartzendruber et al., 1989).

VIII. INFLUENCE OF PENETRATION ENHANCERS ON STRATUM CORNEUM STRUCTURE

The influence of a series of *N*-alkyl-azocycloheptan-2-ones on the structure of human stratum corneum has been studied with x-ray diffraction techniques (Bouwstra et al., 1992a). Stratum corneum was treated with propylene glycol (PG) and *N*-alkyl-azocycloheptan-2-ones in PG, in which the alkyl chain varied between 6 and 16 C atoms. As in the case of water, PG did not result in a shift of the various diffraction peaks in human stratum corneum, implying that no swelling of the intercellular domains occurred. Hexyl-azone only resulted in a decrease of the intensity of the diffraction peaks, while the alkyl azones with 8 or more C atoms in the alkyl chain resulted in a disappearance of the ordering of the lamellae (Fig. 13). These findings agreed with results obtained from electron microscopy, thermal analysis, and penetration studies. Freeze-fracture electron microscopy showed a partial disordering of the lamellar structures for octyl-azone and alkyl-chain azones, with a higher number of carbon atoms in the akyl chain. Treatment with longer alkyl-chain azones resulted in the disappearance of the thermal transition at approximately 70°C, which corresponded to a disordering of the lamellar structure (Bouwstra et al., 1992a). Penetration enhancement of a small peptide, DGAVP, by the whole series of alkyl azones resulted in a jump in the penetration enhancement factor between octyl and decyl azone. These data strongly indicated that alkyl azones with more than six alkyl-chain carbon atoms have an effect on the ordering of the lamellae that results in an increase in penetration of at least hydrophilic drugs. The possible change in lateral packing of the lipids remains to be investigated.

An interesting phenomenon is the influence of alkyl azones on the lamellar ordering after recrystallization of the lipids from 90°C, as shown in Fig. 14. Remarkably, after recrystallization of the lipids, treatment of alkyl azones in PG did not result in a disordering of the lamellar stacking. A possible explanation is that the recrystallization results in large regions of intercellular domains that are free of defects necessary for intercalation of alkyl azones. Another explanation is an irreversible change in the intercellular domain structure after heating to 95°C.

IX. DIFFRACTION STUDIES OF DISEASED SKIN

Very little work has been done to date on the structure of the SC from diseased skin, but this situation will no doubt change in the course of time. Comparisons

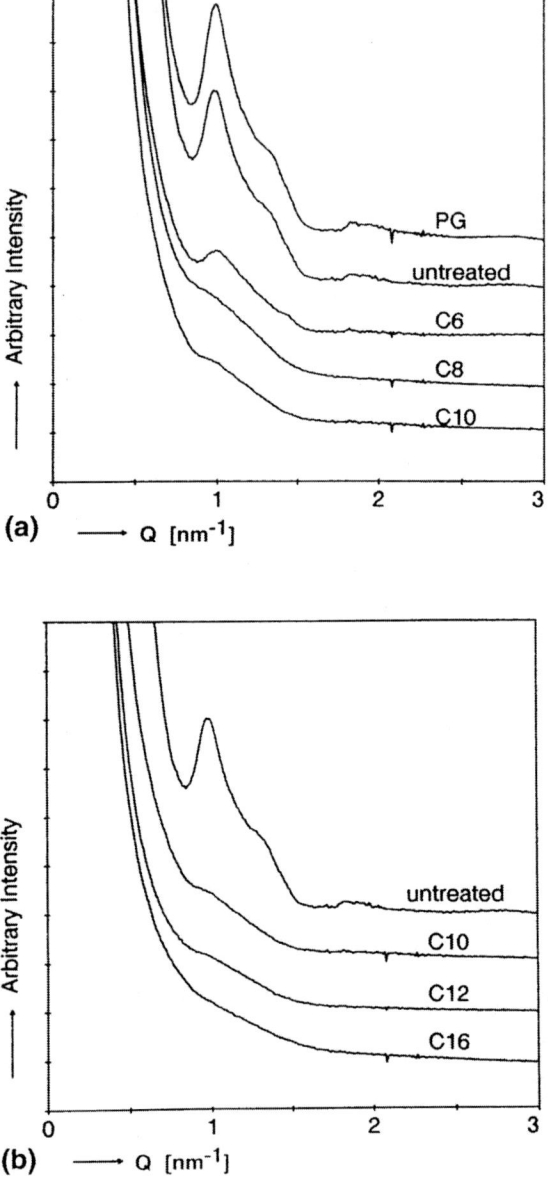

Figure 13 Diffraction patterns from human SC treated with alkyl azones with chain lengths varying between 6 (C6) and 16 (C16). The alkyl azones were solubilized

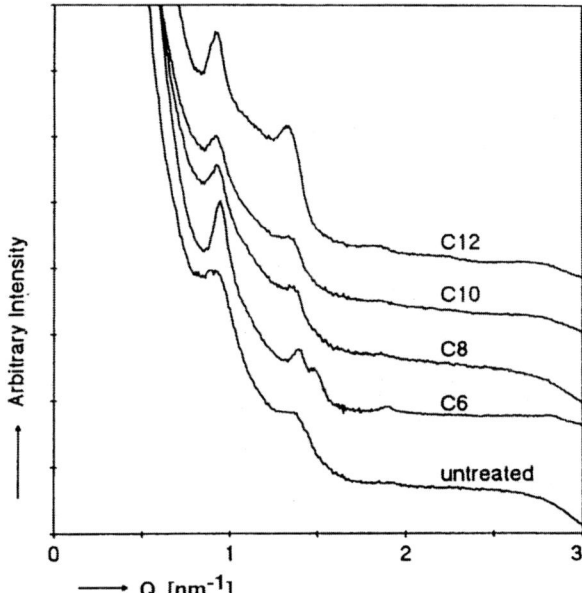

Figure 14 Diffraction patterns from human SC treated with alkyl azones with chain lengths of 6, 8, 10, and 12 carbons. The pattern demonstrates the ordering of the lamellae after recrystallization from 120°C and subsequent treatment with alkyl azones in propylene glycol. (Data from Bouwstra et al., 1992a.)

of diffraction patterns from normal human sunburn scale, x-linked ichthyosis, ichthyosis vulgaris, congenital ichthyosiform erythroderma, and classic lamellar ichthyosis reveal significant differences (S. H. White, M. L. Williams, and P. M. Elias, unpublished). The number of samples was too small to permit generalizations, but the comparisons did demonstrate that the diffraction patterns varied markedly with the pathological state, indicating a clear connection with intercellular domain structure. Hou et al. (1991) compared normal mouse stratum corneum with essential fatty acid deficient (EFAD) stratum corneum and characterized the differences by RuO_4-staining electron micros-

---

in propylene glycol (PG). Untreated and PG-treated SC served as controls. All measurements were carried out at room temperature. The diffraction curve of the untreated SC is similar to that of human SC shown in Fig. 7. (Data from Bouwstra et al., 1992a.)

copy and x-ray diffraction. Using x-ray diffraction, no differences were found in repeat distances between EFAD and normal mouse stratum corneum. Changes in relative intensities of the various diffraction peaks were not taken into consideration. RuO_4-staining electron microscopy revealed changes in the EFAD stratum corneum, displaying regions of either absence of lamellae or excess of lamellae. Interestingly, the EFAD specimens frequently, but not always, displayed diffraction patterns with very strong reflections characteristic of monohydrated cholesterol (S. H. White, unpublished observation).

Recently, the skin barrier properties and SC structure of patients with autosomal recessive lamellar ichthyosis have been examined relative to healthy volunteers (Lavrijsen et al., 1995). Barrier function was found to be impaired, and SC lipid structure was observed to be remarkably different. Normal SC had a repeat period of 64 Å, whereas the diseased SC had values between 50 and 59 Å.

X. CONCLUSIONS

Good progress on the determination of structure of stratum corneum by means of x-ray diffraction has been made in recent years, although much remains to be done. In agreement with electron microscopic measurements, the most fundamental structure of the intercellular lipid domains is lamellar, with a repeat period of about 130 Å. It seems clear that the basic repeating unit is comprised of two or three bilayers and possibly additional components that play a role in maintaining the native structure but that have not yet been identified. Large repeat periods have now been observed in certain ceramide/cholesterol mixtures (McIntosh et al., 1996; Bouwstra et al., 1995b, 1996a, 1996b), similar to that of intact SC. In terms of animal models for transdermal permeation studies, the most important contribution of the diffraction work is the observation that SC from different species have different diffraction patterns. The scattering curves of human stratum corneum suggest the existence of two lamellar structures, with repeat distances of 64 and 134 Å. In mouse stratum corneum, the dominant structure is the one with a repeat distance of 131 Å. Occasionally a second structure, with 60-Å repeat distance, was observed. Pig SC has a very complicated scattering curve, but at least two lamellar structures are present that have repeat periods of 60 and 132 Å. However, one must be very cautious at this time about the number of structures that may be present because of artifacts that can arise from the small number of repeating units in the domains. A particularly striking result is the great improvement in the diffraction pattern obtained from intact SC after recrystallization of the lipids from a high temperature. This procedure invariably led to a single lamellar structure with a repeat period of about 130 Å in pig, human, and mouse SC. The fact that extracted lipids do not invariably have repeat periods of this dimension suggests the possibility of a third component(s) that is able to exert itself more effectively after heating. The component(s) would, however, have to be very robust to withstand heating to 120°C. In all types of stratum corneum, crystalline cholesterol has been observed. However, crystalline cholesterol generally disappears after heating and recrystallization from 120°C, indicating either a nonequilibrium-phase separation of cholesterol at normal temperatures or a very slow recrystallization of cholesterol after the heating/cooling cycle.

ACKNOWLEDGMENTS

S. White acknowledges the research support of the National Institutes of Health (GM37291 and GM46823) and the National Science Foundation (DMB-8412754 and DMB-8807431). J. A. Bouwstra acknowledges the financial support of the Dutch Foundation for Fundamental Research and of the European Economic Community for performance of measurements at Daresbury Synchrotron Station in the United Kingdom. The authors thank J. C. Garson for providing x-ray diffraction photographs.

REFERENCES

Abraham, W. (1995). Deuterium NMR study of structures formed by stratum corneum lipids in vitro. *Proc. Intern. Symp. Control. Release Bioac. Mater. 19*:135.

Abraham, W., Wertz, P. W., Landmann, L. and Downing, D. T. (1987). Stratum corneum lipid liposomes: Calcium-induced transformation into lamellar sheets. *J. Invest. Derm. 88*:212.

Abrahamsson, S., Dahlen, B., Lofgren, H. and Pascher, I. (1978). Lateral packing of hydrocarbon chains. *Prog. Chem. Fats other Lipids 16*:125.

Alonso, A., Meirelles, N. C. and Tabak, M. (1995). Effect of hydration upon the fluidity of intercellular membranes of stratum corneum: An EPR study. *Biochim. Biophys. Acta 1237*:6.

Baden, H. P. and Kubilus, J. (1983). The fibrous proteins of the skin. In: *Stratum Corneum* (R. Marks and G. Plewig, eds.). Berlin, Springer-Verlag, p. 2.

Baden, H. P., Goldsmith, L. A. and Bonar, L. (1973). Conformational changes in the α-fibrous protein of the epidermis. *J. Invest. Derm. 60*:215.

Baden, H. P., McGilvray, H., Lee, L. D., Baden, L. and Kubilus, J. (1980). Comparison of stratum corneum and hair fibrous proteins. *J. Invest. Derm. 75*:311.

Blaurock, A. E. (1982). Evidence of bilayer structure and of membrane interactions from x-ray diffraction analysis. *Biochim. Biophys. Acta 650*:167.

Blaurock, A. E. and Worthington, C. R. (1966). Treatment of low-angle x-ray data from concentric multilayered structures. *Biophys. J. 6*:305.

Bouwstra, J. A., Peschier, L. J. C., Brussee, J. and Boddé, H. E. (1989). Effect of *N*-alkyl-azocycloheptan-2-ones including azones on the thermal behaviour of human stratum corneum. *Int. J. Pharm. 52*:47.

Bouwstra, J. A., Gooris, G. S., Van der Spek, J. A. and Bras, W. (1991). Structural investigations of human stratum corneum by small-angle x-ray scattering. *J. Invest. Derm. 97*:1005.

Bouwstra, J. A., Gooris, G. S., Brussee, J., Salomons-de Vries, M. A. and Bras, W. (1992a). The influence of alkyl-azones on the ordering of the lamellae in human stratum corneum. *Inter. J. Pharamaceut. 79*:141.

Bouwstra, J. A., Gooris, G. S., Salomons-de Vries, M. A., Van der Spek, J. A. and Bras, W. (1992b). Structure of human stratum-corneum as a function of temperature and hydration: A wide-angle x-ray diffraction study. *Inter. J. Pharamaceut. 84*:205.

Bouwstra, J. A., Gooris, G. S., Van der Spek, J. A., Lavrijsen, S. and Bras, W. (1994). The lipid and protein structure of mouse stratum corneum: A wide- and small-angle diffraction study. *Biochim. Biophys. Acta 1212*:183.

Bouwstra, J. A., Gooris, G. S., Bras, W. and Downing, D. T. (1995a). Lipid organization in pig stratum corneum. *J. Lipid Res. 36*:685.

Bouwstra, J. A., Gooris, G. S., Weerheim, A., Cheng, K. and Ponec, M. (1995b). Isolated stratum corneum lipids as a model for the skin barrier. *Proc. Intern. Symp. Control. Release Bioac. Mater. 22*:11.

Bouwstra, J. A., Cheng, K., Gooris, G. S., Weerheim, A. and Ponec, M. (1996a). The role of ceramides 1 and 2 in the stratum corneum lipid organization. *Biochim. Biophys. Acta 1300*:177.

Bouwstra, J. A., Gooris, G. S., Cheng, K., Weerheim, A., Bras, W. and Ponec, M. (1996b). Phase behavior of isolated skin lipids. *J. Lipid Res. 37*:999.

Breathnach, A. S., Goodman, T., Stolinski, C. and Gross, M. (1973). Freeze-fracture replication of cells of stratum corneum of human epidermis. *J. Anatomy 114*:65.

Büldt, G., Gally, H. U., Seeling J. and Zaccai, G. (1979). Neutron diffraction studies on phosphatidylcholine model membranes. I. Head group conformation. *J. Mol. Biol. 134*:673.

Craven, B. M. (1976). Crystal structure of cholesterol monohydrate. *Nature (London) 260*:727.

Elias, P. M., Bonar, L., Grayson, S. and Baden, H. P. (1983). X-ray diffraction analysis of stratum corneum membrane couplets. *J. Invest. Derm. 80*:213.

Finzel, B. C., Poulos, T. L. and Kraut, J. (1984). Crystal structure of yeast cytochrome c peroxidase refined at 1.7-Å resolution. *J. Biol Chem. 259*:13027.

Franks, N. P. and Levine, Y. K. (1981). Low-angle x-ray diffraction. In: *Membrane Spectroscopy* (E. Grell, ed.). Berlin, Springer-Verlag, p. 437.

Franks, N. P., Arunachalam, T. and Caspi, E. (1978). A direct method for determination of membrane electron density profiles on an absolute scale. *Nature (London)* 276:530.

Franks, N. P., Melchoir, V., Kirschner, D. A. and Caspar, D. L. D. (1982). Structure of myelin lipid bilayers: Changes during maturation. *J. Mol. Biol. 155*:133.

Fraser, R. D. B. and MacRae, T. P. (1973). *Conformation in Fibrous Proteins and Related Synthetic Systems.* New York, Academic Press, pp. 1–628.

Friberg, S. E. and Osborne, D. W. (1985). Small-angle x-ray diffraction patterns of stratum corneum and a model structure for its lipids. *J. Dispersion Sci. Tech.* 6:485.

Garson, J. C., Doucet, J., Tsoucaris, G. and Leveque, J. L. (1990). Study of lipid and non-lipid structure in human stratum corneum by x-ray diffraction. *J. Soc. Cosmet. Chem. 41*:347.

Garson, J. C., Doucet, J., Leveque, J. L., and Tsoucaris, G. (1991). Oriented structure in human stratum corneum revealed by x-ray diffraction. *J. Invest. Derm. 96*:43.

Golden, G. M., Guzek, D. B., Harris, R. R., McKie, J. E. and Potts, R. O. (1986). Lipid thermotropic transitions in human stratum corneum. *J. Invest. Derm. 86*:255.

Goldsmith, L. A. (1983). Human epidermal transglutaminase. *J. Invest. Derm. 80*:39s.

Goldsmith, L. A. and Baden, H. P. (1970). Uniquely oriented epidermal lipid. *Nature (London) 225*:1052.

Hosemann, R. and Bagchi, S. N. (1962). *Direct Analysis of Diffraction by Matter.* Amsterdam, North-Holland, pp. 1–734.

Hou, S. Y. E., Mitra, A. K., White, S. H., Menon, G. K., Ghadially, R. and Elias, P. M. (1991). Membrane structures in normal and essential fatty acid deficient stratum corneum—Characterization by ruthenium tetroxide staining and x-ray diffraction. *J. Invest. Derm. 96*:215.

Keith, H. D., Padden, F. J. and Giannoni, G. (1969). Crystal structures of β-poly-L-glutamic acid and its alkaline earth salts. *J. Mol. Biol. 43*:423.

Lampe, M. A., Williams, M. L. and Elias, P. M. (1983). Human epidermal lipids: Characterization and modulations during differentiation. *J. Invest. Derm. 24*:131.

Landmann, L. (1984). The epidermal permeability barrier. Comparison between in vivo and in vitro lipid structures. *Eur. J. Cell Biol. 33*:258.

Lavrijsen, A. P. M., Bouwstra, J. A., Gooris, G. S., Weerheim, A., Boddé, H. E. and Ponec, M. (1995). Skin barrier properties: Stratum corneum lipid structures in patients with autosomal recessive lamellar ichthyosis. *J. Invest. Derm. 105*:619.

Lesslauer, W. and Blasie, J. K. (1972). Direct determination of the structure of barium stearate multilayers by x-ray diffraction. *Biophys. J. 12*:175.

Lewis, B. A. and Engelman, D. M. (1983). Lipid bilayer thickness varies linearly with acyl chain length in fluid phosphatidylcholine vesicles. *J. Mol. Biol. 166*:211.

Löffgren, H. and Pascher, I. (1977). Molecular arrangements of sphingolipids. The monolayer approach. *Chem. Phys. Lipids 20*:273.

Madison, K. C., Swartzendruber, D. C., Wertz, P. W. and Downing, D. T. (1987). Presence of intact intercellular lipid lamellae in the upper layers of the stratum corneum. *J. Invest. Derm. 88*:714.

McIntosh, T. J., Stewart, M. E. and Downing, D. T. (1996). X-ray diffraction analysis of isolated skin lipids: Reconstitution of intercellular lipid domains. *Biochemistry 35*:3649.

Pascher, I., Lundmark, M., Nyholm, P. G. and Sundell, S. (1992). Crystal structures of membrane lipids. *Biochim. Biophys. Acta 1113*:339.

Peterson, L. L., Zettergren, J. G. and Wuepper, K. D. (1983). Biochemistry of transglutaminases and cross-linking in the skin. *J. Invest. Derm. 81*:95s.

Rhodes, G. (1993). *Crystallography Made Crystal Clear.* San Diego, Academic Press, pp. 1–202.

Schoenborn, B. P. (1975). Advantages of neutron scattering for biological structure analysis. *Brookhaven Symp. Biol. 27*:110.

Shah, J., Atienza, J. M., Duclos, R. I., Jr., Rawlings, A. V., Dong, Z. X. and Shipley, G. G. (1995a). Structural and thermotropic properties of synthetic C16:0 (palmitoyl) ceramide: Effect of hydration. *J. Lipid Res. 36*:1936.

Shah, J., Atienza, J. M., Rawlings, A. V. and Shipley, G. G. (1995b). Physical properties of ceramides: Effect of fatty acid hydroxylation. *J. Lipid Res. 36*:1945.

Shieh, H. S., Hoard, L. G. and Nordman, C. E. (1977). Crystal structure of anhydrous cholesterol. *Nature (London) 267*:287.

Small, D. M. (1986). *The Physical Chemistry of Lipids.* New York, Plenum Press, pp. 1–672.

Smith, G. S., Sirota, E. B., Safinya, C. R., Plano, R. J. and Clark, N. A. (1990). X-ray structural studies of freely suspended ordered hydrated DMPC multimembrane films. *J. Chem. Phys. 92*:4519.

Steinert, P. M. and Cantieri, J. S. (1983). Epidermal keratins. In: *Biochemistry and Physiology of the Skin* (L. A. Goldsmith, ed.). New York, Oxford University Press, p. 135.

Swanbeck, G. (1959). Macromolecular organization of epidermal keratin. *Acta Dermato-Venereologica 39*(Supl. 43):5.

Swanbeck, G. and Thyresson, N. (1961). An x-ray diffraction study of scales from different dermatoses. *Acta Dermato-Venereologica 41*:289.

Swanbeck, G. and Thyresson, N. (1962). A study of the state of aggregation of the lipids in normal and psoriatic horny layer. *Acta Dermato-Venereologica 42*:445.

Swartzendruber, D. C., Wertz, P. W., Kitko, D. J., Madison, K. C. and Downing, D. T. (1989). Molecular models of the intercellular lipid lamellae in mammalian stratum corneum. *J. Invest. Derm. 92*:251.

Swartzendruber, D. C., Manganaro, A., Madison, K. C., Kremer, M., Wertz, P. W. and Squier, C. A. (1995). Organization of intercellular spaces of porcine epidermal and palatal stratum corneum: A quantitative study using ruthenium tetroxide. *Cell Tissue Research 279*:271.

van Duzee, B. F. (1975). Thermal analysis of human stratum corneum. *J. Invest. Derm.* 65:404.

van Hal, D. A., Jeremiasse, E., Junginger, H. E., Spies, F. and Bouwstra, J. A. (1996). Structure of fully hydrated human stratum corneum: A freeze-fracture electron microscope study. *J. Invest. Derm.* 106:89.

Warren, B. E. (1969). *X-ray Diffraction.* Reading, MA, Addison-Wesley, pp. 1–381.

Wertz, P. W., Swartzendruber, D. C., Kitko, D. J., Madison, K. C. and Downing, D. T. (1989). The role of the corneocyte lipid envelopes in cohesion of the stratum corneum. *J. Invest. Derm.* 93:169.

Wertz, P. W., Kremer, M. and Squier, C. A. (1992). Comparison of lipids from epidermal and palatal stratum corneum. *J. Invest. Derm.* 98:375.

White, S. H., King, G. I. and Jacobs, R. E. (1986). Solubility of volatile hydrocarbons in lipid bilayers: A new perspective. In: *Molecular and Cellular Mechanisms of Anesthetics* (S. H. Roth and K. W. Miller, eds.). New York, Plenum Press, p. 279.

White, S. H., Mirejovsky, D. and King, G. I. (1988). Structure of lamellar lipid domains and corneocyte envelopes of murine stratum corneum. An x-ray diffraction study. *Biochemistry* 27:3725.

Wiener, M. C. and White, S. H. (1991a). Fluid Bilayer Structure Determination by the Combined Use of X-ray and Neutron Diffraction. I. Fluid Bilayer Models and the limits of Resolution. *Biophys. J.* 59:162.

Wiener, M. C. and White, S. H. (1991b). Fluid bilayer structure determination by the combined use of x-ray and neutron diffraction II. "Composition space" refinement method. *Biophys. J.* 59:174.

Wiener, M. C. and White, S. H. (1992). Structure of a fluid dioleoylphosphatidylcholine bilayer determined by joint refinement of x-ray and neutron diffraction data. III. Complete structure. *Biophys. J.* 61:434.

Wilkes, G. L., Nguyen, A. L. and Wildnauer, R. (1973). Structure-property relations of human and neonatal rat stratum corneum. I. Thermal stability of the crystalline lipid structure as studied by x-ray diffraction and differential thermal analysis. *Biochim. Biophys. Acta* 304:267.

Wilkins, M. H. F., Blaurock, A. E. and Engelman, D. M. (1971). Bilayer structure in membranes; *Nature New Biol.* 230:72.

Woolfson, M. M. (1970). *X-ray Crystallography.* Cambridge, England, Cambridge University Press, pp. 1–380.

Worthington, C. R. and Blaurock, A. E. (1969). A low-angle x-ray diffraction study of the swelling behavior of peripheral nerve myelin. *Biochim. Biophys. Acta* 173:427.

Zaccai, G., Büldt, G., Seelig, A. and Seelig, J. (1979). Neutron diffraction studies on phosphatidylcholine model membranes. II. Chain conformation and segmental disorder. *J. Mol. Biol.* 134:693.

3
Infrared Spectroscopic and Differential Scanning Calorimetric Investigations of the Stratum Corneum Barrier Function

Aarti Naik
Aston University, Birmingham, England

Richard H. Guy
Centre Interuniversitaire de Recherche et d'Enseignement, Archamps, France

I. INTRODUCTION

The lipid and protein mosaic that is the hallmark of stratum corneum architecture, by its very nature, lends itself ideally to biophysical investigation by techniques customarily employed in general biomembrane research.

Among this ensemble of methods, infrared (IR) spectroscopy [1–5] and differential scanning calorimetry (DSC) [6–11] feature prominently in the study of model and natural biomembranes. The functional significance of the lipid bilayer, particularly its polymorphic state, in all biological membranes is well established. The polymorphic nature of membrane lipids, together with the great assortment of lipid and protein structures found in biomembranes, inevitably leads to a melange of diverse membrane states and hence, functionalities, which are evidently exploited by nature. Infrared spectroscopy and DSC have traditionally been used to investigate the thermotropic phase behavior of membrane lipids and can provide considerable insight into membrane structure and function [12,13]. Indeed, for a number of simple prokaryotic and eukaryotic cell membranes, this membrane thermotropism can be elegantly correlated to biological function [6,8]. The anisotropic nature of most mammalian membranes (where composition, structural arrangements, and membrane dynamics can vary from region to region), however, impedes the facile elucidation of such structure–function relationships in the native system. Infrared spectroscopy and, in particular, DSC have therefore been applied to a variety of simple model systems, starting with pure lipids (natural and synthetic) and progressing to well-defined binary and tertiary mixtures, with the result that our understanding of the relationship between lipid structure and thermodynamics has been greatly enhanced. Moreover, these techniques have enabled interactions between the lipid matrix and intrinsic membrane proteins to be monitored [14,15], in addition to the effect of additives such as drugs, anaesthetics, ions, and cholesterol on lipid thermotropism [13,16].

The simplistic portrayal of the stratum corneum as a stratified and heterogenous membrane composed of proteinaceous cells embedded in a lipoidal matrix does not do justice to the structural and functional complexity of this membrane. This model, nevertheless, has been a convenient starting point; the arrangement of these two constituents alone having the potential to control and modify barrier function [17]. Most notably, the extracellular lipids that form the only continuous structure from the exterior to the interior of the SC have been shown to represent the primary pathway (*and* barrier, as a consequence of the inherently high diffusional resistance) for the penetration of water and small compounds [18,19]. Concordantly, the conformational disorder of the lipid domain has been directly correlated with SC water permeability [20,21], as has the removal of SC lipids [22]. The intense application (as evidenced by the literature) of DSC and IR to the stratum corneum, with the attendant emphasis on the lipid network is therefore not surprising, and has yielded, both singularly and in combination, a wealth of information characterizing the organization and dynamics of this cutaneous biomembrane.

It is the goal of this chapter to provide an up-to-date overview of the applications of infrared spectroscopy and differential scanning calorimetry to the study of stratum corneum barrier function. The reader is referred to previous, excellent reviews of the literature upon which this article has its foundation [23–27].

II. INFRARED SPECTROSCOPY

Infrared spectroscopy records the molecular vibrations of absorbing species, occurring as a result of their interaction with electromagnetic energy. The wave–particle duality of electromagnetic radiation generates a number of seminal relationships; those germane to the ensuing discussion are summarized below.

Electromagnetic waves are described by their wavelength (λ) and frequency (Hz), which are inversely related by the following expression:

$$\lambda = \frac{c}{\nu} \tag{1}$$

where λ = the wavelength, in centimeters, c = the velocity of electromagnetic radiation in a vacuum (2.998×10^{10} cm sec^{-1}), and ν = the frequency, in hertz (wave cycles per second).

Electromagnetic energy is quantized, where the amount of energy corresponding to 1 quantum of energy (or 1 photon), ε, of a given frequency is described by the Bohr equation:

$$\varepsilon = h\nu = \frac{hc}{\lambda} \tag{2}$$

where h = Planck's constant (6.626×10^{-34} J sec). Hence, the energy of a photon varies directly with its frequency but inversely with its wavelength. As IR radiation is absorbed, oscillations within the different chemical bonds of constituent groups corresponding to vibrational energies precisely matching the absorbed energy are amplified.

In a dispersive IR instrument, polychromatic radiation from the source is divided into two beams, of equal intensity, and passed, alternately, through the sample and the reference materials. If the energy of any vibrating bond within the sample or the reference coincides with that of the component frequencies of the incident light, radiation corresponding to that wavelength is absorbed by the material. The transmitted beams are then spatially dispersed into their constituent wavelengths by a monochromator before reaching the detector, which views one frequency element at a time, ultimately enabling the relative absorption of the sample to be monitored as a function of wavelength.

The intensity of absorption by a sample varies with the length l of the sample according to the Beer–Lambert law:

$$\log \frac{I}{I_o} - -a[J]l \tag{3}$$

where I_o = the incident intensity (at a particular wavelength); I = the intensity after passage through a sample of length, l; [J] = the molar concentration of the absorbing species; and a = the molar absorption coefficient, also known as the extinction coefficient (L mol^{-1} cm^{-1}).

The dimensionless product

$$A = a[\text{J}]l \tag{4}$$

is referred to as the *absorbance* of the sample (formerly the "optical density"), and the ratio I/I_o is referred to as the *transmittance T*; these two quantities are related by the expression

$$\log T = -A \tag{5}$$

The visual format of an IR spectrum can take one of several forms. The ordinate is expressed in the form of either % transmittance or absorbance. The abscissa, or the location of the absorption band, can be represented by the wavelength of the radiation, or more commonly the wavenumber ($\tilde{\nu}$):

$$\tilde{\nu} = \frac{1}{\lambda} = \frac{\nu}{c} \tag{6}$$

This unit is the reciprocal of wavelength, usually expressed in cm^{-1}, but unlike wavelength has the advantage of being linear with energy (cf. frequency). For this reason, the term *frequency* is commonly used to describe the position of an absorbance, although strictly speaking it is more accurate to use the term *wavenumber*.

Most modern IR spectrometers now utilize Fourier transform (FT) techniques of spectral detection and analysis, offering distinct advantages over the earlier, dispersive instruments [28]. These include increased speed, sensitivity, accuracy, and optical throughput—often allowing sample analysis that would otherwise be impossible with dispersive instruments. The application of FT–IR in the pharmaceutical sciences, together with the basic principles of the technique, has been reviewed by Markovich and Pidgeon [29]. Briefly, the heart of the FT-spectrometer is a Michelson interferometer, a device that replaces the conventional monochromator and enables the simultaneous analysis of all the frequencies, at greatly enhanced resolution, in the polychromatic radiation source [30]. The interferometer bisects and conveys the beam from the IR source via two optical paths: one with a fixed, the other with a variable (regulated by moving mirror), optical path length. The two beams are then recombined, and half the beam passes through the sample, where the non-absorbed radiation continues on to the detector. As a result of the different optical path lengths, a phase difference is introduced when the beams recombine, causing the two beams to interfere either constructively or destructively, depending on the extra distance traveled by the one. This produces a time-dependent optical interference pattern (interferogram) at the detector, now also encoding spectral information about the sample.

Consider a monochromatic beam: The detected signal oscillates as the two components alternately come into and out of phase as the path difference (p) is varied and gives rise to an interference pattern, the ac portion of which is a modulated cosine wave. The simplest equation representing this is

$$I(p) = B(\tilde{v}) \cos 2\pi p\tilde{v} \tag{7}$$

in which $I(p)$ is the intensity of the detector signal as a function of optical retardation p, and $B(\tilde{v})$ is the spectral intensity at a wavenumber, $\tilde{v}$, as modified by instrumental characteristics.

An actual signal consists of radiation spanning a large number of wavenumbers, and the total intensity at the detector is the integral of all their cosine waves:

$$I(p) = \int_0^\infty B(\tilde{v}) \cos (2\pi p\tilde{v}) \, dv \tag{8}$$

Equation 8 mathematically describes the interferogram (intensity versus optical retardation, which is a function of *time*) and that which is physically measured by the spectrometer. It represents one half of a cosine Fourier transform pair, the other being

$$B(\tilde{v}) = \int_{-\infty}^{+\infty} I(p) \cos (2\pi p\tilde{v}) \, dp \tag{9}$$

Equation 9 represents the IR spectrum (intensity versus wavenumber), which can be derived from expression (8) using a mathematical technique known as Fourier transformation. Needless to say, this requires spectrometer-interfaced computing power, which additionally provides the capacity for spectral manipulation such as deconvolution, smoothing, and subtraction.

The mid-IR range of the electromagnetic spectrum, 4000 cm^{-1} (2.5 µm) to 625 cm^{-1} (16 µm), encompasses absorption bands corresponding to the fundamental vibrations of most functional groups. Each band in an IR spectrum can be characterized by the wavenumber (or "frequency") of its absorption maximum, in addition to its intensity and bandwidth. The wavenumber at which an absorbance occurs is characteristic of the underlying molecular motion and consequently of the atoms participating in the chemical bond and on their conformation and immediate environment. The bandwidth, on the other hand, is related to the rates of motion of the molecule, and increases as motional rates increase.

Although an application of both quantum and classical wave theory is necessary for the elucidation of selection rules for vibrational and rotational transitions, much of the infrared spectra of organic molecules is interpreted in terms of classical ideas of characteristic group frequencies. The principles governing the vibrations of an atomic system can be understood by analogy with simpler oscillating systems: Since vibrational frequencies are determined by interatomic distances, bond angles, and force constants of a molecule, they can be readily assigned to functionalities. Since these vibrations are sensitive to the local molecular and physicochemical environment, a series of sequential molecular fingerprints, obtained as a function of varying conditions, will identify not only the characteristic functionalities but also any accompanying structural modifications.

III. DIFFERENTIAL SCANNING CALORIMETRY

Differential scanning calorimetry measures the thermodynamic parameters associated with thermally induced phase transitions. Here, the sample of interest and an inert reference are heated or cooled independently at a programmed rate, and in tandem, such that their temperatures change in unison and the differential temperature is maintained at zero. If the sample undergoes a thermally induced transition, heat must be applied to or withdrawn from the sample in order to maintain the same temperature in both sample and reference compartments. The instrument measures the heat flow into the sample relative to the reference and this *differential* heat flow (or excess specific heat) is recorded as a function of temperature, resulting in a trace, as shown in Fig. 1

Figure 1 is a hypothetical DSC thermogram for a lipid undergoing a typical endothermic phase transition such as a gel to liquid–crystalline phase change. If the experiment were performed from high to low temperature, the peak would be inflected in the opposite direction, indicating an exothermic process. Several important thermodynamic parameters can be derived from the DSC thermogram, and these together with their significance are briefly discussed below.

Differential scanning calorimetry investigations of the SC can involve direct analysis either of the isolated membrane or of the extracted components, often with these materials being examined as a function of hydration or enhancer treatment. The material under investigation is sealed in the sample compartment, while the reference cell is usually left blank (unless the sample is suspended in a solvent, in which case the reference cell will contain an equivalent mass of solvent). As a sample is heated, its internal energy in-

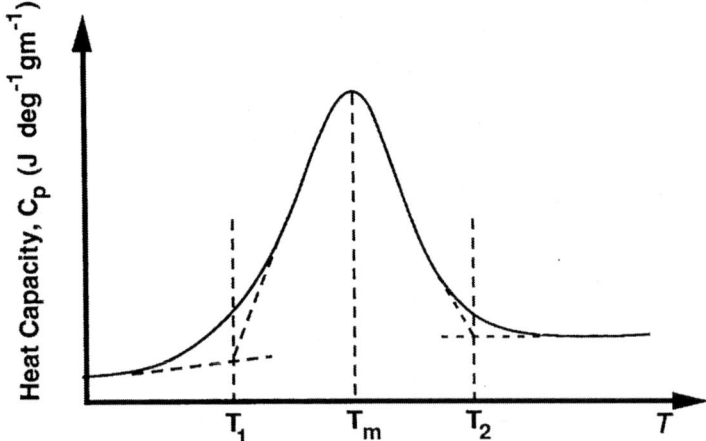

Figure 1 A hypothetical differential scanning calorimetric profile for an endothermic transition, where T_m is the transition midpoint, and T_1 and T_2 are the extrapolated onset and completion phase transition temperatures, respectively.

creases, with a resultant increase in the vibrational and rotational motion of the molecular constituents. The temperature of the sample is raised proportionately, with the magnitude of the increase being governed by the heat capacity of the sample at that temperature. Hence, if the internal energy of the sample is plotted against temperature, then the slope of the curve at any temperature provides the heat capacity (C_p):

$$C_p = \frac{1}{m} \times \frac{\partial H}{\partial T} \tag{10}$$

where m is the mass of substance being heated, H is the heat content, and T is the temperature. That is, an infinitesimal change in internal energy brings about an infinitesimal change in temperature, and the constant of proportionality is the heat capacity. Heat capacities vary with temperature; however, since the variation is quite small over narrow temperature ranges, they are treated as almost independent of temperature, being defined as the amount of heat (per gram or per mole) required to raise the temperature of the sample by $1°C$ (or K). Subsequent to appropriate calibration, the rate of heat input into the sample (J min^{-1} gm^{-1}) is measured by the scanning calorimeter and, given the scanning rate (°C min^{-1}), the parameter recorded is usually C_p (J °C^{-1} gm^{-1}) as a function of temperature. The DSC technique is particularly sensitive to changes in C_p, which may be detected by the displacement of the baseline (for instance, the upward sloping baseline in Fig. 1 is indicative of a larger value of C_p subsequent to the transition).

The phase transition temperature, T_m, represents the temperature at which the heat capacity, and consequently the excess specific heat absorbed by the system, reaches a maximum. This excess heat (*excess* because now the heat supplied does not result in a corresponding temperature rise) is required by the molecule to execute a conformational change—such as the conversion from a lipid gel to the liquid crystalline state. The enthalpy of this transition ΔH_{cal} (per mole or unit mass of material) can be determined directly from the area of the peak. For a symmetric curve, T_m refers to the midpoint of the transition and is the characteristic temperature at which both phases exist in equilibrium. For pure lipids undergoing a first-order transition, this phase change is expected to occur over an infinitely small temperature range corresponding to T_m. However, in practice most transitions occur over a width of several degrees (T_1 to T_2 in Fig. 1). The sharpness of the phase transition (often expressed as the temperature width at half-height, or the difference between T_2 and T_1) is related to the cooperativity of the process. The *cooperativity* is the degree to which the entire sample participates in the phase transition. Generally, pure lipids or homogeneous systems yield sharp peaks and the process is termed cooperative, whereas heterogeneous or impure systems produce broad peaks, denoting a noncooperative process. The size of the cooperative unit may also be estimated from a quantitative analysis of the DSC data, in which the equilibrium constant for the two-state transition is determined as a function of temperature and treated to yield the van't Hoff enthalpy (ΔH_{vH}), defined as the transition enthalpy per mole of the cooperative unit undergoing the phase change [7].

Additionally, we would expect a lipid melting transition to be accompanied by a change in the degree of molecular order and hence accompanied by a change in entropy. For a reversible two-state transition, T_m represents the temperature at which both phases are in equilibrium and hence the free energy change (ΔG) associated with the process is zero. The expression

$$\Delta G = 0 = \Delta H - T_m\,\Delta S$$

$$\Delta S = \frac{\Delta H}{T_m}$$

(11)

can, therefore, be used to determine the change in entropy (ΔS) for the transition from measured calorimetric values of T_m and ΔH.

Finally, experimental parameters such as amount of material, heating rates, and the state of equilibrium of the system under study are of paramount importance to the acquisition of accurate data. These are not specifically discussed here, but the reader should be aware that in order to obtain valid thermodynamic parameters the system must not only be at equilibrium during the run but also be scanned at a rate that does not kinetically limit the thermally induced transitions [14]. With respect to complex, multicomponent membranes such as the SC, ensuring a state of equilibrium between all the constituents of the system (including exogenous additives) is a particularly difficult problem.

IV. IN VITRO LIPID BIOPHYSICS

Both IR and DSC share the advantage of being nonperturbing, compared to techniques such as fluorescence and electron spin resonance spectroscopies, which require probe molecules to discern the makeup of the neighboring milieu. Although DSC, in isolation, cannot directly provide information regarding lipid and/or protein conformation at the molecular level, the bulk thermodynamic parameters it yields (and those cannot be obtained by IR) provide supplementary data; a hypothesis generated by either set of data must, therefore, be compatible with both the conformational model (generated by IR) and the thermodynamic constraints imposed on the system (as measured by DSC). Additionally, IR can be used noninvasively, both in vitro and in vivo, offering substantial versatility. As the reader will note, DSC is a rather more traditional technique compared to IR. While the former is limited to the study of thermotropic phase behavior, IR has found several additional and innovative applications in the study of skin barrier function.

As with other lipid systems, a study of temperature- and hydration-induced alterations of IR spectral parameters, together with parallel DSC studies, has provided essential insight into the biophysical properties of the stratum corneum. Extensive characterization of SC from a variety of mammalian species has been undertaken, and a thorough treatise of these earlier investigations, together with their phospholipid corollaries, has been presented by Potts and co-workers [23,24].

Investigation of intact SC samples by transmission IR was first undertaken in the 1970s by Park and Baddiel [31] and has since become a routine procedure. The thin (10–20 μm) cross section of the SC allows an intact sheet of SC (following isolation from epidermal membranes) to be analyzed directly by transmission IR. The resulting spectrum is typified by absorbances originating from lipids, proteins, and water, which are easily assigned in the spectrum (Fig. 2).

With respect to the SC, the most informative lipid absorbances are those originating from the hydrophobic alkyl chain [27]. Of these, the most extensively studied are the carbon–hydrogen stretching vibrations, which give rise to two prominent peaks near 2850 cm^{-1} and 2920 cm^{-1} as a result of their asymmetric and symmetric stretching modes, respectively. The frequencies of these bands are sensitive to the trans/gauche ratio of the alkyl chain and are thus excellent indicators of the conformational status of the hydrocarbon tails. The asymmetric (~2956 cm^{-1}) and symmetric (~2870 cm^{-1}) stretching modes of the terminal methyl groups are also useful conformational markers, providing information specific to the environment within the interior of the bilayer. The lipid alkyl backbone may be further probed by analyzing the CH$_2$ scissoring (1462–1474 cm^{-1}) and rocking (720–730 cm^{-1}) vibrations, which are descriptors of the lateral packing within the lamellae [5]. Together, then, these vibrational modes provide a multifaceted view of the conformational nature of the lipid domains.

Phase transitions of SC lipids and the accompanying melting of hydrocarbon chains are readily monitored via the CH$_2$ stretching vibrations. Figure 3

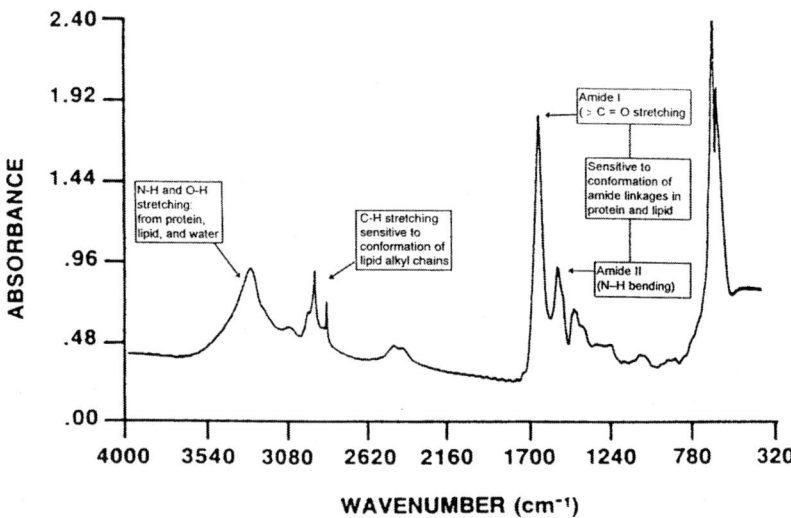

Figure 2 A transmission infrared spectrum of porcine stratum corneum. (Adapted from Ref. 24)

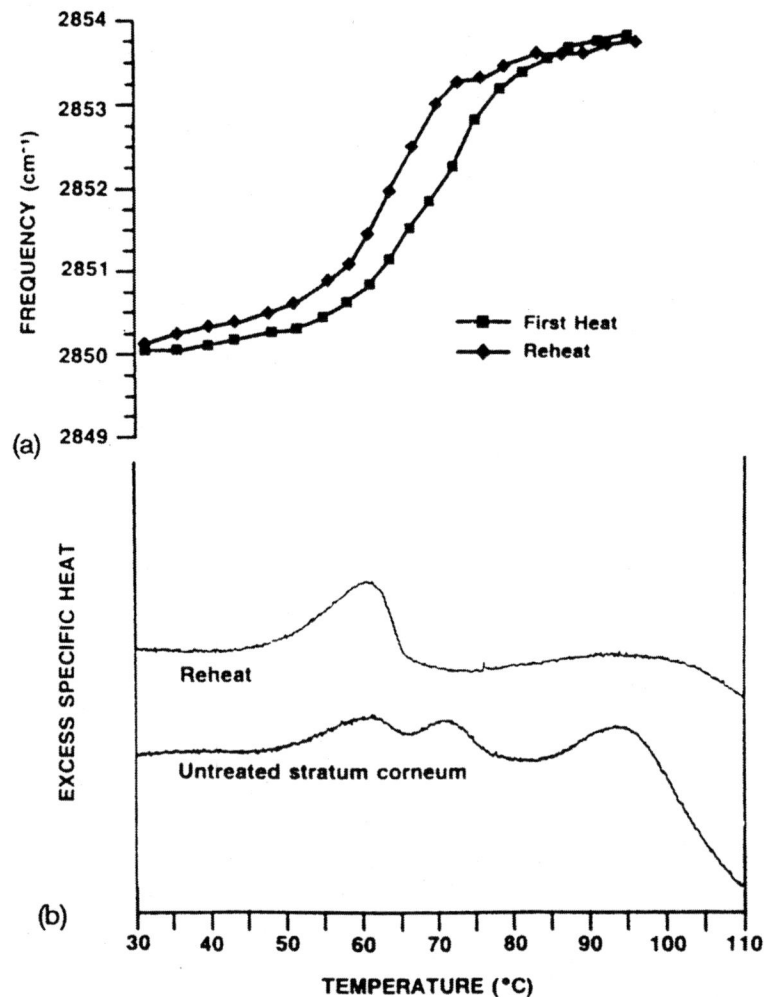

Figure 3   (a) The change in the C–H symmetric stretching frequency [v_s(CH$_2$)] as a function of temperature for porcine SC. (b) The DSC thermal profile for identically treated porcine SC. (From Ref. 25.)

illustrates the thermally generated changes in the CH_2 symmetric stretching frequencies $[v_s(CH_2)]$ of porcine SC; the resultant sigmoidal curve with an abrupt increase in frequency between 60–80°C is typical of SC tissue. The absolute frequencies, in addition to the magnitude of the thermal shift, reflect the degree of hydrocarbon chain order. Depicted by this scheme is a gel to liquid–crystalline phase transition occurring between 60 and 80°C, characterized by a significant increase in gauche rotational isomers along the alkyl chains, now demanding greater vibrational energy and thus occurring at higher IR frequencies. This abrupt increase in vibrational frequency (or, more precisely, the vibrational energy) is accompanied by an increase in bandwidth (data not shown), representing the concomitant increase in motional freedom and in the number of conformational states of the alkyl chains.

For porcine SC, the temperature dependence of the terminal methyl group conformation has also been investigated [32]. By virtue of its location, the terminal methyl group reports on the alkyl chain order pertaining to the interior of the bilayer. In contrast to the methylene stretching frequency, the methyl stretching frequency increased progressively with increasing temperature, with the absence of a distinct phase transition. Based on results from other phospholipid systems, this behavior is considered to be the consequence of a less constrained environment toward the center of the bilayer, compared to the methylene groups closer to the polar headgroups.

While a temperature-dependent IR spectrum allows one to examine specific elements of a transition, a DSC thermogram enables the visualization of transitions in their entirety and the calculation of associated thermodynamic parameters. The IR and DSC thermal profiles for identically treated samples of hydrated porcine SC are shown in Fig. 3. The results of a series of thermograms for intact, delipidized, fractionated, and reheated SC as well as extracted lipids suggest that these three major transitions near 60, 70, and 95°C in intact SC are due to intercellular lipid, a lipid–protein complex associated with the corneocyte membrane, and intracellular keratin, respectively. Evidence supporting these deductions is elegantly presented by Golden et al. [33]. More recently, the presence of a subzero lipid transition at –9°C has also been reported [34].

The complementary nature of DSC and IR is further validated by comparing the profiles obtained by these two techniques (Fig. 3): the C–H stretching frequency transition spans the temperature range seen for the two lipid endotherms in DSC, with a slight inflection at approximately 70°C, suggestive of the two transitions also observed by DSC. Furthermore, this inflection is not apparent upon reheating the membrane, with a singular transition at a slightly decreased temperature, as in the DSC profile, being observed. Studies with murine [35,36] and human SC [37,38] have established similar thermal profiles. Corresponding DSC thermal profiles of human SC depicting major transitions at 68, 80, and 95°C and a small and variable transition near 35°C are shown in Fig. 4.

The minor transition observed at ~35°C in such studies has usually been attributed to lower-melting-point lipids, for example, those of sebaceous origin. However, the evidence for this assignment has been, at best, circumstantial. Despite its designation as a lipid-based transition over two decades ago [39], it is only recently that studies by Gay et al. [40] and Ongpipattanakul et al. [32] have provided novel insights into the possible origin and significance of this and other low-temperature SC lipid transitions. Gay et al. [40] monitored the calorimetric transition temperatures of human SC endotherms as a function of hydration and found that above a water content of 20% (g/100 g dry SC), the temperature of the lowest transition remained essentially constant, with an average value of 35.9°C ($n = 12$, SE = 0.5), whereas further dehydration caused T_m to progressively increase, reaching 43°C in the dry

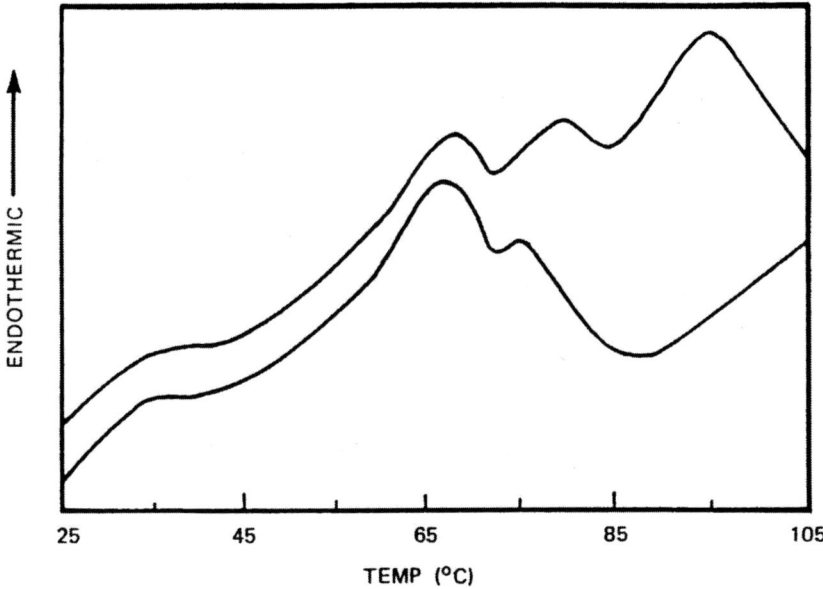

Figure 4 The DSC thermal profiles of human stratum corneum (upper trace) and the same sample reheated (lower trace), both obtained at 50% water content. (From Ref. 37.)

state. This hydration-dependent behavior is consistent with that of other lipid–water systems [41] and, together with the deductions of Van Duzee [39] based on the thermal reversibility and lack of interaction with urea further, substantiates the lipid nature of this transition. Furthermore, this transition (comprising 7–10% of the total measured enthalpy) was observed in 17 of the 19 individual specimens examined, contending the previously stated variability of this transition.

To assess the association of this transition with sebaceous lipids, SC samples were exogenously treated with a model sebum lipid mixture (chiefly comprising triolein, oleyl oleate, palmitic acid, and squalene) and examined calorimetrically. With treatment, there was no significant change in the enthalpies of the endotherms at 37, 68, and 80°C, although a small increase in T_m for the former two transitions was noted. Upon reheating, the 68°C and 80°C peaks coalesced to a single endotherm at 63–65°C, which, for the treated sample, demonstrated a slight increase in the transition temperature, apparent cooperativity, and enthalpy. The 37°C transition, however, remained unchanged, suggesting that the addition of sebum did not have a discernible effect on the lowest transition temperature, even after reheating, which should have further facilitated the incorporation (and any impact) of the lipid material.

This deduction was further corroborated by results of high-performance thin-layer chromatographic (HP-TLC) compositional analysis. Chromatograms of these SC samples showed no detectable bands corresponding to sebum lipids, suggesting that if these samples were indeed contaminated by sebum, it was at a level less than 2% by weight (the detection limit of the technique). These DSC and HP-TLC results, acquired with SC samples from leg tissue (a site known to be sparsely populated with sebaceous glands) that had been hexane washed prior to analysis (a procedure that removes most superficial sebum contamination), strongly suggested that the 37°C transition was not due to the presence of sebum. Inspection of the C–H stretching frequencies in this temperature range offered further clues to the origin of this transition.

Figure 5 shows the thermally induced (10–60°C) changes in the CH_2 stretching frequency of intact human SC plotted as a function of hydration and reheating. Corresponding data for the extracted lipid samples are depicted in Fig. 6. For SC, the frequency increased with temperature and showed a small, but definite, inflection point between 35 and 45°C. Under dry conditions, the midpoint was estimated to be 45°C, decreasing to a constant value of ~35°C as the hydration level was increased. This behavior closely mimicked the calorimetric results described, suggesting that the 35°C inflection observed by IR corresponded to the same endothermic process measured by DSC. However, no evidence of a thermal transition at 35°C was observed by IR in the extracted lipids. Moreover, it is unlikely that this transition is related to variations in lattice packing since an abrupt increase in stretching frequency would not be anticipated for an orthorhombic-to-hexagonal change. Further, since the absolute frequencies of the CH_2 motions assume characteristic values dependent on the conformational state of the lipid chains [5], the data clearly show that the observed $v_s(CH_2)$ of 2849.5–2849.7 cm^{-1} at 10°C reflects lipid predominantly in the gel phase. The increasing value of $v_s(CH_2)$ as the temperature of the system is raised must therefore represent an increasing proportion of gauche conformers along the alkyl chain such that a $v_s(CH_2)$ ranging from 2850.0 to 2850.5 cm^{-1} between 32 and 37°C must denote the existence of a mixed population of both solid and fluid lipids in the physiological temperature range. These observations concerning the 35°C transition have therefore been interpreted in terms of a solid-to-fluid phase change for a discrete subset of lipids. The absence of this transition in extracted lipid samples implies that these lipids are not uniformly present throughout the SC but would appear to be differentially distributed. This concept is further supported by the reported absence of the 35°C transition in cultured SC, the lipid organization of which (as shown by electron microscopy) is significantly different to its human counterpart [42].

Thermal lipid transitions in the physiologic temperature range have also been reported for porcine [32] and neonatal murine [43] SC. Based on arguments similar to those presented above, the transition near 20°C in porcine SC detected by IR has been attributed, not to sebaceous lipids, but to a solid-to-fluid phase change for a small fraction of SC lipids.

Gay et al. [40] also reported the presence of a thermally reversible (and previously undetected) transition at ~55°C in human SC. This endotherm was variable, being detectable by DSC only in 20% of the samples examined and only at low hydration close to the sensitivity limit of the instrument. Once again, the corresponding IR data were able to elaborate further on the nature and significance of this transition. Although, the CH_2 stretching data revealed no discernible change in frequency at 55°C, parallel analysis of the temperature-dependent CH_2 scissoring vibrations demonstrated otherwise.

The IR measurement of the CH_2 vibrations from the scissoring region provides an extremely sensitive means of monitoring qualitative changes in the lattice packing of alkyl lipids [44,45]. These vibrations are influenced by interactions between methylene groups on neighboring alkyl chains. For example, existence of the gel phase lipids in a loosely packed subcell such as that in a hexagonal (HEX) arrangement results in a single peak at a frequency near 1470 cm^{-1}. In contrast, when the alkyl chains are tightly packed in an orthorhombic (OR) crystalline lattice with the planes of the carbon skeletons

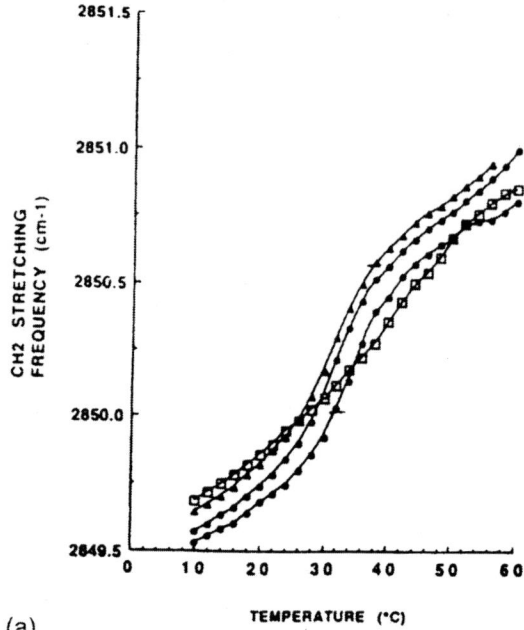

(a)

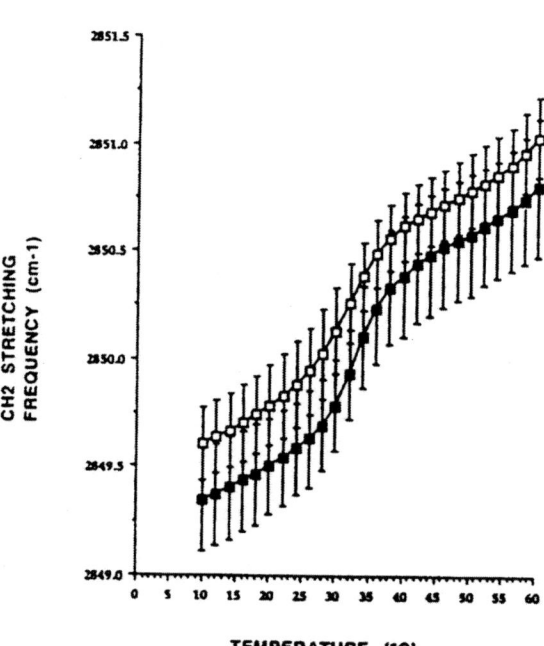

(b)

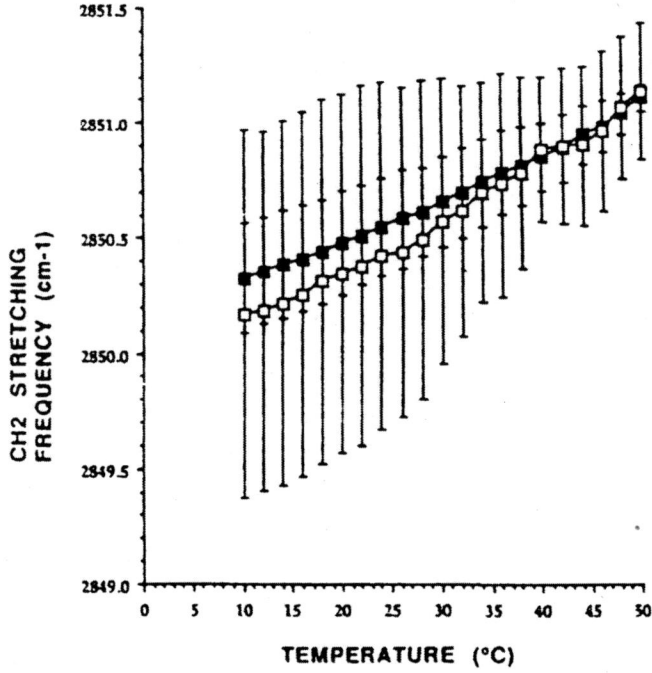

Figure 6 Average CH_2 symmetric stretching frequency of stratum corneum lipids, isolated by chloroform: methanol extraction, plotted as a function of temperature (closed square, first heat; open square, second heat) at constant hydration (95% RH). Error bars, SD. (From Ref. 40.)

perpendicular to each other, lateral chain interactions give rise to factor group splitting of the CH_2 scissoring peak, resulting in two bands replacing, and approximately equidistant from, the original peak.

Figure 7 illustrates the temperature-dependent IR factor group splitting of the alkyl chain CH_2 scissoring mode of human SC as a function of

Figure 5 Thermally induced changes in CH_2 symmetric stretching frequency of intact human SC measured by infrared spectroscopy. (a) First heat as a function of SC hydration (open square, 4%; closed circle, 23%; open circle, 100%; closed triangle, 300%). (b) Average values for first (closed square) and second (open square) heats at constant hydration (95% RH). Error bars, SD. (From Ref. 40.)

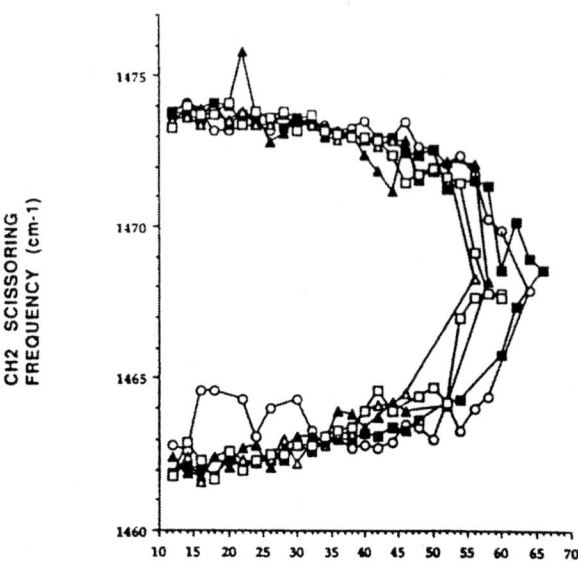

(a)

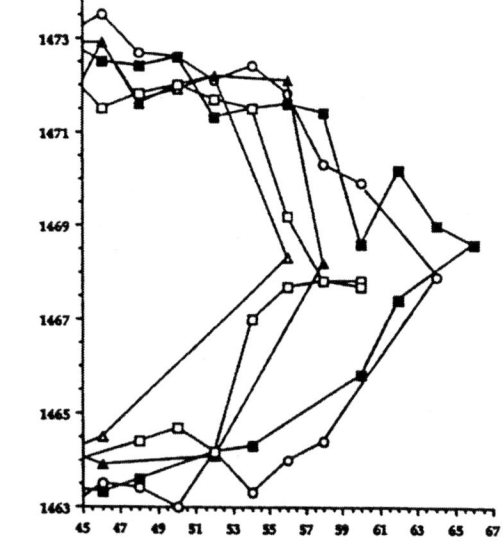

(b)

hydration. Two distinct bands (1462 and 1473 cm^{-1}) were observed from 10 to 45°C, before their rapid collapse to a single value (1468 cm^{-1}) between 45 and 65°C. The temperature at which these peaks coalesced progressively decreased as the hydration state of the SC was increased. This observed thermal profile for the CH$_2$ scissoring vibrations was consistent with lipids, aligned in OR subcells at physiological temperature, undergoing an ortho-rhombic-to-hexagonal transition between 45 and 65°C, prior to the main gel-to-liquid crystalline transition. Moreover, the thermally induced alteration in the lateral packing of the SC lipids observed by IR coincided with the 55°C endotherm detected by DSC, suggesting that this variable calorimetric transition was not artifactual and that the lattice changes were not linked to the 35°C transition. Independent evidence for the existence of OR structures has been found with x-ray diffraction using hairless mouse [46], neonatal rat [47], and human SC [48,49] and with nuclear magnetic resonance studies of porcine SC lipids [50]. (See also Chapters 2 and 4 of this book.)

Infrared examination of porcine SC by Ongpipattanakul et al. [32] has also revealed the existence of OR structures. Notably, through the use of deconvolution and second-derivative techniques in this analysis, resolution of the CH$_2$ scissoring band was further enhanced. As a result, peak positions of the component CH$_2$ scissoring bands could be resolved at each temperature increment, revealing the existence, from –10°C to ~40°C, of three peaks near 1464, 1468, and 1473 cm^{-1}. Based on the rationale presented above, the bands at 1464 and 1473 cm^{-1} were attributed to OR gel phase packing, while the peak near 1468 cm^{-1} was associated with the more mobile chains of the hexagonal subcell. The spectral analysis also showed that all three peaks persisted until ~55–60°C, after which only the 1468 cm^{-1} band remained. Thus, these results indicated the coexistence of orthorhombic and hexagonal gel phases up to just below the main chain melting transition between 60 and 80°C as monitored by the CH$_2$ symmetric stretching frequencies. Analogous lateral packing behavior has been implied for hairless mouse SC with a postulated solid–solid phase change occuring between 31 and 43°C, preceded by the coexistence of both phases [36]. Although, the lack of experimental data below 30°C, together with the absence of a CH$_2$ scissoring doublet in this

---

Figure 7 (a) Temperature-dependent factor group splitting of the infrared-active, CH$_2$ scissoring mode of human stratum corneum as a function of different hydration (open circle, 0%; closed square, 17%; open triangle, 33%; closed triangle, 70%; open square, 300%). (b) The same data plotted on an expanded scale. (From Ref. 40.)

murine study, hinders an explicit conclusion based on the IR data alone, supportive evidence for the coexistence of orthorhombic and hexagonal phases in hairless mouse SC has been obtained by x-ray diffraction studies [46]. Moreover, coexistence of these OR and HEX phase lipids has also been demonstrated for human SC using x-ray diffraction: Though IR studies confirm this view for porcine SC [32], IR analyses of human SC [40] were not able to corroborate this observation. (That is, although the presence of multiple phases in the physiological temperature range is predicated for human SC on the basis of the 35°C transition, the precise nature of these phases is undetermined by IR). This disparity is, very likely, a consequence of the different techniques of spectral analysis utilized in the IR investigations of human and porcine SC, which offered, in the latter study, greater sensitivity to structural resolution.

The IR results with human and porcine SC reveal the existence of a dominant gel-to-liquid-crystalline phase transition for two subsets of lipids, one of which may be associated with a proteinaceous component. Below this main phase transition, the studies demonstrate the presence of multiple phases, which coexist at physiological temperature. Although neither the precise composition nor the quantity of lipids participating in these substructures can be unequivocally defined, these observations, together with those from thermotropic phase behavior studies of other lipid systems, have provided a number of conjectures regarding SC organization [32,40]. The significance of these transitions will naturally be dependent on the location of the contributing lipids. Although it is not clear whether the 35°C transition arises from a small disordering of a large subset of SC lipids or from a large disordering of a smaller subset, the noticeable increase in $v_s(CH_2)$ and decrease in T_m upon hydration intimate how skin hydration might influence skin permeability, particularly if this transition reflects the latter scenario. The absence of this phase change in extracted lipids might suggest the corneocyte envelope as a plausible location.

Indeed, the corneocyte envelope is also an attractive candidate for the OR lipid configuration noted by IR [40]. As articulated by this study, the highly ordered nature of OR lipids requires that the participant alkyl chains be of roughly the same length and orientation to maximize interchain interactions. Introduction of dissimilar molecules (like cholesterol) will rapidly destroy the propensity for such an intimate arrangement. This physicochemical dependence is exemplified by the disappearance of OR structure in phospholipid-based systems after the addition of small molecule perturbants such as anaesthetics and cholesterol [51–53]. Since the corneocyte lipid envelope both lacks cholesterol and consists mainly of covalently bound ceramides, it has been suggested as a good candidate for the site of OR lipids. Furthermore, the occurrence of such a tightly arranged lipid structure could account for the relatively low permeability of the corneocyte as proposed by Potts and Francoeur [17] and as surmised from observations that epidermal tissues deficient in bound lipids are associated with increased water permeability [42,54,55]. Evidence for the presence of OR structure in extracted lipids [32,46], however, suggests that this OR lipid configuration is not restricted to the lipid envelope. More importantly, the existence of a solid–liquid phase transition in human SC in the physiological temperature range, which is notably influenced by the level of hydration, immediately evokes a point of intervention by penetration enhancers.

V. IN VIVO LIPID BIOPHYSICS

In addition to providing information regarding the biophysical properties of SC in vitro, FT-IR has become a widely utilized technique for the in vivo assessment of SC. This has been possible through the use of internal reflectance or attenuated total reflectance-infrared (ATR-IR) spectroscopy. A thorough account describing the principles of this phenomenon and its contemporary applications, which have been expanded through the introduction of Fourier transform techniques, can be found in the literature [56]. Briefly, the ATR effect occurs when radiation propagating through a medium of refractive index, n_1 strikes an interface of a second medium of lower refractive index, n_2, at an angle that is greater than the critical angle, θ_c, [$\theta_c = \sin^{-1}(n_2/n_1)$] (Fig. 8). Under these circumstances, the beam undergoes total internal reflection; as it does so, an evanescent wave established at the interface propagates into the medium of lower refractive index (i.e., sample, such as SC). If the first medium is IR transparent while the second medium has absorption bands in the energy range of the incident radiation, then each propagation will result in energy loss due to absorption, with the effect being amplified by successive reflections within the second medium.

Hence, in contrast to transmission spectroscopy, where the sample intercepts the path of the IR beam, in ATR the sample is placed on an IR-transparent crystal (IRE, internal reflection element), permitting total internal reflection. In vivo (or in situ) experimentation is permitted by virtue of one of several design arrangements: (a) the region of skin under study may be placed directly in contact with the crystal; (b) a remote fiber-optic probe (with IRE head) may be used to transfer the IR beam from the source to the sample and ultimately to the detector; and (c) samples removed from the subject may be placed directly onto the crystal.

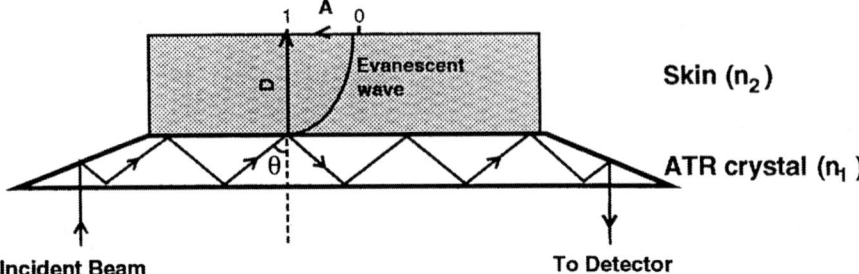

Figure 8 A schematic representation of attenuated total reflectance. An incident beam propagating through an IR transparent crystal of refractive index, n_1 strikes the skin interface of lower refractive index, n_2 at the angle θ which is greater than the critical angle ($\theta_c = \sin^{-1} [n_2/n_1]$). As a result, the beam is totally internally reflected and an evanescent beam established at the interface propagates into the skin. The amplitude (A) of the wave decays exponentially with increasing distance (D) from the interface. A = (intensity at distance, D)/(intensity at interface).

The ability of ATR spectroscopy to detect IR absorbances depends upon a number of factors, including the intensity, wavelength, and entry angle of incident radiation, the absorptivity of the sample, the degree of contact between the two media, and the depth of penetration of the evanescent wave into the sample. The sensitivity of this technique may be enhanced by improving the energy coupling of the evanescent wave to the absorbing medium, which is achieved by choosing an IRE with a refractive index greater than, but close to, that of the sample. Additionally, the depth of penetration of the evanescent beam into the sample may be increased by selecting an incident angle greater than, but close to, the critical angle, θ_c. In practice, standard instruments typically have a fixed beam, and the incident angle is therefore varied through the choice of precision cut IREs. The "depth of penetration" of this beam cannot, however, be defined absolutely since the evanescent wave decreases exponentially with increasing depth into the sample. Consequently, it is more usual to express an "apparent" depth of penetration that approximates the distance into the sample at which the incident intensity decreases to 37% (or $1/e$) of its value at the interface, and is given by the expression

$$\text{depth of penetration} = \frac{\lambda}{2\pi n_1 \, [\sin^2 \theta - (n_2/n_1)^2]^{1/2}} \tag{12}$$

where λ = the wavelength (mm), n_1 = the refractive index of the crystal, n_2 = the refractive index of the sample, and θ = the crystal face angle (degrees).

With respect to skin, this depth is in the order of 0.3–3 μm, depending on the IRE substrate, the wavelength of interest, and the hydration level of the sample. Thus, when the skin is directly analyzed by this technique, the information obtained from a single ATR-IR spectrum pertains only to the immediate layers in contact with the crystal, i.e., the superficial strata of the SC. Information from the deeper regions of the SC may, however, be obtained through sequential tape stripping, where successive layers of the SC are progressively revealed and spectrally examined. Ultimately, a layer-by-layer spectroscopic profile of the SC is assembled into a composite model. A further consideration in ATR-IR spectroscopy concerns the dependence of the magnitude of an IR absorbance on both the degree of contact between the membrane and IRE and the pressure with which the two are apposed. Hence, when spectra are used for quantitative evaluation, the absorbance of interest is normalized to another peak in the spectrum that is not an experimental variable but is equally affected by the experimental conditions—in the same way as an internal standard in chromatographic analysis.

A number of investigators have utilized the technique of reflectance spectroscopy to characterize human skin in vivo [57–60]. In particular, the technique has been extensively used for ascertaining the extent of skin hydration, both in pathological skin conditions and in the evaluation of moisturizing treatments (see later).

More recently, Bommannan et al. [61] used ATR-IR to examine the SC as a function of serial tape stripping. The nonuniform and inhomogeneous nature of the membrane has inevitably led to questions concerning the exact location of the barrier within the SC. With ATR-IR in conjunction with tape stripping, it has been possible to probe, at discrete intervals across the forearm SC in human subjects, spectral features associated with both the intercellular lipids and the hydration level of the membrane, key determinants of skin barrier function. On average, each tape-stripping procedure removed one SC layer per strip and enabled the progressive examination of 50–75% of the SC tissue.

As previously, the CH_2 stretching vibrations in the 2850–2950-cm^{-1} region were the focal point for the lipid-related analyses. Since the area under the curve of an infrared absorbance is directly proportional to the amount of the absorbing species [62,63], the area under the asymmetric stretching band provided an indication of the amount of lipid in the vicinity of each measurement. Similarly, the frequency and bandwidth of these absorbances reported on the conformational order of the SC lipids under study. The water concentration in each successive layer was estimated from a measurement of the area under the O–H stretching band at 2100 cm^{-1}. The sequential IR analyses demonstrated that the amount and degree of disorder of lipids progressively decreased over the outer cell layers, remaining essentially constant after 3–4 tape strips. More precisely, a 60% reduction in lipid quantity was noted as one progressed from the surface inwards, with this reduction occurring over four tape strippings. On the other hand, the lipids near the surface were, on average, more fluid than those deeper in the SC, as demonstrated by the 2-cm^{-1} red shift and 20% reduction in bandwidth following three tape strips. A postulated explanation of this observation was that the lipids near the surface are a mixture of (a) highly ordered intercellular and (b) low-melting sebaceous lipids. Certainly, the modified lipid composition of these outermost desquamating layers might be expected to reflect the differentiating phenomenon responsible for their fate. Although the composition and distribution of lipids as a function of epidermal differentiation and site have been exquisitely characterized [64–66], a detailed analysis of the variation, if any, *within* the SC is absent and, indeed, is not a simple task. The depth-dependent IR profile obtained by these authors portrays, albeit nonspecifically, a membrane that is characterized by a nonuniform distribution of lipid and lipid type as a function of SC depth. The inhomogeneity of the membrane (and the utility of the technique) was further illustrated by the hydration profile, which clearly showed, as expected, an increase in water content from the surface toward the stratum granulosum. The gradation in hydration level was further corroborated by the amide I and amide II absorbances. These bands report on the carbonyl stretching and N–H bending, respectively, of the amide linkages and are consequently influenced by the degree of hydrogen bonding. As the SC was removed, the frequency of the amide I absorbance decreased while that of the amide II absorbance increased, indicating progressively increasing H-bonding and presumably reflecting the increasing availability of water.

VI. PENETRATION ENHANCEMENT

It is of course not only the concentration of water that may be deduced by this methodology; in fact, any penetrant possessing a characteristic IR signature, distinct from the SC components, can be similarly monitored. Consequently, one of the noteworthy uses of reflectance spectroscopy has been the in vivo evaluation of penetration enhancement, both in the assessment of enhancer efficacy and in the investigation of their *mode of action*. The basis of this research, however, lies in the extensive in vitro investigations, by IR and DSC, of penetration enhancer activity and it is therefore pertinent to first review the principal literature.

Substances reputed to enhance skin penetration belong to diverse chemical families [67–70], countering the possibility that they are unified in their action by a singular mode of operation. As discussed by Hadgraft and Walters [71], there are a number of ways in which the pharmaceutical scientist can enhance drug penetration through the skin. Basic physicochemical principles can serve to predict how formulation variables, including drug and vehicle interaction, can modify percutaneous penetration; however, the role of molecules, and indeed physical techniques, that interact with SC components and modify barrier function per se is still a matter of intense research. The investigation of these interactions by DSC and IR spectroscopy has been at the forefront of this work.

One of the best studied and most ubiquitous of penetration enhancers known to man is, of course, water. The effect of this chemical on the thermal transitions of human SC was first systematically investigated by van Duzee (using DSC [39]), who found that both the shape and the position of the four endotherms at 40, 70, 80, and 110°C were dependent on water content, with the peaks sharpening and the transition temperatures decreasing with increasing sample hydration. Analogous hydration-dependent calorimetric behavior for human SC has been reported elsewhere [37,38]. Similarly, IR results have indicated that the thermally induced mesomorphic transitions in human SC near 35 and 55°C [40] are dependent on water (see discussion above), as are the main chain-melting transitions near 70 and 80°C [37]. Examples of such lyotropic mesomorphism are abundant in the phospholipid literature [6,72] and have been attributed to the association of water with polar headgroups, leading to decreased dispersion forces between the hydrocarbon chains and a lowering of T_m. In contrast, IR studies have concluded that water does not modify the lipid alkyl chain order in porcine and human SC at *ambient* temperature [73], a finding substantiated by x-ray diffraction studies of human [74] and murine [75] SC. The hydration-induced lipid fluidization concluded from earlier IR data [35] may be explained on the basis of methodological differences in the two studies. The use of water to hydrate the tissue, as in the earlier investigation, gives rise to a broad O–H stretching absorbance adjacent to the C–H stretching bands (used to indicate alkyl chain order), distorting the peak position of the latter. The most recent work utilized deuterated water to hydrate the membrane, hence replacing the broad O–H stretching band with O–D vibrations at lower energy and thereby eliminating this skewing effect.

Observations of this nature are not unique to water, and a diverse range of penetration enhancers has been found to modify the phase transitions of human SC components, albeit selectively and to varying degrees. What is the significance of these findings, and how might they be interpreted in relation to their effect on barrier function? As discussed earlier, a DSC thermogram furnishes thermodynamic and biophysical data characteristic of the phase transition(s) under study, notably, the transition temperature/midpoint and enthalpy, heat capacity, and cooperativity. These parameters can be modified selectively by "perturbants," providing they interact with the component(s) involved in the transition under study. This is most easily illustrated by studies of well-defined lipid systems but is also demonstrated by studies of mammalian biomembranes [10]. Papahadjopoulos et al. [76] investigated the influence of a series of proteins on the phase behavior of dipalmitoylphosphatidylcholine and dipalmitoylphosphatidylglycerol bilayers, categorizing the interactions into three groups—based on the nature of their effect on the thermal profile. Although later studies have revealed that not all proteins fall neatly into these categories, these classifications are useful in illustrating the types of phase behavior modulation that can be achieved by virtue of hydrophobic and electrostatic interactions within lipid bilayers. Similarly, Jain and co-workers [16,77] studied the influence of over 90 lipid-soluble compounds (including alkanols, fatty acids, detergents, and organic solvents) on the phase transition behavior of dipalmitoylphosphatidylcholine (DPPC) liposomes, classifying the resulting gel to liquid–crystalline transition profile into five categories. These distinct effects were then interpreted in terms of the nature of perturbation and, hence, together with a structural knowledge of the additive, correlated to the postulated location of the perturbant along the bilayer. These seminal arguments have provided the basis for the interpretation of much of the subsequent lipid thermotropic research.

The complexity of the SC membrane hinders such definitive interpretation, but, nevertheless, alterations in endotherms can be used to screen molecules suspected of altering membrane function. Conversely, one should note that the absence of additive-induced alterations in the phase transition profile does not rule out their perturbing effect, but rather indicates that the additive does not modify the gel phase. As described earlier, a DSC thermogram of hydrated but untreated human SC yields four endotherms, the first three of which can be identified as noncooperative lipid-associated phase transitions, while the high-temperature endotherm is attributed to keratin denaturation [33,37].

A.   Azone® and Its Analogs

The interactions of the well-known enhancer Azone® (1-dodecyl azacyclo-heptan-2-one) and its analogs [69] on SC have been examined calorimetrically by a number of investigators. Goodman and Barry [38,78] studied the effect of Azone treatment (3% Azone in 0.1% Tween 20 in normal saline, for 24 hours) on SC prehydrated to a level of 20%. The subsequent DSC scan revealed the eradication of all lipid endotherms, with no noticeable effect on the protein transition, relative to the control experiment (0.1% Tween 20 in normal saline) and has been interpreted in terms of the "solubilization" of lipids, accomplished by insertion of the entire Azone molecule directly into the lipid lattice [79,80].

This hypothesis may not appear to be entirely consistent with the physicochemical characteristics of the enhancer; although extremely lipophilic (octanol-water log P, 6.21), the structure of Azone involves a long alkyl chain bounded by a polar azacycloheptan-2-one ring (which is freely soluble in water as well as organic solvents), thereby rendering it amphiphilic. The log P of Azone and its all-carbon analog differ by four orders of magnitude, indicating the extent to which the lactam group influences the polarity of the molecule [81]; hence, this polar group would be expected to interact with the hydrophilic headgroup regions of the lipid lamellae, while the carbon side chain inserts into the structured alkyl chains of the lipid matrix. Molecular modeling calculations [82,83] have suggested that the adoption of a "spoon" conformation by the Azone molecule, with the azacycloheptan-2-one ring in the plane of the lipid polar headgroup region, and in a bent conformation relative to the alkyl chain, would both accommodate the enhancer at the hydrocarbon/polar headgroup interface and perturb the lipid structure (hence, increasing permeability) (Fig. 9). Additionally, this structural conformation is also able to account for the concentration-dependent surface expansions observed as a result of the interaction of Azone with DPPC [82] and ceramide [84] monolayers at the air–water interface. Although the interaction of azone with monomolecular films of model SC lipids [85] and ceramide/cholesterol mixtures [84] does not lead to lateral expansion, the conversion to liquid-expanded films indicates the introduction of acyl chain disorder.

On the other hand, studies with three-dimensional isotropic lamellar matrices have shown that Azone is a weakly polar molecule, which can occupy the interfacial region as well as the hydrocarbon interior of bilayers [86,87]. The contrasting observations of Azone promoting the assembly of reversed-type liquid–crystal phases (e.g., reversed hexagonal and reversed micellar) in simple model lipid systems [88–90], while also favoring the formation of lamellar structures in one of these mixtures [91], adds further confusion to the discussion [92]. This notwithstanding, the studies by Schückler and co-workers [91] emphasize the differences in the calorimetric profiles of intact human stratum corneum (HSC) and model SC lipid mixtures: Although these systems are clearly useful and versatile, extrapolation of inferences from model lipids to the intact membrane must be performed with caution.

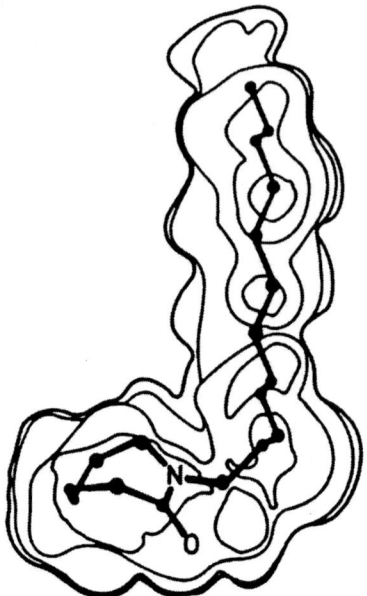

Figure 9 "Soup spoon" conformation with van der Waals contours of *N*-dodecylaza-cycloheptan-2-one, obtained through torsion of the peptide bond over 10°, with $\varphi_{C1\text{-}C2\text{-}C3\text{-}C4} = 62°$. Refer to original reference for computational details. (From Ref. 83. Reprinted from *International Journal of Pharmaceutics*, 76(1-2), Hoogsraate et al, Kinetics, ultrastructural aspects and molecular modelling of transdermal peptide flux enhancement by *N*-alkylazacycloheptanones, pp. 37–47, 1991, with kind permission from Elsevier Science, NL, Sara Burgerhartstraat 25, 1055 KV, Amsterdam, The Netherlands.)

Similar DSC findings with respect to the lipid endotherms have been reported by Hirvonen et al. [93] following treatment of hydrated HSC (45%) for 1 hour with neat Azone. In contrast to the studies by Goodman and Barry [38,78], the enthalpy of the protein transition was also significantly lowered. Bouwstra and co-workers [74,94,95] studied the influence of *N*-alkyl-aza-cycloheptan-2-ones, with carbon chain lengths (C_6–C_{16}), on human stratum corneum by DSC and small-angle x-ray scattering (SAXS). Hydrated HSC samples were preheated at 47°C for 10 hours, cooled to 0°C, and subsequently treated with a solution of the alkyl-azone in propylene glycol, PG (10% w/w) for 24 hours. The resulting thermal profiles were chain-length dependent, with the hexyl-azone not affecting the peak shapes of the lipid endotherms near 70 and 85°C but lowering their T_ms by about 15°C relative to the untreated SC, and by 4–5°C relative to the control PG treatment (i.e., PG alone lowered the T_m by ~10°C). With further increases in alkyl chain length, the two lipid endotherms became less separated, gradually merging into one peak with a lower total enthalpy. All treatments, including PG alone, abolished the protein denaturation peak. This latter observation was attributed to extraction of water from the protein regions by PG, rather than direct intervention by the solvent, based on the facts that (a) the protein endotherm is highly dependent on water, (b) PG is a known humectant, and (c) PG did not cause the two lipid endotherms to coalesce as might be anticipated in the event of protein interaction. Incidentally, at higher concentrations, PG has been reported to broaden the protein transition [79]. Although the influence of alkyl-azones alone on the protein endotherm could not be directly determined from these SAXS/DSC experiments, the SAXS data suggested that the alkyl-azones in combination with PG influence only the lipids *not* associated with proteins; i.e., alkyl-azones with more than six C atoms in their alkyl chain obliterate the 70°C endotherm while lowering the T_m of the 85°C transition. Experiments on denatured and delipidized SC may be useful in probing this postulated selectivity of Azone. Parenthetically, Schückler and Lee [96] investigated the concentration-dependent effect of Azone subsequent to reheating. That is, hydrated samples were treated with methanolic solutions of Azone, heated to ~130°C at a rate of 10°C/min, cooled, and then reheated, with calorimetric analysis being performed on the second thermogram. Although no information regarding the first scan was reported (thus not enabling inferences regarding proteinaceous domains), the reheat data demonstrated a concentration-dependent reduction in the T_m of the 80°C endotherm, with progressive diminution of the peak above an enhancer loading of 12% w/w.

Although the calorimetric investigations with Azone have been performed under a variety of treatment regimes, the prevailing observation is that of a reduced lipid transition enthalpy, the degree of which is dependent on treatment. Jain and Wu [16] suggested that amphipaths with strong polar groups could be expected to behave differently from moderately amphipathic solutes, such as *n*-alkanols and alkanoic acids. The latter molecules cause broadening of the main transition, with an attendant change in T_m, consistent with their localization in the vicinity of the methylene groups nearer to the polar headgroup in the bilayer, involving a significant change in both the packing and the size of the cooperative unit. In contrast, strongly polar groups such as that of the surfactant sodium dodecyl sulphate, SDS (and that of Azone, we might speculate; Fig. 10), would repel adjacent polar groups and thus modify or disrupt the cooperative unit completely, forming a liquid–crys-

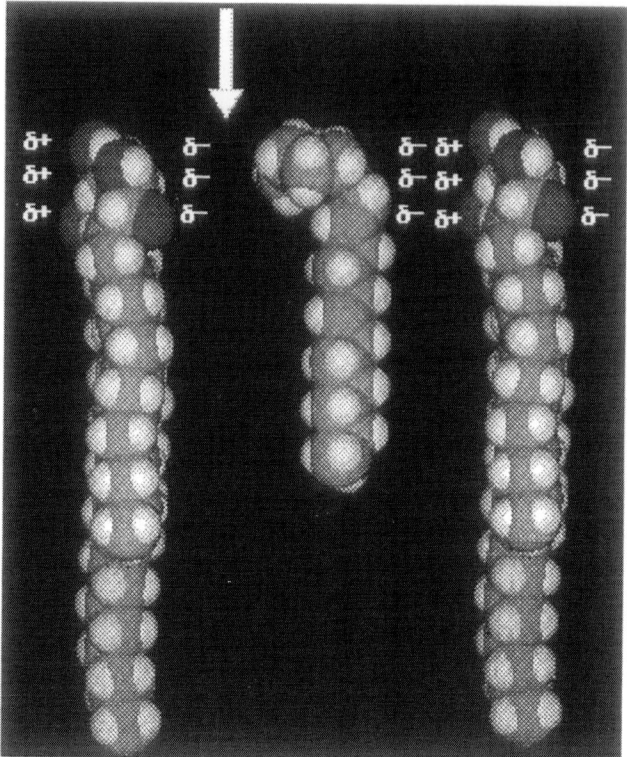

Figure 10 A molecular model representation of discontinuity in a ceramide bilayer, in the presence of Azone due to the "soup spoon" conformation and imbalance in electrostatic potential of the head group region. (From Ref. 197.)

talline phase at ambient temperature (above the temperature range of the reported scans) and consistent with a reduced enthalpy for the main gel–liquid-crystalline transition, as noted for SDS (0.1–10 mM).

B. Surfactants

In view of the experimental model in the above studies by Jain and Wu [16], the effect of SDS on protein domains cannot be surmised; however, similar thermal behavior has been reported for human SC following treatment with the surfactants SDS and cetyl trimethyl ammonium bromide, both of which

(1.5% w/v, i.e., at 10-fold-higher concentrations) eliminated the lipid-associated transitions, with little modification of the protein endotherm [97]. By contrast, Goodman and Barry [79] have reported a concentration-dependent effect for SDS (0.2–1% w/v); 1% SDS caused the lipid (~80°C) and protein T_ms to decrease and the peaks to coalesce with the lower (~70°C) lipid endotherm, with a reduction in the total enthalpy.

The effect of a number of other surfactants on human skin has also been investigated calorimetrically [97–99]. However, interpretation of the results, as well as correlation to the enhancing capacity, is often obscured by the simple fact that the penetration-enhancing ability of surfactants is strongly dependent on their concentration and on their physicochemical nature (cationic, anionic, or nonionic). That is, the total enhancing effect is dependent not only on the membrane interaction of the surfactant, but also on thermodynamic considerations dictated by the interplay of the permeant with the micellar surfactant [68,100].

C. Alkyl Sulfoxides

Of the alkyl sulfoxides, dimethyl sulfoxide (DMSO) is perhaps the best-known, though now seldom-used, penetration enhancer. Its application to skin has been associated with a number of phenomena, some of which have been demonstrated by DSC and IR. Reported effects include extraction of lipid, lipoprotein, and nucleoprotein structures [101,102], protein denaturation [103], and lipid fluidization [104], all of which have been implicated in its mode of action [105]. DMSO at ≥ 60% v/v is required to promote significantly the penetration of solutes [106], and a similar thermal dependence has been illustrated by DSC [38,79]. At 60% and below, subsequent to a 1-hour soaking regimen, the two lipid endotherms remained unaffected, whereas at 80% and 100% DMSO levels, the temperatures of both transitions were lowered significantly. Above 40% DMSO, the protein transition was also absent, although treatment of delipidized skin for 30 seconds revealed a concentration-dependent reduction in the protein T_m and concurrent endotherm broadening, rather than elimination of the peak. As a consequence, although one might postulate the masked presence of the protein endotherms in the thermograms following the soaking regimen [38,79], the use of two different experimental protocols does not allow an unambiguous inference. Certainly, immersion of HSC in 100% DMSO for 24 hours results in significant protein denaturation and lipid extraction, as shown by DSC and IR [107,108]. The modulation of both protein and lipid domains by alkyl sulfoxides was elegantly demonstrated by Oertel [109] using IR spectroscopy, which showed that similar soaking treatments of

HSC in vitro with DMSO caused a reversible α-helical to β-sheet conversion, of a fraction of the keratin, probably by displacement of bound water. This α-to-β conversion was also accompanied by lipid extraction, although a causal link between the two could be excluded on the basis that lipid extraction with organic solvents was not accompanied by this protein alteration. Additionally, a direct correlation between this conformational change in keratin and permeability enhancement cannot be put forward, on the basis that DMSO concentrations ($< 60\%$) that induce protein transitions are not associated with significant flux increases [79] and that, among a series of sulfoxide homologs, the order of enhancement [110] is not correlated to the extent of α-to-β conversion induced [109]. The greater importance of lipid interaction in the process of DMSO-induced enhancement might be inferred from the concentration-dependent results of Goodman and Barry [79]. Although lipid fluidization was not observed in another IR study [108], this effect cannot be ruled out on the basis that the spectral wavenumber resolution ($2~\mathrm{cm}^{-1}$) utilized does not allow the detection of frequency changes of a smaller magnitude.

The more hydrophobic homolog, decylmethylsulfoxide (DCMS), has been shown to produce a greater level of α-to-β-keratin conversion, compared to DMSO, and as deduced by FT-IR [109]. Correspondingly, DSC studies have revealed that DCMS has a similar effect to DMSO on the stratum corneum thermogram, but at greatly reduced concentrations [79].

D. Alkanols

In Vitro Studies with Alkanols

Ethanol, an extensively used cosolvent in pharmaceutical formulations, was the first enhancer to be incorporated into transdermal devices [115,116]. The mode of action of this alcohol, and that of its congeners, is the subject of ongoing research. Kai et al. [117] examined the interaction of a homologous series of *n*-alkanols (C_2–C_{12}) with hairless mouse skin (HMS) using conventional in vitro penetration studies in conjunction with reflectance IR spectroscopy. All alkanols, following pretreatment of skin, enhanced the flux of the polar and poorly permeable solute, nicotinamide. The degree of enhancement varied parabolically with alkanol chain length, with *n*-hexanol generating maximal enhancement. Similarly, alkanol flux through HMS also varied parabolically with carbon number, with butanol permeating most efficiently, although alkanol *uptake* by skin increased linearly with increasing lipophilicity. The examination of additive-induced protein and lipid changes by IR spectroscopy requires that the excipient not absorb IR radiation in the region of study. For example, scrutiny of the lipid domains by IR relies predominantly on the frequencies associated with the methylene groups from the lipid alkyl chains. If the exogenous agent under study also possesses methylene groups, and is present at a level similar to that of the endogenous component, the IR signal cannot distinguish between the two entities. For this reason, skin samples were pretreated with ethanol and perdeuterated analogs of butanol and octanol (alkanols with elevated skin uptake compared to ethanol, and thus with a greater likelihood of confounding SC lipid absorbances) and examined by reflectance IR. The value of this approach is that the C–H absorbances from the SC lipids are separated from the C–D absorbances of the alkanols. The resulting spectra revealed radical attenuation of the area under the C–H stretching vibration bands (attributed to the lipid hydrocarbon tails), implying significant lipid extraction by the alkanols, while IR analysis of the alkanols used for the pretreatment disclosed the presence of lipids. Comparably, calorimetric studies with human and rabbit pinna SC have reported the elimination of all lipid endotherms subsequent to treatment with *n*-dodecanol [93]. Although the effect of the alkanols on the protein domains cannot be discerned from these studies, the severe lipid extraction observed must play an important role in the enhancement action of alkanols. Ethanol has also been shown to be capable of modifying the gel–liquid-crystalline phase transition temperature in model phospholipid systems [16,118–120]. Indeed, a mechanism involving lipid "fluidization" has been suggested for the enhancing action of ethanol [121], a hypothesis that has been the subject of further investigation in later studies.

The effect of ethanol on the lipid phase behavior of hairless mouse SC and model phospholipid systems [DPPC/dipalmitoylphosphatidic (DPPA) and distearoylphosphatidylcholine (DSPC)/distearoylphosphatidic (DSPA) multilamellar vesicles (MLV's)] was explored by Krill et al. [122]. Transmission FT-IR studies (where each sample served as its own control) revealed that perdeuterated ethanol neither caused an increase in lipid chain order nor increased chain mobility of the SC lipids at physiological temperature, as would be expected of a fluidizing agent. Rather, there was evidence of decreased hydrocarbon chain mobility (reflected by a decrease in CH_2 symmetric and asymmetric stretching bandwidths) in the presence of ethanol. However, this decreased chain mobility was not accompanied by increased conformational order, contrary to that observed in the model lipid systems. The assessment of ethanol effects on the lipid-phase transitions of murine SC (requiring progressive heating of samples and thus necessitating different SC samples to be used for control and treatment protocols) was rendered difficult by intermouse variability. Nevertheless, the model lipid systems demonstrated an ethanol-induced decrease in chain mobility and an increase in conformational order *below* the gel–liquid-crystalline phase transition temperature, in contrast to a reduction in chain mobility and an increase in conformational disorder at temperatures *above* the phase transition. Similarly, it has been shown that iso-propanol, *n*-propanol, and *n*-butanol, at concentrations that promote penetration enhancement, do not alter the lipid chain order of hairless mouse SC at physiological temperature [123]. Because the amplified ordering of lipids cannot explain the permeability-enhancing properties of these alkanols, alternative mechanisms to explain their action must be considered.

The possibility of ethanol-induced alterations in the protein domains of SC was considered by Kurihara-Bergstrom et al. [124], who examined human SC treated with perdeuterated ethanol–water systems by FT-IR. The penetration studies showed that the maximal permeability coefficient for salicylic acid and ethanol from saturated ethanol–water delivery systems was achieved at 0.63 volume fraction of ethanol. Infrared spectra of SC samples immersed in EtOD-D_2O systems for 6 hours revealed the presence of keratin, predominantly in the α-helical conformation, up to 0.25 volume fraction EtOD. Above this concentration, the appearance of shoulders at 1688 and 1615 cm^{-1} near the Amide I band at 1650 cm^{-1} was interpreted as the formation of extended chains or distorted β-strands within the protein domain. An evaluation of lipid extraction was also made by comparing the intensities of the infrared bands arising primarily from stratum corneum proteins to those associated with lipid domains. A decreased absorbance of the C–H stretching bands relative to the N–H stretching band would indicate that some degree of lipid extraction had occurred. The ratio of these two bands decreased from 0.96 to 0.76 as volume fraction ethanol increased from 0.4 to 1.00, respectively, indicating lipid extraction.

In Vivo Studies with Ethanol

The inclusion of ethanol in commercially available transdermal systems has naturally provoked curiosity concerning its role as an enhancer in human skin, particularly in vivo. The mechanism by which ethanol compromises the human stratum corneum in vivo was investigated by Bommannan et al. [125] using ATR-IR in studies analogous to those described previously in this chapter [61]. Those in vivo studies on the untreated ventral forearm of healthy adults had revealed a depth-dependent ordering and reduction of the intercellular lipids relative to the superficial layers. Consequently, in the ethanol experiments, the measurement site (about 20 cm^2) was tape stripped four times prior to ethanol treatment in order to isolate the effect of ethanol from the inherent lipid changes in untreated SC. The examination site was treated for 30 minutes with absolute ethanol (10 ml) and then spectrally examined periodically over the next 4 hours and at 24 hours posttreatment. The resulting spectra indicated the permeation of ethanol into the treated SC by virtue of the augmented C-C skeletal and C-O stretching vibrations (arising from ethanol) compared to the control. Figure 11 illustrates the shift in $v_a(CH_2)$ as a function of the treatment protocol. Subsequent to the pretreatment spectrum (assigned a shift of 0 cm^{-1}), the site was tape stripped four times and $v_a(CH_2)$ decreased by ~2 cm^{-1}, as previously reported [61]. Following ethanol treatment there was a further net decrease by (~1 cm^{-1}) in $v_a(CH_2)$, indicating a slight ordering (rather than *disordering*) of the lipid alkyl chains. Furthermore, because the ethanol that had partitioned into the SC also contributed to the C–H absorbances, and

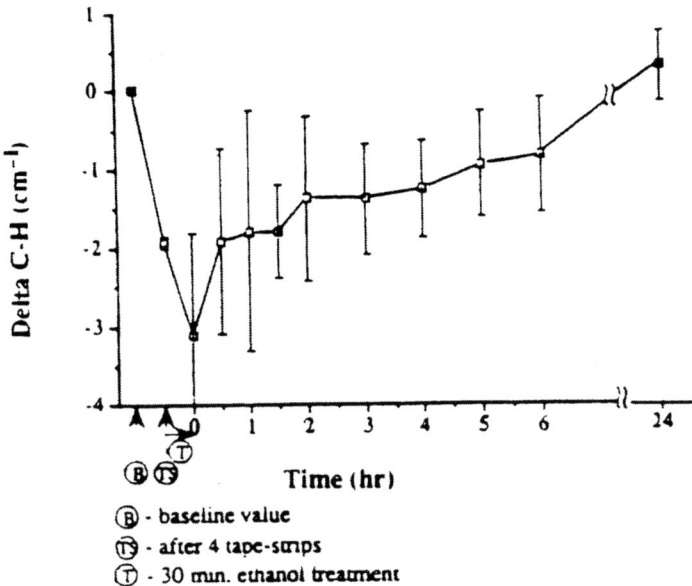

Figure 11 Average values ($n = 6$, error bars = SD) of the shift in the peak maximum of the C–H asymmetric stretching absorbance plotted as a function of time during the ethanol liquid treatment protocol. ANOVA followed by Scheffe's F-test revealed a statistically significant difference ($P < 0.05$) between the location of the peak maximum before and after the 30-min ethanol exposure. There was no statistically significant difference between the baseline value and that at 24 hr. (From Ref. 125. Reprinted from *Journal of Controlled Release, 16*, Bommannan et al. Examination of the effect of ethanol on human stratum corneum in vivo using infrared spectroscopy, pp. 299–304, 1991, with kind permission from Elsevier Science, NL, Sara Burgerhartstraat 25, 1055 KV, Amsterdam, The Netherlands.)

because $v_a(CH_2)$ for ethanol is approximately 10 cm^{-1} higher than that for SC lipids, the change observed following ethanol treatment may be an underestimate of the ordering effect perceived. The bandwidth at half-height of the C–H asymmetric stretching absorbance indicated the identical ordering pattern. Notably, DSC data have shown that 40% ethanol in water increase the T_ms of porcine SC lipid transitions [126]. Such ethanol-induced ordering has been observed in other lipid systems, with reports being accompanied by a number of explanatory hypotheses. These include the promotion of interdigitation of the hydrocarbon chains by displacement of bound water molecules at the lipid headgroup/membrane interface region [127] and by intercalation of ethanol between the headgroup regions of lipid molecules [128].

The experiments by Bommannan et al. [125] were also able to discern the extent of lipid extraction occurring in vivo in the presence of ethanol. The area under the C–H asymmetric stretching absorbance, being indicative of the SC lipid level, was assessed as a function of treatment (Fig. 12). Tape stripping caused a decrease in the lipid content relative to the pretreatment value, in accordance with previous observations [61]; ethanol treatment elicited a further, highly significant, decrease—which recovered to the pretreatment value in a manner very similar to that shown by $v_a(CH_2)$. The results suggested, therefore, that ethanol had indeed extracted an appreciable amount of SC lipid. Once again, as the ethanol present in the SC contributed to the C–H stretching absorbance, the perception of reduced lipid content may be an underestimate of the total effect. Furthermore, evaporation of the ethanol treatment liquid and subsequent IR analysis of the residue revealed large lipid-associated absorbances in all samples. Finally, to confirm that the lipid extraction phenomena was not masking a true lipid disordering action (i.e., there was not sufficient lipid remaining for the effect to be detected by IR), the experiments were repeated with ethanol-saturated vapor. In this case, no lipids could be extracted into the solvent phase. Once again, ethanol uptake into the SC was apparent but no disordering effects were observed. These results, therefore, concluded that in vivo, in humans, ethanol did not induce lipid disordering. However, the significant lipid extraction observed may be responsible for rendering the barrier more permeable in the presence of ethanol.

E. Fatty Acids

In Vitro Studies

The fatty acids have received extensive interest as potential penetration enhancers [129]. Over the years, in addition to studies investigating the potential

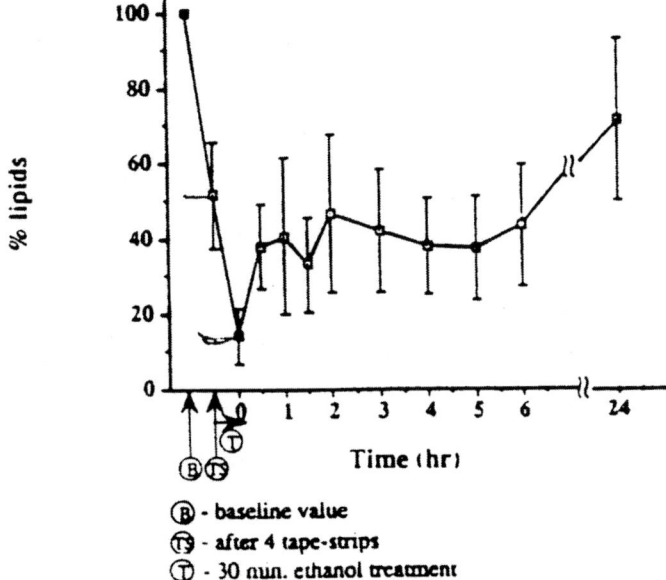

Figure 12 Average values ($n = 6$, error bars = SD) of the amount of ATR-IR detected SC lipids plotted as a function of time during the ethanol liquid treatment protocol. ANOVA followed by Scheffe's F-test revealed a statistically significant difference ($P < 0.05$) between the amount of lipids before and after the 30-min ethanol exposure. There was no statistically significant difference between the baseline value and that at 24 hr. (From Ref. 125. Reprinted from *Journal of Controlled Release*, *16*, Bommannan et al. Examination of the effect of ethanol on human stratum corneum in vivo using infrared spectroscopy, pp. 299–304, 1991, with kind permission from Elsevier Science, NL, Sara Burgerhartstraat 25, 1055 KV, Amsterdam, The Netherlands.)

enhancer activity of these agents, structure–activity correlations, studying in particular the dependence of their efficacy on chain length, degree/position, and configuration of unsaturation and the extent of branching, have been undertaken. In general, the penetration-enhancing effects of saturated fatty acids are greatest for C_{10} and C_{12} fatty acids [130,131], while unsaturated long-chain fatty acids are more effective enhancers compared to their saturated counte parts [132]. Golden et al. [133] investigated the effect of a series of isomeric C_{18} fatty acids on porcine SC by DSC and transmission IR, in parallel with their ability to enhance salicylic acid flux; these results are summarized in Table 1.

For the DSC experiments, SC was incubated for 2 hr in a 0.15M solution of the fatty acid in ethanol, after which samples were rehydrated to a water content of ~30% w/w. Treatment with (saturated) octadecanoic acid resulted

Table 1 Summary of Spectral, Thermal, and Flux Changes Following Treatment of Porcine Stratum Corneum with Fatty Acids of 18 Carbon Length

Treatment	IR frequency,[a] cm^{-1}	DSC T_m [b] (°C)	Flux of salicylic acid $(mg \cdot cm^{-2} \cdot hr^{-1})$
Octadecanoic acid	2918.1 ± 0.4	62.5 ± 1.0	1.21
cis-6-Octadecenoic acid	2919.0 ± 0.4	60.5 ± 0.9	0.79
trans-6-Octadecenoic acid	2919.0 ± 0.3	62.0 ± 0.9	0.97
cis-9-Octadecenoic acid	2920.0 ± 0.5	59.0 ± 1.5	3.81
trans-9-Octadecenoic acid	2919.4 ± 0.4	61.5 ± 0.9	2.35
cis-11-Octadecenoic acid	2920.1 ± 0.4	57.0 ± 1.1	5.53
trans-11-Octadecenoic acid	2918.8 ± 0.5	61.0 ± 1.0	1.11
Ethanol	2918.8 ± 0.4	62.0 ± 1.0	1.31
No treatment	2918.8 ± 0.4	62.0 ± 1.0	—

[a]Value represents the average ± SEM of three samples.
[b]Differential scanning calorimetry (DSC) determination of the temperature of the transitions maximum (T_m); values represent the average ± SEM of three samples.
Source: From Ref. 133. Reproduced with permission of the American Pharmaceutical Association.

in no change in the T_ms of the lipid endotherms relative to the untreated and ethanol-treated controls. Introduction of a *trans* olefinic bond had little or no effect on the T_ms relative to the controls, regardless of the position of the double bond along the chain. However, introduction of a *cis* olefinic bond both decreased T_m and broadened the transitions near 65 and 75°C, with no effect on the protein endotherm. Furthermore, these effects were more pronounced for the $18:1^{\Delta 11cis}$ isomer compared to the $18:1^{\Delta 9cis}$ isomer. Finally, the reduction in T_m produced by the series of fatty acids was highly correlated to the enhancement of salicylic acid flux across porcine skin. These combined results were therefore suggestive of lipid disruption as a possible mechanism for the fatty acid–induced flux enhancement. On the other hand, the IR data from these studies are difficult to interpret due to the contribution of the fatty acid backbone to the C–H stretching frequencies reported (that is, the data do not report solely on the SC lipid order, but on the average order of the SC lipids and the incorporated enhancer). Although similar positional effects of un-saturation ($18:1^{\Delta 11cis}$ vs. $18:1^{\Delta 9cis}$) have been reported in the literature [132], the striking difference in enhancing ability noted between *cis* and *trans* configurational isomers by Golden et al. [133] has not been consistently observed [134]. Nevertheless, *cis*-9-octadecenoic acid (oleic acid, OA) has been the subject of numerous investigations, having been shown to be an effective enhancer for a wide range of compounds [132,133,135–138].

More specifically, studies to elucidate the mechanism of action of this popular agent have arrived at the general conclusion that OA primarily modulates the extracellular lipid domain of the SC [126,133,139–141]. Once again, DSC and IR spectroscopic studies have been central to these inferences. Francoeur et al. [126] examined the effect of OA (0.25% v/v in a series of ethanol:water vehicles) on porcine SC as a function of temperature. The results of these calorimetric studies indicated that OA significantly reduced the T_m values of the two lipid transitions near 60 and 70°C, with the effect being greatest for the first lipid peak and no modification being noted for the higher-temperature protein transition. Although, a reduction in the enthalpy of these lipid transitions was also observed subsequent to OA treatment, this effect was equally recorded for the ethanol:water control; a similar reduction in enthalpy has been observed following treatment with 5% w/v OA in ethanol [79]. Moreover, the extent to which OA decreased the T_m value was highly correlated to the amount of fatty acid taken up by the SC, with the largest reduction in T_m being produced by exposure to vehicles containing 40–50% ethanol, the same vehicles that delivered the greatest amount of OA to the SC (Fig. 13). This correlation could be extended further: The decrease in T_m for porcine SC was linearly related ($r = 0.95$) to the flux of piroxicam across human and hairless mouse skin following treatment with identical formulations, in a manner similar to that previously noted for salicylic acid [133]. These data, therefore, were indicative of a powerful correlation between enhanced transport and OA-induced perturbation of the SC lipids, although the nature of this perturbation remained unclear. Such downward shifts in T_m following the incorporation of "lipid-perturbants" have been observed for phospholipid systems and explained on the basis of melting point depression [118,142]. However, Jain and Wu [16] have argued that "such a treatment cannot a priori explain qualitatively different behaviour of the various additives" since the colligative effect is dependent on (a) equimolar amounts of different solutes inducing equal effect, and (b) the approximation of biomembranes as a bulk solvent. Moreover, even if colligative phenomena were to explain the OA-induced lowering of SC lipid T_ms, the relevance of this effect to the actual mechanism of enhanced permeation is unclear, since at physiological temperature the SC lipids are predominantly in the gel phase, even in the presence of OA.

Further insightful observations concerning the mechanistic role of OA were provided by a series of experiments in which the flux of piroxicam (an anionic antiinflammatory agent) across OA-treated hairless mouse skin was

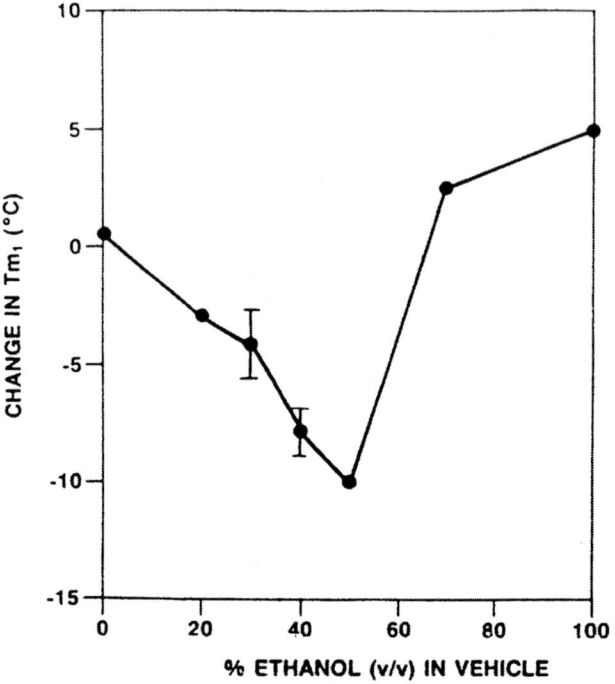

Figure 13 The change in the transition temperature (T_m) for the second lipid endotherm (near 70°C) in porcine stratum corneum as a function of the vehicle ethanol concentration. All vehicles contained 0.25% (v/v) oleic acid. Error bars depict SE ($n =$ 3); for those points with no error bars, $n = 2$. (From Ref. 126.)

studied as a function of pH [126]. The donor vehicle comprised a saturated solution or suspension of piroxicam in a 50% ethanol:buffer vehicle containing 0.25% OA, except for the controls (in which OA was absent). According to the pH-partition hypothesis, permeation across the skin is expected to be a function of only the neutral drug concentration, which, through the use of saturated systems in these experiments, remained essentially constant over the pH range of the study (while that of the ionised species increased). Piroxicam flux across untreated skin obeyed this precept in that it was independent of donor pH. However, for the OA-containing vehicles, an increase in pH from ~4 to ~7 significantly enhanced the flux of piroxicam relative to the controls. The data, therefore, suggested, that in the presence of OA, enhanced transport was dependent on the total drug concentration, including the anion and neutral drug species, and that this fatty acid appeared to alter the properties of the SC such that diffusion of ionized molecules was facilitated. Notably, several parallels could be drawn with observations of enhanced ion transport in phospholipid systems. For example, unexpectedly high diffusion rates for small ions such as Na^+ and K^+ have been reported for various phospholipid systems that were heated to their phase-transition temperature [143,144], where the gel and liquid-crystalline phases would be in equilibrium. The enhanced flux of these ions was thought to be related to their elevated diffusion across permeable defects at the phase boundaries. In addition, enhanced ion transport has been observed in two-component lipid systems exhibiting lateral phase separation [145,146]. In view of the possible existence of separate fluid–solid domains in porcine [32] and murine [46] SC at physiological temperatures, and the analogies with facilitated ion diffusion through phase-separated phospholipid systems, Francoeur et al. postulated that penetration enhancement may result from similar interfacial "defects" in the SC lipids following treatment with OA.

This hypothesis was probed further by transmission IR investigations of OA-treated porcine SC [147]. Figure 14 shows an infrared spectrum, spanning

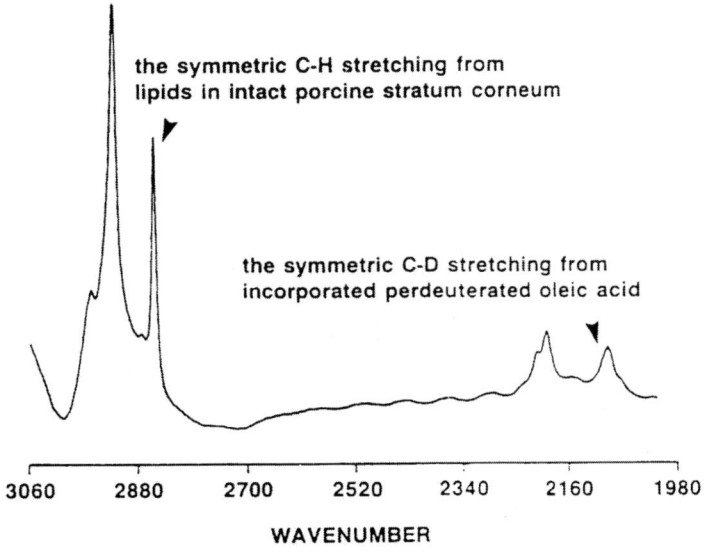

Figure 14 Transmission infrared spectrum of porcine stratum corneum treated with perdeuterated oleic acid. (From Ref. 147.)

from about 3000 to 1900 cm^{-1}, for a porcine SC sample that had been treated with perdeuterated oleic acid. In a separate set of experiments, samples were identically treated with ^{3}H-oleic acid in order to quantitate the level of uptake by the SC. Of particular interest for these studies were the C–H and C–D symmetric stretching frequencies at approximately 2850 and 2090 cm^{-1}, respectively. As discussed earlier, the significance of these particular bands is that changes in width and frequency reflect, on a molecular level, conformational changes of the contributory groups. In this case, the C–H vibrations originated primarily from the extracellular SC lipids, whereas the C–D bands reported on the behavior of the OA by virtue of the chemical substitution of deuterium for hydrogen in this fatty acid. The use of deuterated analogs in the study of lipid biophysics is well established [4,148]; more recently, use of the perdeuterated analog of Azone as a model for the underivatized enhancer was validated using both model lipid and human SC systems [149].

Figure 15 illustrates the changes in $v_s(CH_2)$ for the OA-treated and the untreated SC as a function of temperature. In these experiments, the average concentration of OA taken up by the SC was determined to be 60 μg/mg SC. The incorporation of OA had no significant effect on the conformational order of the endogenous lipids below the T_m. Treatment with OA did, however, lower the T_m of the SC lipids by 7.7°C, in agreement with results obtained by DSC [126]. At temperatures above T_m, higher values ($p > 0.95$) for $v_s(CH_2)$ were found in the treated samples, indicating that the melted lipids were further disordered in the presence of OA. Similar effects were observed in the extracted SC lipid samples, for which T_m of the extracted lipids was lowered by 9.5°C. Hence, these results indicated that OA did not modify the conformational order of the gel-phase endogenous lipids at physiological temperature, but did generate further disorder in the already-melted SC lipids above the transition temperature. Additionally, separate studies showed that OA had no effect on $v_s(CH_3)$, that is the alkyl residues toward the center of the bilayer, which are inherently more disordered than the rest of the chain, were unaffected by OA over the same temperature range [150].

Moreover, an analysis of $v_s(CD_2)$ and $v_s(CH_2)$ as a function of temperature (Table 2) revealed that while $v_s(CH_2)$ for the SC lipids increased by 4–5 cm^{-1}, the corresponding change in $v_s(CD_2)$ was negligible. That is, the OA incorporated in the SC or extracted lipids did not undergo a cooperative-phase transition; in fact, the value of $v_s(CD_2)$ at physiological skin temperature (~32°C) corresponded to OA, which was more or less fully disordered (i.e., melted). Although the technique was not able to deduce the precise composition or conformation of the lipid phase containing the liquid OA, the results unequivocally emphasized, *at physiological temperature*, the presence of

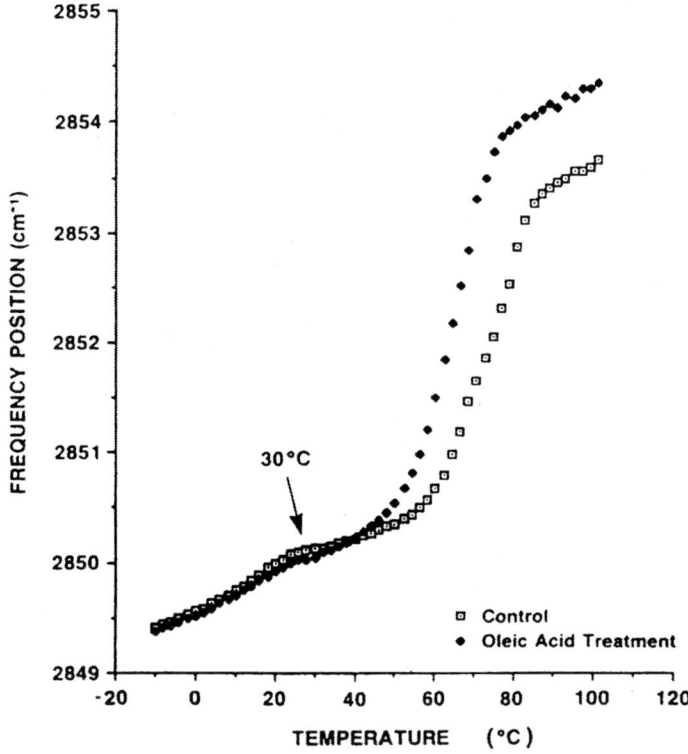

Figure 15 The symmetric CH_2 stretching vibration frequency $[(v_s(CH_2)]$ as a function of temperature for untreated and perdeuterated oleic acid-treated porcine SC. (From Ref. 147.)

OA in a liquid state and, therefore, phase-separated from the endogenous solid lipids. The penetration-enhancing properties of OA have frequently been ascribed to the fatty acid–induced fluidization of endogenous SC lipids [151,152]. The IR data here suggested that while lipid fluidization could perhaps account for the reduced diffusional resistance of the SC at elevated temperatures, it could not explain the barrier modification observed at physiological temperatures. In contrast, the heterogeneous insertion of oleic acid throughout the lipid bilayer would create numerous solid–fluid interfacial defects without necessarily fluidizing the lipids, and yet explain the enhancement of permeability, including that of ionized species.

Table 2 Selected Symmetric Stretching Frequencies, $v_s(CH_2)$ and $v_s(CD_2)$, for Stratum Corneum and Extracted Lipids Treated with ^2H-Oleic acid. For $v_s(CH_2)$ Values, Selected Temperatures Represent Values Above and Below the Transition

Temperature (°C)	Stratum corneum		Extracted lipids	
	$v_s(CH_2)^a$	$v_s(CD_2)^b$	$v_s(CH_2)^b$	$v_s(CD_2)^b$
20		2096.9 ± 0.5	2849.7 ± 0.0	2097.1 ± 0.0
30	2850.1 ± 0.0	2097.2 ± 0.6		2097.4 ± 0.2
40		2097.5 ± 0.4		2097.6 ± 0.1
50		2097.8 ± 0.2		2098.3 ± 0.4
60		2098.3 ± 0.2		2098.7 ± 0.0
70		2098.0 ± 0.1		2098.4 ± 0.0
75			2854.2 ± 0.2	
80		2098.0 ± 0.1		2098.3 ± 0.1
90	2854.2 ± 0.2	2097.6 ± 0.3		
100		2097.8 ± 0.1		

[a]Mean ± SE where n = 4.
[b]Mean ± SE where n = 2.
Source: Adapted from Ref. 147.

In Vivo Studies with Oleic Acid

The nature of OA interaction with SC lipids in vivo was of significant interest, particularly in light of the IR results above. Reflectance IR spectroscopy in conjunction with the use of a deuterated probe once again proved to be a valuable approach for the noninvasive evaluation of this enhancer in humans [153]. Prior to treatment, test sites on the inner ventral forearm of volunteers were cleansed with water, after which the subject remained at constant temperature and relative humidity, while three pretreatment spectra were collected. The experimental site on one arm was treated with a 5% v/v solution of perdeuterated oleic acid (^2H-OA) in ethanol, while the control site, on the contralateral arm, was treated with ethanol alone. Both formulations were applied under occlusion for 16 hours; posttreatment, the sites were swabbed clean with ethanol and then air-exposed for 2 hours to allow the occluded skin to dry. An ATR-IR spectrum of the dosed site was then obtained. This site was then tape stripped once and a second spectral examination was made. This sequential tape stripping and spectral acquisition was repeated ~20 times in order to obtain an incremental spectral profile as a function of SC depth (defined by the cumulative weight of SC removed with tape stripping). IR spectra thus collected yielded the following information: (a) the distribution profile of ^{2}H-OA across the SC (by virtue of the normalized area under the C–D stretching absorbances), (b) the conformational order of the SC lipids as a function of depth, and (c) the phase behavior of the enhancer in the SC (through analysis of the C–D stretching frequencies). An in vivo assessment of ^{2}H-OA uptake into human skin and its subsequent effect on SC lipids, at discrete intervals across the membrane, was thereby facilitated.

The concentration profile of ^{2}H-OA in the SC was evaluated by measuring the CD_2 stretching absorbances; this signal was detected at all levels of the SC examined and decreased with increasing mass of SC removed, reaching a limiting value near zero in the deepest layers of the SC probed. Figure 16 illustrates the $v_{as}(CH_2)$ originating from the SC lipids plotted as a function of the average cumulative SC mass removed by tape stripping (or SC depth). The first measurement represents the baseline value of SC prior to treatment, for the ^{2}H-OA-treatment and control sites. These data (Fig. 16 and Table 3) show that the subsequent two measurements (pre- and post-first tape strip) for the

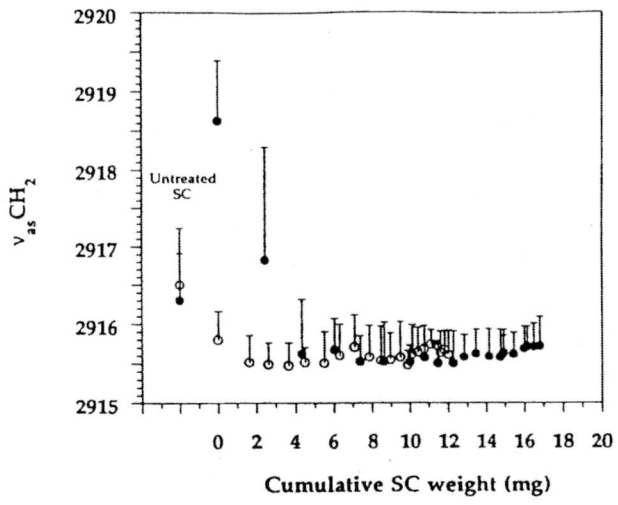

Figure 16 CH_2 asymmetric stretching frequencies, $v_{as}CH_2$ (originating from the SC lipids), as a function of SC weight removed, following treatment with ethanol alone ($\bigcirc$) or 5% (v/v) [^{2}H] oleic acid in ethanol ($\bullet$). Mean ± SD, $n = 7$ or 8. (From Ref. 153. Reprinted from *Journal of Controlled Release*, *37*, Naik et al. Mechanism of oleic acid-induced skin penetration enhancement in vivo in humans, pp. 299–306, 1995, with kind permission from Elsevier Science, NL, Sara Burgerhartstraat 25, 1055 KV, Amsterdam, The Netherlands.)

Table 3 Asymmetric [v_{as}(CH$_2$)] and Symmetric [v_{sy}(CH$_2$)] Stretching Frequencies for [^{2}H]-Oleic-Acid–Treated Human Stratum Corneum

	v_{as}(CH$_2$)	v_{sy}(CH$_2$)
Untreated SC	2916.40 ± 0.68[a]	2849.00 ± 0.29[a]
Control		
Prestripping[b]	2915.80 ± 0.37	2848.48 ± 0.21
Poststripping[c]	2915.48 ± 0.27	2848.41 ± 0.16
OA-treated		
Prestripping[b]	2918.63 ± 0.77	2849.93 ± 0.37
Poststripping[c]	2915.62 ± 0.70	2848.64 ± 0.39

[a]Values represent mean ± SD, for n = 8 or n = 16.
[b]Measurement of SC surface, prior to tape stripping.
[c]Measurement of SC surface, following two tape strippings.
Source: From Ref. 153.

^{2}H-OA-treated group were significantly ($p < 0.01$) elevated with respect to the background (untreated skin) and control (ethanol-treated) measurements. Thereafter, all v_{as}(CH$_2$) data conformed to a common mean value (± SD) of 2915.60 (± 0.33) cm^{-1}, identical to the corresponding control group mean frequency of 2915.60 (± 0.31) cm^{-1}, characteristic of "solid" alkyl chains in a predominantly *trans* configuration. Hence, the deduction from this profile was that following topical administration of ^{2}H-OA, lipid disordering was sustained only by the surface and uppermost layers, where the concentration of ^{2}H-OA and intrinsic fluidity of the SC lipids are greatest [61]. The lipid viscosity in the remainder of the membrane was essentially unaffected by ^{2}H-OA treatment.

These results were consistent with the previous in vitro data derived from ^{2}H-OA-treated porcine SC [147], demonstrating that the average conformational order of SC lipids was unaffected by ^{2}H-OA. The frequency reported by an IR spectrum represents a weighted average for the population of methylene groups undergoing stretching oscillations, the precise value of which will be dependent on the relative contribution (amount and conformational state) of each subpopulation. Since transmission IR spectroscopy (used to scan the sample in vitro) examines and reports on the distribution of vibrational frequencies encountered across the entire membrane intersecting the path of the beam, the technique is insensitive to any localized or depth-dependent variations. By contrast, the in vivo approach, using reflectance IR spectroscopy, facilitates the differentiation of any depth-dependent variation, though not lateral disparities. Interestingly, the CH_2 frequency shifts incurred by the superficial SC layers following [2]H-OA treatment were significantly smaller than those typically accompanying thermotropic phase transitions of human [37] and porcine [20,33] SC, and thus indicative of a lower degree of perturbation.

The small decrease in $v_{as}(CH_2)$ observed in both control and [2]H-OA-treated sites (excluding surface layers), relative to untreated skin, most likely reflects the combined outcome of two phenomena: (a) a heterogeneous gradient of lipid composition as revealed by repeated tape stripping, and (b) the extraction of surface lipids (sebaceous in origin and predominantly liquid at physiological temperature) by prolonged contact with ethanol. In support of these inferences, the findings of Bommannan et al. [61,125] reported (a) a stratal gradient of lipid concentration and conformational order, with a predominance of less structured lipids near the surface, and (b) the concurrent percutaneous penetration of ethanol, extraction of SC lipids, and decrease in the intensity, bandwidth, and frequency of the CH_2 stretching vibrations, following in vivo dermal treatment with ethanol.

The phase behavior of the topically administered oleic acid within the SC could be similarly discerned from a survey of the CD_2 stretching absorbance maxima (Fig. 17). This value remained essentially constant across the membrane, with a mean ($\pm$ SD) frequency of 2196.60 ($\pm$ 0.3) cm^{-1}. Furthermore, comparison of this measurement with the $v_{as}(CD_2)$ value of 2197.17 cm^{-1} for neat (and therefore fluid) [2]H-OA at 25°C indicated that the [2]H-OA within the membrane existed in a predominantly liquid phase. The results demonstrated, therefore, that upon application to human skin in vivo, under conditions that enhance transdermal permeability, [2]H-OA did not globally modify the conformational order of SC lipids; rather, it appeared to decrease lipid viscosity only in the superficial layers. Furthermore, while the SC lipids existed in a solid state, [2]H-OA incorporated into the SC was present in fluid domains. As reviewed by Ongpipattanakul et al. [147], lipid-phase separation can result in substantially enhanced permeability in mammalian SC, as in other lamellar lipid barriers. Additionally, studies with simpler lipid systems have shown the propensity of cis-unsaturated fatty acids (like oleic acid) to distribute inhomogeneously or to form a phase-separated liquid–crystalline domain when introduced into a solid, saturated lipid mixture [154], epidermal lipids [155], model SC lipids [156], and DPPC liposomes [157]. Based on these collective observations, and the in vivo IR data, we can conclude that OA-induced enhanced transdermal permeability may occur through a dual mechanism involving lipid perturbation via both conformational disordering and phase separation, with the latter effect predominating.

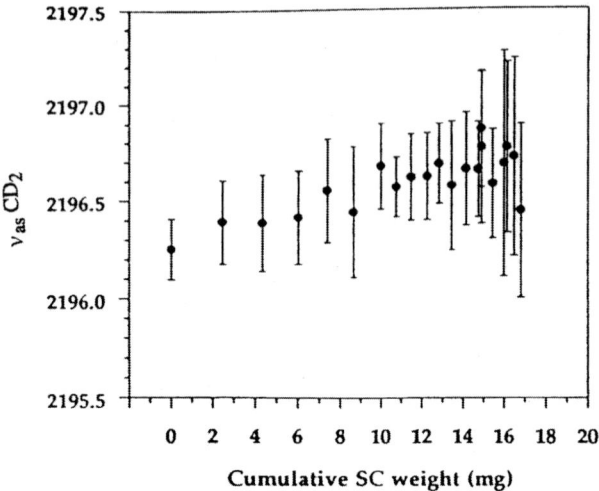

Figure 17 CD_2 asymmetric stretching frequencies, ($v_{as}(CD_2)$, originating from the topically applied [^{2}H] oleic acid) as a function of SC weight removed, following treatment with 5% (v/v) [^{2}H] oleic acid in ethanol. Mean ± SD; $n = 7$ or 8. (From Ref. 153. Reprinted from *Journal of Controlled Release, 37,* Naik et al. Mechanism of oleic acid-induced skin penetration enhancement in vivo in humans, pp. 299–306, 1995, with kind permission from Elsevier Science, NL, Sara Burgerhartstraat 25, 1055 KV, Amsterdam, The Netherlands.)

Selective deuteration, however, is not the only means by which an exogenous chemical (such as OA) can be observed within the SC using IR spectroscopy. For example, Mak et al. [158] monitored the concentration of OA within the superficial SC layers in humans in vivo by studying the absorbance at 1710 cm^{-1}, arising from C=O stretching vibrations in the molecule. This absorbance is well separated from that of C=O stretching oscillations occurring in *esterified* carboxyl residues such as those predominating in SC lipids. In fact, the ratio of the OA-specific absorbance at 1710 cm^{-1} to that of endogenous SC lipids at 1741 cm^{-1} (to normalize the results for variations in the degree of contact between subjects' arms and IREs) was used as an indicator of the level of OA within the tissue following treatment with increasing concentrations of the enhancer. These results demonstrated that OA uptake was proportional to the enhancer treatment concentration, and hence in agreement with the results of in vitro experiments quantifying ^{14}C-OA uptake into excised SC. By use of three different IREs of varying optical configuration, data were obtained from the skin surface to a maximum of 2 μm into the SC. Exposure of human skin to 1.0% OA for 30 minutes caused an increase in $v_{as}(CH_2)$ of ~3 cm^{-1}, indicating that the presence of fatty acid caused an *overall* increase in the lipid hydrocarbon chain disorder. However, in this instance the $v_{as}(CH_2)$ reflected contributions from both SC lipids *and* OA; therefore, as progressively increasing levels of OA were incorporated into the SC, the measured value of $v_{as}(CH_2)$ would be expected to approach that of the pure OA component. Similarly, reflectance IR spectroscopic studies investigating the effect of OA on rat stratum corneum in vitro have concluded that the fatty acid disorders the SC lipid matrix [152,159]. Once again, the measured $v_{as}(CH_2)$ reflects contributions from OA as well as SC lipids. Although in these studies with rat SC, the authors hypothesized that the contribution to $v_{as}(CH_2)$ from the penetrant was minimal, it should be recalled that OA uptake into SC lipids has been reported to be ~20% w/w for human SC [158] and > 40% w/w for porcine SC [150] following treatment with similar concentrations of OA. Hence, contamination of the $v(CH_2)$ signal by OA cannot be ruled out and can be discerned only by selective labeling techniques. Clearly though, since the spectral data obtained by the reflectance technique pertain only to the surface layer in contact with the IRE, and in view of the in vivo results with deuterated OA, the effect observed by Mak et al. [158] and Takeuchi et al. [152,159] may, at least in part, be a consequence of SC lipid disordering of the outer layers.

F. Effect of Iontophoresis

The remarkable resistance of the SC intercellular lipid network to the passive penetration of therapeutic agents has intensified the search for devices, chemical and physical, with the ability to perturb this lipid environment. Of the many physical techniques investigated, iontophoresis (or electrically enhanced transdermal transport) has become an important focal point [160–162]. Unparalleled in its ability to deliver (noninvasively) ionized drugs across the skin, its modus operandi appears to be largely dependent on transcutaneous ion-conducting pathways (which may be paracellular), rather than a function of direct interaction with the lipid infrastructure [163]. Nevertheless, the effect of the applied current on the lipid (and protein) domains is a matter of interest with respect to both safety considerations (i.e., does the applied current induce structural alterations?) and mechanistic insight. ATR-FTIR has been used in a number of studies to discern the effect of iontophoresis on SC lipid and protein structures, both in vivo and in vitro. In separate studies, human SC was examined in vivo following the delivery of current at 0.1–0.2 mA/cm^2 for 30 minutes [164,165]. Neither study found measurable changes in the CH_2 symmetric and asymmetric stretching frequencies, reporting on lipid order, though both noted, as expected, increased SC hydration subsequent to iontophoresis. The in vitro iontophoresis (1.25 mA/cm^2 for 60 minutes) of human SC samples also failed to produce changes in the lipid spectrum when examined by reflectance spectroscopy, or in the protein endotherm when examined by DSC [108]. The possibility of transient structural changes *during* iontophoresis (which might be reversible upon suspension of current flow) was also investigated, by collecting ATR-FTIR spectra while applying a voltage in the range of 5–30 V for 60 minutes across the membrane positioned on the reflection element. Again, no spectral changes in the intercellular lipid matrix were observed; nevertheless, the examination of SC in vivo during iontophoresis would be of considerable interest in this instance. The absence of observable frequency changes reported in these experiments should, however, be viewed in light of some of the caveats of IR and, in particular, of reflectance spectroscopy, discussed earlier. First, the wavenumber resolution employed (1–2 cm^{-1}) in some of these experiments is, without further spectral analysis, not sufficient to discern conformational changes that result in frequency shifts of less than 1–2 cm^{-1}; as we have seen, the induction of lipid disorder can involve frequency shifts of a smaller magnitude. Second, in the reflectance mode, spectra are collected from the immediate layers (1–2 µm) in contact with the crystal; as such, the spectral data (and, consequently, the inferences therefrom) do not pertain to the entire SC thickness but are limited to the surface layers.

G. In Vivo Studies with Model Permeants to Demonstrate Penetration Enhancement

In vivo studies of the type described above have been further extended to demonstrate enhanced percutaneous absorption in man. These studies have relied on the use of a model permeant that gives rise to a distinct IR absorbance, in a region where the SC is effectively "IR transparent." This, in turn, allows facile spectroscopic detection of the compound upon application to the skin. Incorporation of the "IR active" permeant into a formulation system comprising a test penetration enhancer thus allows the effect of this enhancer on the transport kinetics of the permeant to be investigated. An example of such a probe molecule is 4-cyanophenol (CP), possessing an intense IR absorbance at 2230 cm^{-1} due to the C≡N bond stretching vibrations. Mak et al. [166] administered CP topically as a 10% w/v solution, either in propylene glycol or in propylene glycol containing 5% v/v oleic acid, to the forearm of human subjects. The absorbance at 2230 cm^{-1}, representing a measure of the CP level within the superficial SC layers, diminished significantly faster when CP was codelivered with OA, indicating the facilitated throughput of the penetrant in the presence of OA. Similarly, the fate of the vehicle, propylene glycol, was followed via measurement of the peak at 1040 cm^{-1} (C–O stretch) and, as for CP, demonstrated the enhanced clearance of PG from the skin in the presence of OA.

Subsequent studies have attempted to quantitatively evaluate the effect of OA on the *distribution* of CP in human skin by simultaneous spectroscopic and radiochemical assays [167]. Cyanophenol was administered for periods of 1, 2, or 3 hours, either (a) as a 10% w/v solution in propylene glycol or (b) in an identical vehicle also containing 5% v/v oleic acid. Radiochemical quantification of CP penetration was achieved by incorporating a known amount of ^{14}C-CP into the above solutions. At the end of the treatment periods, SC at the application site was progressively removed by tape stripping, and IR spectra were obtained at each newly exposed skin surface, thus generating a spectroscopic distribution profile as a function of SC depth (Fig. 18a). Meanwhile, the tape strips were analyzed by liquid scintillation counting to determine the absolute amount of CP in each layer removed. The presence of OA in the applied formulation significantly increased the rate and extent of CP delivery as evaluated by either spectroscopy or radiochemical analysis. Furthermore, the ATR-IR and direct ^{14}C analysis of CP as a function of SC position were highly correlated (Fig. 18b). This degree of correlation between two independent analytical methods, therefore, provided initial validation for reflectance IR spectroscopy as a tool for quantitative analysis in vivo.

The illustration of OA-induced skin penetration enhancement in vivo by reflectance IR has been similarly achieved with the model permeant *m*-azidopyrimethamine ethanesulphonate (MZPES), bearing the intensely IR-active functionality, N_3 [168]. Other molecules that have been successfully utilized as IR probes include 4-nitrophenol [169,170] and 4-cyanonaphthalene [171].

VII. TRANSPORT KINETICS

The ability of ATR-FTIR spectroscopy to identify and quantify permeant concentrations within a membrane in situ so effortlessly has had a tremendous impact on its versatility. For example, the technique has long been used to determine the diffusivity and transport kinetics of a solute in polymer matrices [56], and offers distinct advantages over more conventional methods [172]. With the advent of controlled-release dosage forms, including transdermal devices, the diffusion characteristics of therapeutic agents across polymeric systems are of particular relevance. In addition, conventional topical drug delivery is dominated by semisolid formulations, diffusion of drugs through which has important consequences for their therapeutic efficacy. Recently, ATR-IR spectroscopy has been used in situ to deduce the diffusion coefficient

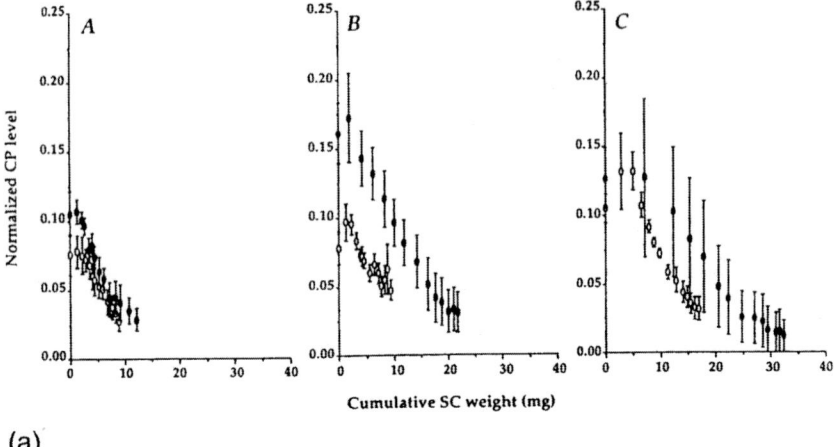

(a)

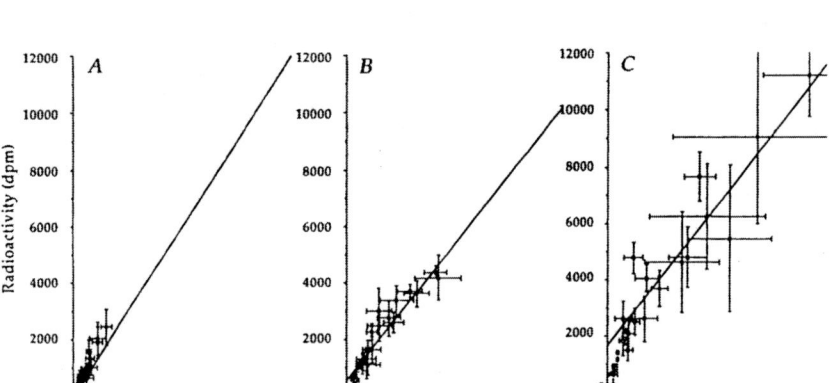

(b)

Figure 18 (a) Normalized CP level as a function of SC weight following treatment with either a 10% (w/v) solution of CP in propylene glycol (○) or the identical solution containing 5% (v/v) oleic acid (●) for (A) 1-hr, (B) 2-hr, and (C) 3-hr. Mean ± SE; n = 4 or 5. (b) Correlation between the absolute radiochemical measurement of CP distribution across the SC and the corresponding spectroscopically determined level, following (A) 1-hr, (B) 2-hr, and (C) 3-hr application of the control (○) and OA treatment (●) formulations. Mean ± SE; n = 4 or 5. The IR absorbance has been normalized to account for the different depths of SC sampled by the radiochemical and spectroscopic techniques. (From Ref. 167.)

of molecules through semisolids [173], polymers [171], and stratum corneum [174], with the objective of acquiring mechanistic insight into topical and/or transdermal delivery.

Essentially, the in vitro spectroscopic experiment involves positioning a membrane of known thickness in contact with the horizontal IRE, above which the test formulation is applied via a trough. The spectrophotometer then records the appearance of the permeant/vehicle (*any* diffusant with a unique IR signal) as it diffuses towards the crystal–membrane interface and into the zone "accessed" by the evanescent wave. This distance *within* the membrane at which the diffusant is monitored is defined by the optical characteristics of the IRE and membrane, being usually on the order of 1 μm. The IR absorbance increases with time as the permeant concentration rises, finally plateauing as membrane saturation is approached. The time dependence of the diffusant IR absorbance can then be analyzed using a Fickian diffusion model, yielding, for a membrane of known thickness (L) the diffusion coefficient (D), or for a membrane of unknown thickness (such as the SC) a composite parameter D/L^2; in addition, the relative membrane solubility is obtained from the "plateaued" absorbance.

To investigate the effect of the known penetration enhancers Azone and transcutol (monoethyl ether of diethylene glycol) on permeant diffusivity and solubility in human SC, enhancer-induced changes in these parameters for the model permeant, 4-cyanophenol, were monitored by ATR-IR and compared to the overall effects of the enhancers on flux as measured by conventional in vitro permeation studies [174]. Both techniques demonstrated enhancement of CP flux across human skin in vitro in the presence of the enhancers. However, ATR-IR enabled further deconvolution of the diffusional and partitioning steps involved in the permeation process. Fickian analysis of the ATR-IR absorbance profiles suggested that while Azone reduced the diffusional resistance of the SC to the permeation of CP, transcutol increased the solubility of the penetrant in this membrane. Although both these effects explain the enhanced flux of CP across human SC, it is clear that only the ATR-IR technique was able to differentiate between the two contributing physicochemical phenomena and thus offer mechanistic insight into enhancer action. In addition, the technique enables the rapid and accurate measurement of solute diffusion through a one-step approach where analysis of the solute(s) is an integral part of the methodology. Further, the transport of multiple species, as well as membrane-solute interactions, can be simultaneously monitored when the individual components have distinct IR absorbances.

More recently, this approach has been further extended to in vivo application in man, with a view to developing a general model to predict the rate and extent of chemical absorption for diverse exposure scenarios from simple, and safe, short-duration studies [175]. Access to such a model is central to the reliable prediction of topical and transdermal bioavailabilities of cutaneously applied drugs and to the accurate estimation of risk from environmental dermal exposure to potentially toxic chemicals. Measurement of the concentration profile of a permeant (4-cyanophenol) in the SC was achieved by ATR-IR in a similar fashion to that described previously; in this instance, however, tape strips themselves, as opposed to the skin surface, were analyzed directly on the IRE, thus minimizing intersubject contact/pressure variations and preventing chemical loss by transfer to the IRE. Following exposure to the formulation for 15 minutes, the measured concentration profile was analyzed using the Fickian unsteady-state diffusion equation. The derived parameters D/L^2 (ratio of the diffusivity to the diffusion path length squared) and K (partition coefficient of CP between SC and vehicle) were then used to predict (and experimentally confirm) concentration profiles, in addition to estimating the flux, cumulative transport, and the permeability coefficient following longer exposure times.

A representative ATR-FTIR–assessed concentration profile of CP across human SC in vivo following a 15-minute exposure to a saturated aqueous solution, together with the best fit of the unsteady-state equation to the data, is shown in Fig. 19. The values of D/L^2 and K are presented in Table 4, together with parameters from other subjects. These values were then used to predict the concentration profile subsequent to a 1-hour exposure of the identical formulation; these theoretical data along with the measured profile are shown in Fig. 20 and illustrate the excellent agreement of the predicted and measured profiles. Furthermore, the linear concentration profile, consistent with steady-state diffusion, is in agreement with the estimated time to reach steady-state diffusion (~2.3 $L^2/6D = 1.0$–1.5 h) as deduced from the mean D/L^2 (from 15-min data). Typically, the thickness of the SC (assumed to represent the diffusional path length, L) is found to be in the order of 10–20 μm; in these analyses, a value of 15 μm was arbitrarily chosen to calculate the in vivo values for the steady-state flux (J_{ss}) and permeability coefficient (K_p) and subsequently compared with the fitted parameters from the experimentally determined profiles (Table 4). The similarity of the predicted and measured parameters, together with their concordance with values derived from disparate theoretical models and experimental systems lends considerable support to the model employed here and to the predictive nature of the in vivo methodology. In a separate series of experiments, the applied formulation was spiked with ^{14}C-radiolabeled chemical, and the tape strips were analyzed by accelerator mass spectrometry (AMS), a highly sensitive radioisotope detection technique, and by conventional liquid scintillation, in addition to ATR-FTIR. The total uptake of CP into human SC in vivo, as determined by these different techniques, is shown in Table 5. Correlation between the totality of IR and AMS measurements is given in Fig. 21.

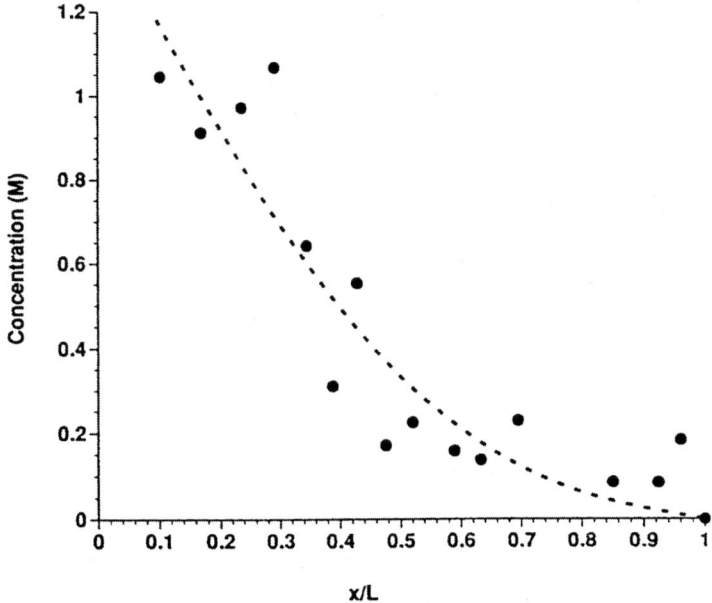

Figure 19 A representative concentration profile of 4-cyanophenol transport across human stratum corneum in vivo following exposure of the skin to an aqueous solution of the chemical for 15 minutes. The values on the abscissa (x/L) are calculated from the ratio

$$\left(\sum_{i=1}^{j} M_i\right) \Bigg/ \left(\sum_{i=1}^{n} M_i\right)$$

where M_i is the SC mass removed by the ith tape-strip and $\sum_{i=1}^{n} M_i = M_T$, the total SC mass removed by all n tape strips combined. Nonlinear regression was used to obtain the best fit of Equation § from Table 4 (p. 142) (dashed line; $r^2 = 0.84$) to the data. From this analysis, it can be deduced that $D/L^2 = 9.90 \times 10^{-5}$ s^{-1} and K = 5.5. (From Ref. 175.)

VIII. STRATUM CORNEUM HYDRATION

This review has considered the utility of IR spectroscopy in monitoring both endogenous components of the SC as well as the transport of exogenous additives, and ultimately the interaction of these permeants with the membrane constituents. A molecule that is embraced by all these aspects of investigation is water. DSC studies investigating the uptake and binding of water have been reviewed by Potts [23] and will not be dealt with further in this chapter. As alluded to at the beginning of this review, one of the nascent applications of IR spectroscopy to the study of barrier function pertains to the estimation of

Table 4 Measured, Fitted, and Predicted Parameters Characterizing CP Transport Across Human Stratum Corneum in Vivo, Following Application of an Aqueous 4-Cyanophenol (CP) Solution for 15 and 60 Minutes

Subject	[CP] in SC at 15 min[a] (M)	15-min fitted parameters[b]				[CP] in SC at 60 min[a] (M)
		K	D/L^2 $(10^5 s^{-1})$	$C_{x=0}$ (M)	T_{lag} (min)	
Mean	0.45	8.4	8.4	1.64	32.5	0.63
SD ($n = 3$)	0.15	3.6	1.5	0.70	6.2	0.24

[a]Measured experimentally.

[b]From the fit of equation § (below) to the 15-min in vivo data.

[c]From the fit of the steady-state form of equation § to the 60-min in vivo data.

[d]Calculated from the gradient of the fitted in vivo data to the steady-state form of equation § (below), assuming $L = 15$ μm.

[e]Predicted using the values of K and D/L^2 from the 15-min exposure experiments, and assuming $L = 15$ μm.

K = partition coefficient of CP between SC and vehicle; D/L^2 = ratio of the diffusivity to the diffusion pathlength squared; $C_{x=0}$ = CP concentration at the skin surface = $K \cdot C_{veh}$; T_{lag} = Lag time = $L^2/6D$; J_{ss} = Steady-state flux = $(K \cdot D/L) \cdot C_{veh}$; K_p = Permeability coefficient = $K \cdot D/L$.

Equation § represents the concentration profile of the chemical (i.e., C(x) as a function of position x and time t):

$$C(x) = KC_{veh}\left[1 - \frac{x}{L}\right] - \frac{2}{n\pi}\sum_{n=1}^{\infty} KC_{veh} \sin\left(\frac{n\pi x}{L}\right)\exp\left(\frac{-Dn^2\pi^2 t}{L^2}\right)$$

Source: From Ref. 175.

water content (free and/or bound) in the uppermost layers of the stratum corneum. These in vitro and in vivo studies range from the examination of ichthyotic conditions to the evaluation of occlusion, moisturizing treatments, dermatological/cosmetic formulations, and wound dressings. A chronological account of these earlier ATR-IR studies, together with those of other noninvasive methods, has been presented by Potts [176,177]. These reviews elegantly describe the methodological (and technological) progression of ATR-IR to skin hydration studies. Several regions of the IR spectrum have been used to determine the concentration of water, including the broad OH stretching asorbance near 3400 cm^{-1} [60], the ratio of Amide I (1650 cm^{-1}) to Amide II 1550 cm^{-1}) bands [178–180], a combination band near 2100 cm^{-1} [181], as well as OD oscillations following hydration with D_2O [182]. One of the drawbacks of reflectance spectroscopy in the in vivo quantitation of SC hydration is that the measurement itself, as a result of occlusion while the skin is in contact with the IRE, can alter the water content of the test site. More recently, near-infrared diffuse reflectance spectroscopy, comprising a non-

	60-minute fitted parameters[c]			60-minute predicted parameters[e]	
K (cm)	$C_{x=0}$ (M)	J_{ss}^d (nmol·cm^{-2}·sec^{-1})	$10^7 \times K_p$ (cm·sec^{-1})	J_{ss} (nmol·cm^{-2}·sec^{-1})	$10^7 \times K_p$ (cm·sec^{-1})
7.4	1.44	0.18	9.4	0.20	10.4
2.6	0.52	0.04	1.9	0.05	2.6

occlusive optical probe, has been employed to evaluate skin moisture through the measurement of water bands near 6900 cm^{-1} and 5200 cm^{-1} [183,184].

IX. NOVEL APPROACHES

The range of IR bands that can be utilized to assess hydration alludes to the pervasiveness of water absorbance in an IR spectrum: Water is a strong IR absorber and thus can pose a particular difficulty in the spectral examination of aqueous samples. The advent of computer-interfaced FT systems allowing spectral manipulation (such as band subtraction) can circumvent these difficulties, as can the use of specialized accessories such as ATR elements [3] and even alternative vibrational spectroscopic techniques, e.g., FT-Raman spectroscopy. FT-Raman spectroscopy, providing complementary information to IR, has in recent years been employed for the characterization of human SC [185–190] and model SC lipids [191], as well as for the noninvasive monitoring of topically applied compounds [192] and the in vitro evaluation of SC–enhancer interactions [193].

The Raman effect is observed when a sample is irradiated with a beam of intense monochromatic light, typically from a laser, and the radiation, which is scattered perpendicular to the beam, is recorded. Light is scattered by the sample molecules in a number of ways, producing a characteristic spectrum. Most of the incident photons are scattered with unchanged energy and thus at the same frequency as the incident radiation, v_0 (Rayleigh scattering). Additionally, radiation may be either (a) absorbed, exciting the molecule into higher vibrational energy states, with consequent scattering at lower frequencies relative to the parent line, termed Stokes lines, or (b) re-emitted as the molecule returns to its ground vibrational state, with resultant

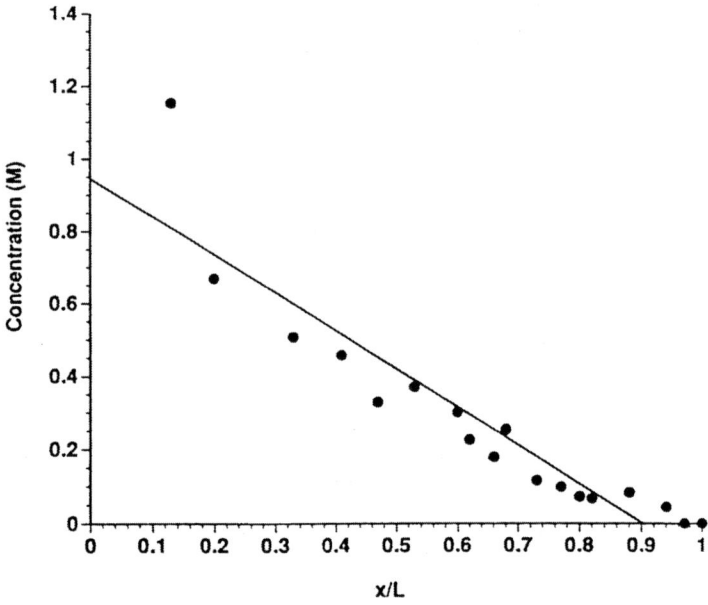

Figure 20 A representative concentration profile of 4-cyanophenol across human stratum corneum following exposure of the skin to an aqueous solution of the chemical for 1 hour. The values on the abscissa (x/L) are calculated from the ratio

$$\left(\sum_{i=1}^{j} M_i\right) \Bigg/ \left(\sum_{i=1}^{n} M_i\right)$$

where M_i is the SC mass removed by the ith tape strip and $\sum_{i=1}^{n} M_i = M_T$, the total SC mass removed by all n tape strips combined. The slope and intercept of the line of linear regression through the data are -1.05 M and 0.95 M, respectively. The values predicted from the 15-minute exposure data are -1.43 M and 1.43 M, respectively. (From Ref. 175.)

scattering at higher frequencies relative to the incident radiation, and termed anti-Stokes lines.

The difference in frequency between the incident radiation and each scattered Raman line represents the frequency of the corresponding vibration, producing the vibrational spectrum of interest. As already mentioned, IR and Raman spectroscopy are complementary techniques; the selection rules for each are distinct and many modes of vibration that produce strong IR absorbances in fact, give rise to weak Raman scattering signals (e.g., water). In order for a vibration to be IR-active, there must be a change in dipole moment during the vibration: The larger the change, the more intense the absorbance. As a re-

Table 5 CP Concentrations in 20 Tape Strips of SC Measured by ATR-FTIR Spectroscopy, LSC, and AMS After 15-min Exposure to Aqueous Solution

Subjects	Applied concentration		Total amount in SC[a] $(nmol \cdot cm^{-2} \cdot mg^{-1})$		
	mM	$nmol \cdot cm^{-2}$	ATR-FTIR	LSC	AMS
1	196	4410	84	62	129
2	196	4410	40	32	37
3	196	4508	64	51	69
		Mean	63	48	78
		SD	22	15	47

[a]The average total amounts of CP in the stratum corneum as determined by the three methods were statistically indistinguishable ($p = 0.05$, Kruskall-Wallis test). In a fourth subject, for whom AMS data were not available, the ATR-FTIR and LSC measurements were 66 and 40 $nmol \cdot cm^{-2} \cdot mg^{-1}$, respectively. For a fifth subject, to whom a lower CP concentration (149 mM) was applied, ATR-FTIR, LSC, and AMS values were 13, 15, and 26 $nmol \cdot cm^{-2} \cdot mg^{-1}$, respectively.

Source: From Ref. 175.

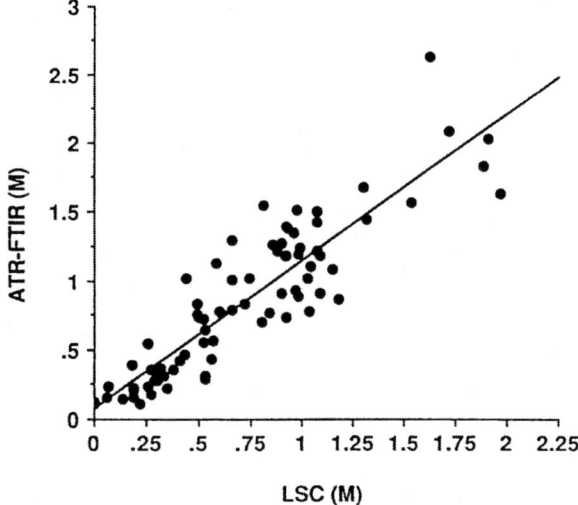

Figure 21 Correlation between the concentrations of CP in the SC, following a 15-minute exposure to an aqueous solution of the chemical, as measured by ATR-FTIR spectroscopy and by liquid scintillation counting (LSC). The accumulated data from four different subjects (78 measurements) are shown. The line of linear regression drawn through the data is $y = 1.07x + 0.08$ ($r^2 = 0.796$, p < 0.0001). The values of the slope and intercept are not significantly different from 1 and 0 (p < 0.05), respectively. (From Ref. 175.)

sult, polar chemical groups are strong IR absorbers. On the other hand, Raman scattering is dependent on the molecular polarizability (constant of proportionality relating the induced dipole moment to the electric field strength) and more sensitive to hydrophobic groups. The most important consequence of these selection rules is that in a molecule with a center of symmetry (e.g., CO_2), those vibrations symmetrical about the center of symmetry (e.g., C=O symmetric stretching) are IR-inactive but Raman-active; those vibrations that are not centrosymmetric (e.g., C=O asymmetric stretching) are usually Raman-inactive and IR-active. The routine use of IR rests with the fact that most functional groups are not centrosymmetric. Additionally, Raman scattering is a relatively inefficient process, necessitating intense excitation sources (usually 300–500 mW). Furthermore, the intensity of the scattering is inversely proportional to the wavelength raised to the fourth power ($\propto \lambda^{-4}$); hence, although longer wavelengths (typically in the near-IR range, e.g., 1064 nm) are desirable to avoid fluorescence and thermal decomposition (of particular relevance, in vivo), this advantage is offset by attenuation of the scattering intensity. Fortunately, as with FT-IR, the multiplex and throughput advantages of the Fourier transform technique are able to overcome much of this inherent disadvantage. The superiority, with respect to sample quality and data-acquisition time, of the FT-Raman system (350-mW laser operating at 1064 nm) over its dispersive counterpart (20–100-mW laser in the visible range at 488 nm) in the study of human SC has been demonstrated [187].

A practical advantage of FT-Raman over FT-IR spectroscopy in skin analysis is undoubtedly the insensitivity of the former technique to the hydration state of the SC (Fig. 22), which in an IR spectrum can confound neighboring bands of interest; on the other hand, FT-Raman has limited application in the evaluation of skin moisture. As part of their analyses of human SC, Williams et al. [187] compared the intra- and interdonor variability of the FT-Raman spectra. Intradonor variability was assessed by recording spectra of four samples of excised abdominal SC from the same donor (repeated for three donors), while interdonor variability was determined from spectra of abdominal SC from three different donors. Both intra- and intercadaver variations in FT-Raman spectra were found to be minimal: although the band intensities of the lipid C–H vibrations differed between donors (accounted for by natural variation in SC lipid content between donors), their peak positions (frequencies) remained constant. These results have been contrasted with those from a large-scale (59 subjects) in vivo ATR-FTIR study [194]. The latter study reported a broad variation in the surface C–H stretching frequencies (up to 10 cm^{-1}) between subjects, possibly reflecting the presence of variable amounts of sebaceous lipids in the superficial layers. As indicated

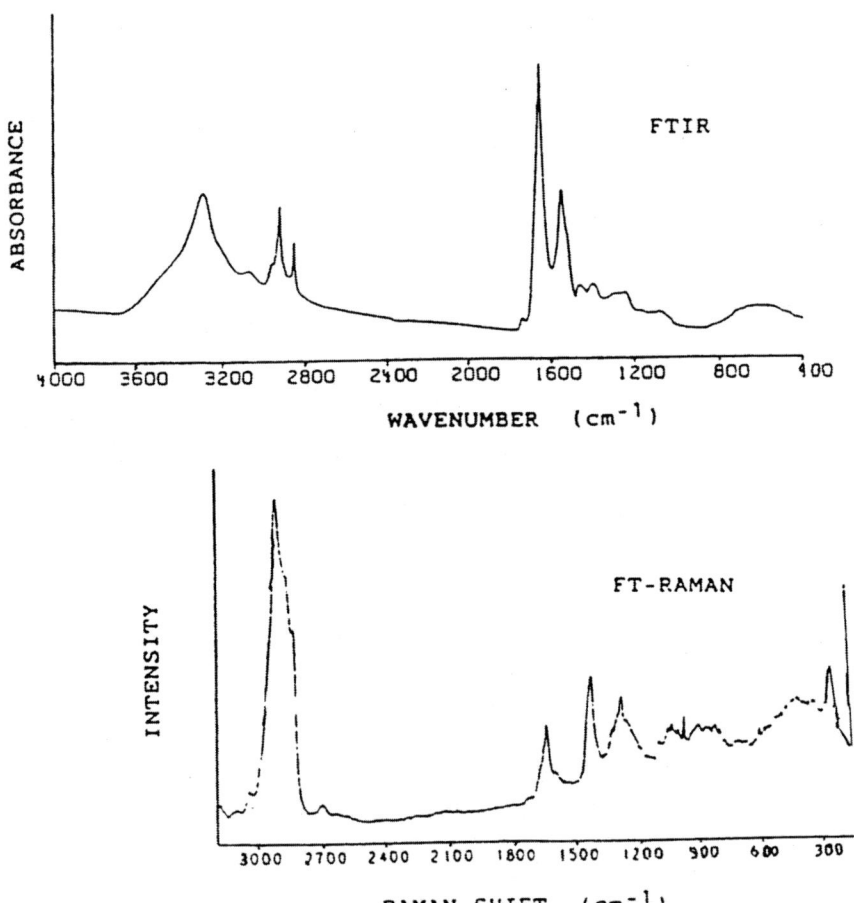

Figure 22 Vibrational spectra of human stratum corneum. FTIR: Fourier transform infrared spectrum; FT-Raman; Fourier transform Raman spectrum. (From Ref. 185. Reprinted from *International Journal of Pharmaceutics, 81* (2–3), Williams et al. Fourier transform Raman spectroscopy: A novel application for examining human stratum corneum, pp. R11–R14, 1992, with kind permission from Elsevier Science, NL, Sara Burgerhartstraaat 25, 1055 KV, Amsterdam, The Netherlands.)

by Williams et al., the disparity between the IR and Raman data may demonstrate a technical difference between the two techniques: Raman spectra are obtained from the surface of the sample, whereas ATR-IR spectra (pertaining to the C–H stretching information) are collected from within the sample (to a depth of < 1 μm). However, and in addition, other important differences between the two studies should also be considered. First, sample preparation of the excised SC is significantly more aggressive than that in the in vivo study; and second, the different sample sizes of the two studies (3 donors vs. 59 subjects) is worth noting. Indeed, significant differences between FT-Raman spectra of human SC collected in vitro and in vivo have been observed [187]. In view of the reported in vivo variation of C–H stretching frequencies, a comparative study of identical samples, examining this feature, with both FT-Raman and FT-IR, would appear to be judicious.

Further recent developments in DSC and IR techniques, with respect to the study of SC barrier properties, include step-scan FT-IR photoacoustic spectroscopy [195] and combined microscopic differential calorimetry–Fourier transform infrared (DSC-FTIR) spectroscopy [196]. The former allows depth profiling of the membrane; the latter enables the simultaneous detection of calorimetric and structural modifications during a thermal transition. Technological advances in DSC and IR will, no doubt, continue to expand the application of these techniques to the study of skin barrier function.

X. SUMMARY

The substantial contributions of calorimetry and infrared spectroscopy to our knowledge base of SC biophysics speaks for themselves. Most notably, the pivotal role of the intercellular lipid domains in SC barrier function has been elucidated and has elevated the understanding of this complex membrane to a new level. In turn, this has allowed mechanisms of permeation and mechanisms of penetration enhancement to be examined and identified. Furthermore, the opportunity to monitor the uptake and distribution of topically administered chemicals into and within the SC offers a level of detail and quantification of the permeation process, in vivo in humans, that was unimaginable a decade ago. The variety of potential applications of these findings is considerable and will form the basis of substantial further work.

Challenges for the use of biophysical techniques remain, however, not the least of which is whether they can be developed to unravel the structural heterogeneity of the SC. To what extent will it be possible to define the different lipid domains within the intercellular spaces and at the corneocyte surface? Is the keratin within the cornified cells completely inactive with respect to the permeation process, or does it have a role as "reservoir" for molecules other than water? Are permeation enhancers capable of "exposing" parts of the SC to penetrating molecules that are passively inaccessible? Ultimately, then, the issue is whether DSC and IR, which are sensitive to the molecular properties of ensembles of molecules, can in addition probe microscopic domains of the membrane.

ACKNOWLEDGMENTS

Our own work in this field has been supported by the U.S. National Institutes of Health (HD-23010) and by Pfizer, Inc. We have benefited enormously from the substantial efforts of our colleagues and collaborators over the last 10 years.

REFERENCES

1. Lee, D. C. and Chapman, D. Infrared spectroscopic studies of biomembranes and model membranes. *Bioscience Reports* 6(3):235–256, 1986.
2. Amey, R. L. and Chapman, D. Infrared spectroscopic studies of model and natural biomembranes. In: *Biomembrane Structure and Function*. D. Chapman, ed. Verlag Chemie, 1989.
3. Fringeli, U. P. and Gunthard, H. H., Infrared membrane spectroscopy. In: Membrane Spectroscopy: Molecular Biology, Biochemistry and Physics, E. Grell, ed. 1981, Springer Verlag.
4. Mantsch, H. H. and McElhaney, M. J. Phospholipid phase transitions in model and biological membranes as studied by infrared spectroscopy. *Chemistry and Physics of Lipids* 57(2–3):213–226, 1991.
5. Casal, H. L. and Mantsch, H. H. Polymorphic phase behavior of phospholipid membranes studied by infrared spectroscopy. *Biochimica et Biophysica Acta* 779:381–401, 1984.
6. Bach, D., Calorimetric studies of model and natural biomembranes. In: *Biomembrane Structure and Function*. D. Chapman, ed. Verlag Chemie, 1984.
7. Gennis, R. B., The structures and properties of membrane lipids. In: *Biomembranes: Molecular Structure and Function*. R. B. Gennis, Ed. Springer-Verlag: New York, 1989.
8. Lewis, R. N. A. H. and McElhaney, R. N. The mesomorphic phase behavior of lipid bilayers. In: *The Structure of Biological Membranes*. P. Yeagle, ed. CRC Press, 1992.
9. Mabrey-Gaud, S., Differential scanning calorimetry of liposomes. In: *Lipo-

somes: From Physical Structure to Therapeutic Applications. Knight, ed. Elsevier/North-Holland Biomedical Press, 1981.

10. Donovan, J. W., Scanning calorimetry of complex biological structures. In: *Trends in Biological Sciences*, 1984; pp. 340–344.

11. Wolf, D. E. Microheterogeneity in biological membranes. *Current Topics in Membranes 40*:143–165, 1994.

12. Melchior, D. L. and Steim, J. M. Thermotropic transitions in biomembranes. *Annual Reviews of Biophysics and Bioengineering 5*:205, 1976.

13. Melchior, D. L. and Steim, J. M. Lipid-associated thermal events in biomembranes. *Progress in Surface and Membrane Science 13*:211–296, 1979.

14. McElhaney, R. N. Differential scanning calorimetric studies of lipid–protein interactions in model membrane systems. *Biochimica et Biophysica acta 864*:361–421, 1986.

15. Mouritsen, O. G. and Bloom, M., Models of lipid–protein interactions in membranes. *Annual Review of Biophysics and Biomolecular Structure 22*:145–171, 1993.

16. Jain, M. K. and Wu, N. M. Effect of small molecules on the dipalmitoyl lecithin liposomal bilayer. *Journal of Membrane Biology 34*:157–201, 1977.

17. Potts, R. O. and Francoeur, M. L. The influence of stratum corneum morphology on water permeability. *Journal of Investigative Dermatology 96*(4):495–499, 1991.

18. Elias, P. M. et al., Percutaneous transport in relation to stratum corneum structure and lipid composition. *Journal of Investigative Dermatology 76*(4):297–301, 1981.

19. Grubauer, G. et al. Lipid content and lipid type as determinants of the epidermal permeability barrier. *Journal of Lipid Research 30*(1):89–96, 1989.

20. Potts, R. O. and Francoeur, M. L. Lipid biophysics of water loss through the skin. *Proceedings of the National Academy of Science 87*:3871–3873, 1990.

21. Denda, M. et al. Stratum corneum lipid morphology and transepidermal water loss in normal skin and surfactant-induced scaly skin. *Archives of Dermatological Research 286*:41–46, 1994.

22. Blank, I. H. Factors which influence the water content of the stratum corneum. *Journal of Investigative Dermatology 18*:433–439, 1952.

23. Potts, R. O. Physical characterization of the stratum corneum: The relationship of mechanical and barrier properties to lipid and protein structure. In: *Transdermal Drug Delivery: Developmental Issues and Research Initiatives*. J. Hadgraft and R. H. Guy, eds. Marcel Dekker: New York, 1989, pp. 23–57.

24. Potts, R. O. et al. Strategies to enhance permeability via stratum corneum lipid pathways. *Advances in Lipid Research 24*:173–210, 1991.

25. Potts, R. O. et al. Mechanism and enhancement of solute transport across the stratum corneum. *Journal of Controlled Release 15*:249–260, 1991.

26. Potts, R. O. and Francoeur, M. L. Physical methods for studying stratum corneum lipids. *Seminars in Dermatology 11(2)*:129–138, 1992.

27. Potts, R. O. and Francoeur, M. L. Infrared spectroscopy of stratum corneum lipids. In: *Pharmaceutical Skin Penetration Enhancement*. K. A. Walters and J. Hadgraft, eds. Marcel Dekker: New York, 1993.

28. Perkins, W. D. Fourier transform—Infrared spectroscopy Part II. Advantages of FT-IR. *Journal of Chemical Education 64*(11):A269–A271, 1987.

29. Markovich, R. J. and Pidgeon, C. Introduction to Fourier transform infrared spectroscopy and applications in the pharmaceutical sciences. *Pharmaceutical Research 8*(6):663–675, 1991.

30. Griffiths, P. R. and de Haseth, J. A. Fourier transform infrared spectroscopy. In: *Chemical Analysis*. Wiley: New York, 1986.

31. Park, A. C. and Baddiel, C. B. Rheology of stratum corneum II: A physico-chemical investigation of factors influencing the water content of the corneum. *Journal of Society of Cosmetic Chemists 23*:13–21, 1972.

32. Ongpipattanakul, B., Francoeur, M. L. and Potts, R. O. Polymorphism in stratum corneum lipids. *Biochimica et Biophysica Acta 1990*:115–122, 1994.

33. Golden, G. M. et al. Stratum corneum lipid phase transitions and water barrier properties. *Biochemistry 26*(8):2382–2388, 1987.

34. Tanojo, H. et al. Subzero thermal analysis of human stratum corneum. *Pharmaceutical Research 11*(11):1610–1616, 1994.

35. Knutson, K. et al. Macro- and molecular physical-chemical considerations in understanding drug transport in the stratum corneum. *Journal of Controlled Release 2*:67–87, 1985.

36. Krill, S. L., Knutson, K. and Higuchi, W. I. The stratum corneum lipid thermotropic phase behavior. *Biochimica et Biophysica Acta 1112*(2):281–286, 1992.

37. Golden, G. M. et al. Lipid thermotropic transitions in human stratum corneum. *Journal of Investigative Dermatology 86*:255–259, 1986.

38. Goodman, M. and Barry, B. W. Differential scanning calorimetry of human stratum corneum: effects of penetration enhancers azone and dimethyl sulphoxide. *Analytical Proceedings 23*:397–398, 1986.

39. van Duzee, B. F. Thermal analysis of human stratum corneum. *Journal of Investigative Dermatology 65*(4):404–408, 1975.

40. Gay, C. L. et al. Characterization of low-temperature (i.e., < 65 deg C) lipid transitions in human stratum corneum. *Journal of Investigative Dermatology 103*:233–239, 1994.

41. Small, D. M. *The Physical Chemistry of Lipids*. New York: Plenum Press, 1986.

42. Kennedy, A. H. et al. Stratum corneum lipids of human epidermal keratinocyte air–liquid cultures: Implications for barrier function. *Pharmaceutical Research 13*(8):1162–1167, 1996.

43. Rehfeld, S. J. and Elias, P. M. Mammalian stratum corneum contains physiologic lipid thermal transitions. *Journal of Investigative Dermatology 79*(1):1–3, 1982.

44. Cameron, D. G., Gudgin, E. F. and Mantsch, H. H. Dependence of acyl chain packing of phospholipids on the head group and acyl chain length. *Biochemistry 20*:4496–4500, 1981.

45. Cameron, D. G., Casal, H. L. and Mantsch, H. H. Characterization of the pretransition in 1,2-dipalmitoyl-sn-glycero-3-phosphocholine by Fourier transform infrared spectroscopy. *Biochemistry 19*:3665–3672, 1980.

46. White, S. H., Mirejovsky, D. and King, G. I. Structure of lamellar lipid domains and corneocyte envelopes of murine stratum corneum. An x-ray diffraction study. *Biochemistry 27*(10):3725–2732, 1988.

47. Wilkes, G. L., Nguyen, A. L. and Wildnauer, R. Thermal stability of the crystalline lipid structure as studied by x-ray diffraction and differential thermal analysis. *Biochimica et Biophysica Acta 304*:267–275, 1973.

48. Bouwstra, J. A. et al. Structural investigations of human stratum corneum by small-angle x-ray scattering. *Journal of Investigative Dermatology 97*(6):1005–1012, 1991.

49. Garson, J.-C. et al. Oriented structure in human stratum corneum revealed by x-ray diffraction. *Journal of Investigative Dermatology 96*:43–49, 1991.

50. Abraham, W. and Downing, D. T. Deuterium NMR investigation of polymorphism in stratum corneum lipids. *Biochimica et Biophysica Acta 1068*(2):189–194, 1991.

51. Mendelsohn, R., Sunder, S. and Bernstein, H. J. Deuterated fatty acids as Raman spectroscopic probes of membrane structure. *Biochimica et Biophysica Acta 443*:613–617, 1976.

52. Asher, I. M. and Levin, I. W. Effects of temperature and molecular interactions on the vibrational infrared spectra of phospholipid vesicles. *Biochimica et Biophysica Acta 468*:63–72, 1977.

53. Pringle, M. J. and Miller, K. W. Differential effects on phospholipid phase transitions produced by structurally related long-chain alcohols. *Biochemistry 18*:3314–3320, 1979.

54. Kitajima, Y. et al. Freeze-fracture cytochemical study of membrane systems in human epidermis using filipin as a probe for cholesterol. *Journal of Investigative Dermatology 84*:149–153, 1985.

55. Golden, G. M. et al. Comparison of skin permeability and thin layer chromatographic analysis of lipids isolated from various stratum corneum. *Journal of Investigative Dermatology 98*:642, 1992.

56. Mirabella, F. M., ed. *Internal Reflection Spectroscopy: Theory and Practice.* Marcel Dekker, 1993.

57. Puttnam, N. A. and Baxter, B. H. Spectroscopic studies of skin in situ by attenuated total reflectance. *Journal of the Society of Cosmetic Chemists 18*:469–472, 1962.

58. Comaish, S. Infra-red studies of human skin by multiple internal reflection. *British Journal of Dermatology 80*:522–528, 1968.

59. Puttnam, N. A. Attenuated total reflectance studies of the skin. *Journal of the Society of Cosmetic Chemists 23*:209–226, 1972.

60. Baier, R. E. Noninvasive, rapid characterization of human skin chemistry in situ. *Journal of the Society of Cosmetic Chemists 29*:283–306, 1978.

61. Bommannan, D., Potts, R. O. and Guy, R. H. Examination of stratum corneum barrier function in vivo by infrared spectroscopy. *Journal of Investigative Dermatology 95*(4):403–408, 1990.

62. Keighley, J. H. In: *Introduction to the Spectroscopy of Biological Polymers.* Jones, ed. Academic Press: New York, 1976, pp. 17–80.

63. Byler, D. M. and Susi, H. Examination of the secondary structure of proteins by deconvolved FTIR spectra. *Biopolymers 25*:469–487, 1986.

64. Gray, G. M. and Yardley, H. J., Lipid compositions of cells isolated from pig, human, and rat epidermis. *Journal of Lipid Research 16*:343–440, 1975.

65. Gray, G. M. and White, R. J. Glycosphingolipids and ceramides in human and pig epidermis. *Journal of Investigative Dermatology 70*(6):336–341, 1978.

66. Lampe, M. A., Williams, M. L., and Elias, P. M. Human epidermal lipids: Characterization and modulations during differentiation. *Journal of Lipid Research 24*:131–140, 1983.

67. Walters, K. A. Penetration enhancers and their use in transdermal therapeutic systems. In: *Transdermal Drug Delivery Developmental Issues and Research Initiatives.* J. Hadgraft and R. H. Guy, eds. Dekker: New York, 1989, pp. 197–246.

68. Walters, K. A. and Hadgraft, J., Eds. *Pharmaceutical Skin Penetration Enhancement.* Dekker: New York, 1993.

69. Smith, E. W. and Maibach, H. I., Eds. *Percutaneous Penetration Enhancers.* CRC Press: Boca Raton, 1995.

70. Walker, R. B. and Smith, E. W. The role of percutaneous penetration enhancers. *Advanced Drug Delivery Reviews 18*:295–301, 1996.

71. Hadgraft, J. and Walters, K. A. Skin penetration enhancement. In: *Drug Absorption Enhancement: Concepts, Possibilities, Limitations and Trends*, A. B. G. de Boer, Ed. Hardwood, 1994, pp. 177–198.

72. Kodama, M., Kuwabara, M., and Seki, S. Successive phase-transition phenomena and phase diagram of the phosphatidylcholine-water system as revealed by differential scanning calorimetry. *Biochimica et Biophysica Acta 689*:567, 1982.

73. Mak, V. H., Potts, R. O., and Guy, R. H. Does hydration affect intercellular lipid organization in the stratum corneum? *Pharmaceutical Research 8*(8):1064–1065, 1991.

74. Bouwstra, J. A. et al. Thermodynamic and structural aspects of the skin barrier. *Journal of Controlled Release 15*:209–220, 1991.

75. Hou, S. Y. E., et al. Membrane structures in normal and essential fatty acid-deficient stratum corneum: characterization by ruthenium tetroxide staining and x-ray diffraction. *Journal of Investigative Dermatology 96*(2):215–223, 1991.

76. Papahadjopoulos, D., et al. Effects of proteins on thermotropic phase transitions of phospholipid membranes. *Biochimica et Biophysica Acta 401*:317–335, 1975.

77. Jain, M. K., Wu, N. Y.-M., and Wray, L. V. Drug-induced phase change in bilayer as possible mode of action of membrane expanding drugs. *Nature 255*:494–496, 1975.

78. Goodman, M. and Barry, B. W. Differential scanning calorimetry (DSC) of human stratum corneum: Effect of azone. *Journal of Pharmacy and Pharmacology 37*:80P, 1985.

79. Goodman, M. and Barry, B. W. Action of penetration enhancers on human stratum corneum as assessed by differential scanning calorimetry. In: *Percutaneous Absorption. Mechanisms, Methodology, Drug Delivery*. R. L. Bronaugh and H. I. Maibach, ed. Dekker: New York, 1989, pp. 567–593.

80. Barry, B. W. Lipid-protein-partitioning theory of skin penetration enhancement. *Journal of Controlled Release 15*:237–248, 1991.

81. Hadgraft, J., Williams, D. G., and Allan, G., Azone: Mechanism of action and clinical effect. In: *Pharmaceutical Skin Penetration Enhancement*. K. A. Walters and J. Hadgraft, eds. Dekker: New York, 1993.

82. Lewis, D. and Hadgraft, J. Mixed monolayers of dipalmitoyl-phosphatidylcholine with Azone or oleic acid at the air–water interface. *International Journal of Pharmaceutics 65*:211–218, 1990.

83. Hoogstraate, A. J. et al. Kinetics, ultrastructural aspects and molecular modelling of transdermal peptide flux enhancement by *N*-alkylazacycloheptanones. *International Journal of Pharmaceutics 76*(1–2):37–47, 1991.

84. Harrison, J. E., Brain, K. R. and Hadgraft, J. The effect of Azone® on structured lipid monolayers. In: *Prediction of Percutaneous Penetration*. K. R. Brain, V. J. James, and K. A. Walters, eds. STS Publishing: Cardiff. pp. 174–182, 1993.

85. Schückler, F. and Lee, G. The influence of Azone on monomolecular films of some stratum corneum lipids. *International Journal of Pharmaceutics 70*(1–2):173–186, 1991.

86. Engblom, J. The bicontinuous cubic phase—A model for investigating the effects on a lipid bilayer due to a foreign substance illustrated by the skin penetration enhancer Azone. *Chemistry and Physics of Lipids 84*(2):155–164, 1996.

87. Ward, A. and Tallon, R., Penetration enhancer incorporation in bilayers. *Drug Development and Industrial Pharmacy 14*:1155, 1988.

88. Engblom, J. and Engström, S. Azone and the formation of reversed mono- and bicontinuous lipid–water phases. *International Journal of Pharmaceutics 98*:173–179, 1993.

89. Engblom, J., Engström, S. and Fontell, K. The effect of the skin penetration enhancer Azone on fatty-acid soap–water mixtures. *Journal of Controlled Release 33*:299–305, 1995.

90. Engblom, J. On the phase behaviour of lipids with respect to skin barrier function. Ph.D. thesis. Department of Food Technology, Lund, Sweden, 1996.

91. Schückler, F. et al. An x-ray diffraction study of some model stratum corneum lipids containing Azone and dodecyl-L-pyroglutamate. *Journal of Controlled Release* 23(1):27–36, 1993.

92. Lee, G. Interaction of Azone® with model lipid systems. In: *Percutaneous Penetration Enhancers.* E. W. Smith and H. I. Maibach, eds. CRC Press: Boca Raton, 1995, pp. 277–287.

93. Hirvonen, J. et al. Mechanism and reversibility of penetration enhancer action in the skin. *European Journal of Pharmaceutics and Biopharmaceutics* 40(2):81–85, 1994.

94. Bouwstra, J. A. et al. Effect of N-alkyl-azocycloheptan-2-ones including Azone on the thermal behavior of human stratum corneum. *International Journal of Pharmaceutics* 52:47–54, 1989.

95. Bouwstra, J. A. et al. The influence of alkyl-azones on the ordering of the lamellae in human stratum corneum. *International Journal of Pharmaceutics* 79:141–148, 1992.

96. Schückler, F. and Lee, G. Relating the concentration-dependent action of Azone and dodecy-L-pyroglutamate on the structure of excised human stratum corneum to changes in drug diffusivity, partition coefficient and flux. *International Journal of Pharmaceutics* 80:81–89, 1992.

97. Ashton, P. et al. Surfactant effects in percutaneous absorption. 2. Effects of protein and lipid structure of the stratum corneum. *International Journal of Pharmaceutics* 87(1–3):265–269, 1992.

98. Eagle, S. C., Barry, B. W. and Scott, R. C. Differential scanning calorimetry and permeation studies to examine surfactant damage to human skin. *Journal of Toxicology—Cutaneous and Ocular Toxicology* 11(1):77–92, 1992.

99. de Vos, A. M. and Kinget, R. Study of the penetration-enhancing effect of two nonionic surfactants (Cetiol HE and Eumulgin B3) on human stratum corneum using differential scanning calorimetry. *European Journal of Pharmaceutical Sciences* 1:89–93, 1993.

100. Ashton, P., Hadgraft, J. and Walters, K. A. Effects of surfactants in percutaneous absorption. *Pharmaceutica Acta. Helvetica* 61(8):228–235, 1986.

101. Allenby, A. C. et al. Mechanism of action of accelerants on skin penetration. *British Journal of Dermatology* 81(Supplement 4):47–55, 1969.

102. Embery, G. and Dugrad, P. H. The isolation of DMSO soluble components from human epidermis preparations: A possible mechanism of action of dimethylsulfoxide in effecting percutaneous migration phenomena. *Journal of Investigative Dermatology* 57:308–311, 1971.

103. Montes, L. F. et al. Ultrastructural changes in the horny layer following local application of dimethyl sulfoxide to guinea pig skin. *Journal of Investigative Dermatology* 48(2):184–196, 1967.

104. Chandrasekaran, S. K., Campbell, P. S. and Michaels, A. S. Effect of dimethyl sulfoxide on drug permeation through human skin. *American Institute of Chemical Engineers' Journal 23*(6):810–816, 1977.

105. Kurihara–Bergstrom, T., Flynn, G. L. and Higuchi, W. I. Physicochemical study of percutaneous absorption enhancement by dimethyl sulfoxide: Kinetic and thermodynamic determinants of dimethyl sulfoxide mediated mass transfer of alkanols. *Journal of Pharmaceutical Sciences 75*(5):479–486, 1986.

106. Hadgraft, J., Penetration enhancers in percutaneous absorption. *Pharmacy International 5*(10):252–254, 1984.

107. Khan, Z. U. and Kellaway, I. W. Differential scanning calorimetry of dimethyl-sulphoxide-treated human stratum corneum. *International Journal of Pharmaceutics 55*:129–134, 1989.

108. Clancy, M. J., Corish, J. and Corrigan, O. I. A comparison of the effects of electrical current and penetration enhancers on the properties of human skin using spectroscopic (FTIR) and calorimetric (DSC) methods. *International Journal of Pharmaceutics 105*:47–56, 1994.

109. Oertel, R. P. Protein conformational changes induced in human stratum corneum by organic sulfoxides: An infrared spectroscopic investigation. *Biopolymers 16*:2329–2345, 1977.

110. Sekura, D. L. and Scala, J. The percutaneous absorption of alkyl methyl sulfoxides. In: *Pharmacology and the Skin*. Appleton-Century-Crofts: New York, 1972, pp. 257–268.

111. Carelli, V. et al. Bile acids as enhancers of steroid penetration through excised hairless mouse skin. *International Journal of Pharmaceutics 89*(2):81–89, 1993.

112. Yamane, M. A., Williams, A. C. and Barry, B. W. Effects of terpenes and oleic acid as skin penetration enhancers towards 5-fluorouracil as assessed with time; permeation, partitioning and differential scanning calorimetry. *International Journal of Pharmaceutics 116*:237–251, 1995.

113. Cumming, K. I. and Winfield, A. J. In vitro evaluation of a series of sodium carboxylates as dermal penetration enhancers. *International Journal of Pharmaceutics 108*:141–148, 1994.

114. Leopold, C. S. and Lippold, B. C. An attempt to clarify the mechanism of the penetration enhancing effects of lipophilic vehicles with differential scanning calorimetry. *Journal of Pharmacy and Pharmacology 47*:276–281, 1995.

115. Gale, R. M. et al. Device for Delivering Fentanyl Across the Skin at a Constant Rate to Maintain Analgesia over a Long Period 1986: U.S. 4,588,580.

116. Good, W. R. et al. A new transdermal delivery system for estradiol. *Journal of Controlled Release 2*:89–97, 1985.

117. Kai, T. et al. Mechanism of percutaneous penetration enhancement: effect of *n*-alkanols on the permeability barrier of hairless mouse skin. *Journal of Controlled Release 12*:103–112, 1990.

118. Rowe, E. S. The effects of ethanol on the thermotropic properties of dipalmitoylphosphatidylcholine. *Molecular Pharmacology* 22:133–139, 1982.

119. Rowe, E. S. Lipid chain-length and temperature-dependence of ethanol phosphatidylcholine interactions. *Biochemistry* 22:3299–3305, 1983.

120. Wood, G. W. and Schroeder, F. Membrane effects of ethanol: Bulk lipid versus lipid domains. *Life Sciences* 43(6):467–475, 1988.

121. Ghanem, A.-H. et al. The effects of ethanol on the transport of B-estradiol and other permeants in hairless mouse skin II. A new quantitative approach. *Journal of Controlled Release* 6:75–83, 1987.

122. Krill, S. L., Knutson, K. and Higuchi, W. I. Ethanol effects on the stratum corneum lipid phase behavior. *Biochimica et Biophysica Acta* 1112(2):273–280, 1992.

123. Krill, S. L., Knutson, K. and Higuchi, W. I. The influence of iso-propanol, *n*-propanol and *n*-butanol on stratum corneum lipid phase behavior. *Journal of Controlled Release* 25:31–42, 1993.

124. Kurihara-Bergstrom, T. et al. Percutaneous absorption enhancement of an ionic molecule by ethanol–water systems in human skin. *Pharmaceutical Research* 7(7):762–766, 1990.

125. Bommannan, D., Potts, R. O. and Guy, R. H. Examination of the effect of ethanol on human stratum corneum in vivo using infrared spectroscopy. *Journal of Controlled Release* 16:299–304, 1991.

126. Francoeur, M. L., Golden, G. M. and Potts, R. O. Oleic acid: Its effects on stratum corneum in relation to (trans)dermal drug delivery. *Pharmaceutical Research 1990* 7(6):621–627, 1990.

127. Lewis, E. N., Levin, I. W. and Steer, C. J. Infrared spectroscopic study of ethanol-induced changes in rat liver plasma membrane. *Biochimica et Biophysica Acta* 986:161–166, 1989.

128. Simon, S. A. and McIntosh, T. J. Interdigitated hydrocarbon chain packing causes the biphasic transition behavior in lipid alcohol suspensions. *Biochimica et Biophysica Acta* 773(1):169–172, 1984.

129. Aungst, B. J. Fatty acids as skin permeation enhancers. In: *Percutaneous Penetration Enhancers.* E. W. Smith and H. I. Maibach, eds. CRC Press: Boca Raton, 1995; pp. 277–287.

130. Aungst, B. J., Rogers, N. J. and Shefter, E. Enhancement of naloxone penetration through human skin in vitro using fatty acids, fatty alcohols, surfactants, sulfoxides and amides. *International Journal of Pharmaceutics* 33:225–234, 1986.

131. Ogiso, T. and Shintani, M. Mechanism for the enhancement effect of fatty acids on the percutaneous absorption of propranolol. *Journal of Pharmaceutical Sciences* 79(12):1065–1071, 1990.

132. Cooper, E. R. Increased skin permeability for lipophilic molecules. *Journal of Pharmaceutical Sciences* 73(8):1153–1156, 1984.

133. Golden, G. M., McKie, J. E. and Potts, R. O. Role of stratum corneum lipid fluidity in transdermal drug flux. *Journal of Pharmaceutical Sciences 76*(1):25–28, 1987.

134. Aungst, B. J. Structure/effect studies of fatty acid isomers as skin penetration enhancers and skin irritants. *Pharmaceutical Research 6*(3):244–247, 1989.

135. Cooper, E. R., Merritt, E. W. and Smith, R. L. Effect of fatty acids and alcohols on the penetration of acyclovir across human skin in vitro. *Journal of Pharmaceutical Sciences 74*(6):688–689, 1985.

136. Barry, B. W. and Bennett, S. L. Effect of penetration enhancers on the permeation of mannitol, hydrocortisone and progesterone through human skin. *Journal of Pharmacy and Pharmacology 39*(7):535–546, 1987.

137. Touitou, E. and Fabin, B. Altered skin permeation of a highly lipophilic molecule: Tetrahydrocannabinol. *International Journal of Pharmaceutics 43*:17–22, 1988.

138. Bond, J. R. and Barry, B. W. Hairless mouse skin is limited as a model for assessing the effects of penetration enhancers in human skin. *Journal of Investigative Dermatology 90*(6):810–813, 1988.

139. Gay, C. L. et al. An electron spin resonance study of skin penetration enhancers. *International Journal of Pharmaceutics 49*:39–45, 1989.

140. Goodman, M. and Barry, B. W. Action of skin permeation enhancers azone, oleic acid and decylmethyl sulphoxide: permeation and DSC studies. *Journal of Pharmacy and Pharmacology 38*:71, 1986.

141. Walker, M. and Hadgraft, J. Oleic acid—A membrane "fluidiser" or fluid within the membrane? *International Journal of Pharmaceutics 71*:R1–R4, 1991.

142. Hill, M. W. The effect of anaesthetic-like molecules on the phase transition in smectic mesophases of dipalmitoyl lecithin. I. The normal alcohol up to $C = 9$ and three inhalation anesthetics. *Biochimica et Biophysica Acta 356*:117, 1974.

143. Papahadjopoulos, D. et al. Phase transitions in phospholipid vesicles. Fluorescence polarization and permeability measurements concerning the effect of temperature and cholesterol. *Biochimica et Biophysica Acta 311*:330–348, 1973.

144. Blok, M. C. et al. The effect of chain length and lipid phase transitions on the selective permeability properties of liposomes. *Biochimica et Biophysica Acta 406*:187–196, 1975.

145. Wu, S. H. W. and McConell, H. M. Lateral phase separations and perpendicular transport in membranes. *Biochemical and Biophysical Research Communications 55*:484, 1973.

146. Shimshick, E. J. et al. Lateral phase separations in membranes. *Journal of Supramolecular Structure 2*:285–295, 1973.

147. Ongpipattanakul, B. et al. Evidence that oleic acid exists in a separate phase within stratum corneum lipids. *Pharmaceutical Research 8*(3):350–354, 1991.

148. Mendelsohn, R. et al. Quantitative determination of conformational disorder in

the acyl chains of phospholipid bilayers by infrared spectroscopy. *Biochemistry* 28:8934–8939, 1989.

149. Harrison, J. E., Brain, K. R. and Hadgraft, J. Validation of the use of the per-deuterated analogue of azone (D-azone) as a suitable model for the penetration enhancer azone. In: *Prediction of Percutaneous Penetration.* K. R. Brain, V. J. James, and K. A. Walters, eds. STS Publishing: Cardiff, Vol. 4b. 1996, pp. 127–130.

150. Ongpipattanakul, B., The perturbation of stratum corneum lipids by perdeuter-ated oleic acid and its implication for the enhancement of skin permeability. Ph.D. thesis. School of Pharmacy. University of Wisconsin Press: Madison, 1991.

151. Barry, B. W. Mode of action of penetration enhancers in human skin. *Journal of Controlled Release* 6:85–97, 1987.

152. Takeuchi, Y. et al. Effects of fatty acids, fatty amines and propylene glycol on rat stratum corneum lipids and proteins in vitro measured by fourier transform infrared/attenuated total reflection (FT-IR/ATR) spectroscopy. *Chemical and Pharmaceutical Bulletin* 40(7):1887–1892, 1992.

153. Naik, A. et al. Mechanism of oleic-acid induced skin penetration enhancement in vivo in humans. *Journal of Controlled Release* 37:299–306, 1995.

154. Ortiz, A. and Gomez-Fernandez, J. C. A Differential scanning calorimetry study of the interaction of free fatty acids with phospholipid membranes. *Chemistry and Physics of Lipids* 45:75–91, 1987.

155. Walker, M. et al. Influence of oleic acid on the physical and chemical properties of the human epidermal barrier. In: *Prediction of Percutaneous Penetration.* R. C. Scott et al., eds. IBC: London, 1991, pp. 86–96.

156. Lieckfeldt, R. et al. Influence of oleic acid on the structure of a mixture of hydrated model stratum corneum fatty acids and their soaps. *Colloids and Surfaces* 90:225–234, 1994.

157. Watkinson, A. C. et al. Evidence of phase separation of oleic acid in DPPC liposomes and excised stratum corneum from a small angle neutron scattering study. In: *Prediction of Percutaneous Penetration.* R. C. Scott et al., eds. IBC: London, 1991, pp. 380–385.

158. Mak, V. H. W., Potts, R. O. and Guy, R. H. Oleic acid concentration and effect in human stratum corneum: Non-invasive determination by attenuated total reflectance infrared spectroscopy in vivo. *Journal of Controlled Release* 12:67–75, 1990.

159. Takeuchi, Y. et al. Effects of oleic acid/propylene glycol on rat abdominal stratum corneum: lipid extraction and appearance of propylene glycol in the dermis measured by Fourier transform infrared/attenuated total reflectance (FT-IR/ATR) spectroscopy. *Chemical and Pharmaceutical Bulletin* 41(8):1434–1437, 1993.

160. Burnette, R. R. Iontophoresis. In: *Transdermal Drug Delivery: Developmental Issues and Research Initiatives.* J. Hadgraft and R. H. Guy, eds. Dekker: New York, 1989, pp. 247–291.

161. Guy, R. H., ed. *Advanced Drug Delivery Reviews*. Vol. 9. Elsevier Science Publishers, 1992.

162. Singh, P. and Maibach, H. I. Iontophoresis in drug delivery: Basic principles and applications. *Critical Reviews in Therapeutic Drug Carrier Systems* 11(2&3):161–213, 1994.

163. Cullander, C. What are the pathways of iontophoretic current flow through mammalian skin? *Advanced Drug Delivery Reviews* 9:119–135, 1992.

164. Green, R. D. and Hadgraft, J. FT-IR investigations into the effect of iontophoresis on the skin. In: *Prediction of Percutaneous Penetration*. K. R. Brain, V. J. James, K. A. Walters, eds. STS Publishing, Cardiff, Vol. 3b, pp. 37–43, 1993.

165. Thysman, S., Vanneste, D. and Preat, V. Noninvasive investigation of human skin after in vivo iontophoresis. *Skin Pharmacology* 8(5):229–236, 1995.

166. Mak, V. H., Potts, R. O. and Guy, R. H. Percutaneous penetration enhancement in vivo measured by attenuated total reflectance infrared spectroscopy. *Pharmaceutical Research* 7(8):835–841, 1990.

167. Higo, N. et al. Validation of reflectance infrared spectroscopy as a quantitative method to measure percutaneous absorption in vivo. *Pharmaceutical Research* 10(10):1500–1506, 1993.

168. Guy, R. H. et al. Mechanism and enhancement of skin penetration in vivo. In: *Prediction of Percutaneous Penetration*. R. C. Scott et al. eds. IBC: London, 1991, pp. 1–12.

169. Naik, A., Keating, G. and Guy, R. H. Assessment of dermal exposure in humans. In: *Prediction of Percutaneous Penetration: Methods, Measurements, Modelling*. La Grande Motte: STS Publishing Ltd., Cardiff, 1995.

170. Keating, G. et al. Assessment of dermal exposure to drinking water contaminants—New measurements and models. In: *Assessing and Managing Health Risks from Drinking Water Contaminants: Approaches and Applications*. E. G. Riechard and G. A. Zapponi, eds. IAHS Press: Wallingford, 1995, pp. 235–244.

171. Watkinson, A. C. et al. The influence of vehicle on permeation from saturated solutions. *International Journal of Pharmaceutics* 121:27–36, 1995.

172. Farinas, K. C. et al. Characterisation of solute diffusion in a polymer using ATR-FTIR spectroscopy and bulk transport techniques. *Macromolecules* 27(18):5220–5222, 1994.

173. Wurster, D. E., Buraphacheep, V. and Patel, J. M. The determination of diffusion coefficients in semisolids by Fourier transform infrared (FT-IR) spectroscopy. *Pharmaceutical Research* 10(4):616–620, 1993.

174. Harrison, J. E. et al. The relative effect of Azone® and Transcutol® on permeant diffusivity and solubility in human stratum corneum. *Pharmaceutical Research* 13(4):542–546, 1996.

175. Pirot, F. et al. Characterization of the permeability barrier of human skin in vivo. *Proceedings of the National Academy of Science* 94:1562–1567, 1996.

176. Potts, R. O. In vivo measurement of water content of the stratum corneum using infrared spectroscopy: A review. *Cosmetics and Toiletries 100*:27–31, 1985.

177. Potts, R. O. Stratum corneum hydration: Experimental techniques and interpretations of results. *Journal of the Society of Cosmetic Chemists 37*:9–33, 1986.

178. Gloor, M. et al. Water content of the horny layer and skin surface lipids. *Archives of Dermatological Research 268*:221–223, 1980.

179. Gloor, M., Hirsh, G. and Willebrandt, U. On the use of infrared spectroscopy for the in vivo measurement of the water content in the horny layer after application of dermatological ointments. *Archives of Dermatological Research 271*:305–314, 1981.

180. Triebskorn, A., Gloor, M. and Greiner, F. Comparative investigations on the water content of the stratum corneum using different methods of measurement. *Dermatologica 167*:64–69, 1983.

181. Potts, R. O. et al. A noninvasive, in vivo technique to quantitatively measure water concentration of the stratum corneum using attenuated total-reflectance infrared spectroscopy. *Archives of Dermatological Research 277*:489–495, 1985.

182. Hansen, J. R. and Yellin, W. NMR and infrared spectroscopic studies of stratum corneum hydration. In: *Water Structure at the Water–Polymer Interface.* H. H. G. Jellinek, ed. Plenum Publishing: New York, 1972, pp. 19–28.

183. Walling, P. L. and Dabney, J. M. Moisture in skin by near-infrared reflectance spectroscopy. *Journal of the Society of Cosmetic Chemists 40*:151–171, 1988.

184. de Rigal, J. et al. Near-infrared spectroscopy: A new approach to the characterization of dry skin. *Journal of the Society of Cosmetic Chemists 44*:197–209, 1993.

185. Williams, A. C., Edwards, H. G. M. and Barry, B. W. Fourier transform Raman spectroscopy. A novel application for examining human stratum corneum. *International Journal of Pharmaceutics 81*(2–3):R11–R14, 1992.

186. Barry, B. W., Edwards, H. G. M. and Williams, A. C. Fourier transform Raman and infrared vibrational study of human skin: Assignment of spectral bands. *Journal of Raman Spectroscopy 23*:641–645, 1992.

187. Williams, A. C., et al., A critical comparison of some Raman spectroscopic techniques for studies of human stratum corneum. *Pharmaceutical Research 10*(11):1642–1647, 1993.

188. Williams, A. C., Edwards, H. G. M. and Barry, B. W. Raman spectra of human keratotic biopolymers—Skin, callus, hair and nail. *Journal of Raman Spectroscopy 25*(1):95–98, 1994.

189. Williams, A. C., Edwards, H. G. M. and Barry, B. W. The iceman—Molecular structure of 5200-year-old skin characterized by Raman spectroscopy and electron microscopy. *Biochimica et Biophysica Acta—Protein Structure and Molecular Enzymology 1246*(1):98–105, 1995.

190. Edwards, H. G. M., Williams, A. C., and Barry, B. W., Potential applications of

FT-Raman spectroscopy for dermatological diagnostics. *Journal of Molecular Structure 347*:379–387, 1995.

191. Wegener, M. et al. Structure of stratum corneum lipids characterized by FT-Raman spectroscopy and DSC. 1. Ceramides. *International Journal of Pharmaceutics 128*(1–2):203–213, 1996.

192. Schallreuter, K. U. et al. Oxybenzone oxidation following solar irradiation of skin—Photoprotection versus antioxidant inactivation. *Journal of Investigative Dermatology 106*(3):583–586, 1996.

193. Anigbogu, A. N. C. et al. Fourier-transform Raman spectroscopy of interactions between the penetration enhancer dimethyl-sulfoxide and human stratum corneum. *International Journal of Pharmaceutics 125*(2):265–282, 1996.

194. Boddé, H. E., Pechtold, L. A. R. M. and de Haan, F. H. N. A large scale, noninvasive in vivo screening of human skin barrier and water holding properties recording infrared spectra, TEWL, skin impedance and temperature. *Pharmaceutical Research 9*:S186, 1992.

195. Baesso, M. L., Snook, R. D. and Andrew, J. J. Fourier transform infrared photoacoustic spectroscopy to study the penetration of substances through skin. *Journal de Physique IV 4*:449–451, 1994.

196. Lin, S.-Y., Liang, R.-C. and Lin, T.-C. Lipid and protein thermotropic transition of porcine stratum corneum by microscopic calorimetry and infrared spectroscopy. *Journal of the Chinese Chemical Society 41*:425–429, 1994.

4

Investigation of Membrane Structure and Dynamics by Deuterium NMR: Application to the Stratum Corneum

William Abraham
Cygnus, Inc., Redwood City, California

Neil Kitson, Myer Bloom, Jenifer L. Thewalt*
University of British Columbia, Vancouver, British Columbia, Canada

I. BROAD IS BEAUTIFUL: THE NATURE OF INFORMATION AVAILABLE FROM WIDE-LINE NMR

A. Introduction

The diffusion of small molecules into the skin from the external world is limited by the stratum corneum (SC). There is now considerable evidence that a major pathway for such diffusion through the stratum corneum itself consists of the intercellular spaces and, in particular, the lipid component of the intercellular spaces. Such lipids are arranged in lamellae that may well be bilayers and that in other respects also resemble biological membranes. In addition, there are other components within the intercellular spaces (e.g., proteins and an aqueous phase) that, although not well understood, mean that the intercellular diffusion path is a heterogeneous material. Within such material, lipids appear to play a very important role (Potts and Guy, 1992), and

---

Current affiliation: Simon Fraser University, Burnaby, British Columbia, Canada

if a predictive model for in vitro testing is to be developed, then the organization and function of SC lipids should be an important consideration.

In this context, there are several principles that determine our experimental approach and that are also more generally applicable to experimental studies of membranes. These are: (a) lipid composition determines important physical properties of membranes; (b) such physical properties (e.g., lipid packing, lipid motion) play a large part in determining other properties of interest such as permeability. These principles are the basis of the "model membrane approach." Since lipid compositions of the stratum corneum intercellular spaces have been extensively studied (Gray and Yardley, 1975a,b; Gray and White, 1978; Gray et al., 1982; Wertz et al., 1987; Downing et al., 1987; Squier et al., 1991a,b; Wertz et al., 1992; Lampe et al., 1983a,b; Elias and Menon, 1991; Schurer and Elias, 1991), the relationship between these and membrane structure can be determined using various methods of model preparation.

Membrane structure and dynamics may be studied by various physical methods, as is illustrated in this volume. In our view, these methods are complementary, and the composite of such information can yield a comprehensive view of membrane lipid organization. A persistent problem, however, has been the difficulty of communication across biophysical tribal boundaries, often due to a lack of understanding of techniques other than one's own, but also because other tribes use languages of their own invention that must be understood even before the techniques themselves can be grasped. A further problem is communication with the larger biomedical world, which may view biophysical studies as being both arcane and irrelevant, a view exacerbated by the "tower of Babel" problem previously described. With these difficulties in mind we present some basic information on nuclear magnetic resonance (NMR), and in particular "wide-line" deuterium NMR, that we hope will be useful to those in other fields in understanding why such a technique may yield useful information about membranes.

B. NMR Basics

Nuclear Spins and the NMR Signal

All nuclei are composed of particles, protons and neutrons, which possess a property called spin that mathematically resembles angular momentum. The sum of the individual particles' spins is characterized by the nuclear spin quantum number I. If I is nonzero, the nucleus will behave like a weak magnet and will display $2I + 1$ energy levels when placed in a magnetic field. Such nuclei can be studied with NMR.

At equilibrium in a magnetic field (at room temperature, say) the nuclei will distribute themselves among the available energy levels according to the Boltzmann distribution. For $I = 1/2$ (for protons, for example), there will be a small excess population (typically one part in 10^4) of nuclei aligning parallel (spin up, or $m = 1/2$, where m is the nuclear spin quantum number) to the magnetic field and the rest pointing antiparallel (spin down, or $m = -1/2$) to the field. Thus the net magnetization of the sample, which is very small, is aligned with the magnetic field. Since this sample magnetization is so small, NMR is a fairly insensitive technique requiring roughly 10^{17} nuclei per sample for reasonable signal strength. For the deuteron, where $I = 1$, there are three energy levels in the magnetic field: up, down and "sideways." The separation between the nuclear spin energy levels is

$$\Delta E = \frac{\gamma h B}{2\pi}$$

where γ is the gyromagnetic ratio, a constant for a given nucleus that relates the resonant frequency to the magnetic field strength, h is Planck's constant, and B is the magnetic field. ΔE is very small: for a proton in a 2-Tesla magnetic field, for instance, $\Delta E = 6 \times 10^{-26}$ joules. This ΔE is vey much smaller than bond energies, so NMR is completely nondestructive.

To excite transitions between the nuclear spin system's energy levels, the sample must be irradiated with photons having the appropriate frequency. NMR frequencies lie within the radio-frequency (rf), or megahertz, band. In the pioneering days of NMR, a spectrum was acquired bit by bit by irradiating the sample with different rf frequencies and measuring the resulting signal at each frequency. Most of the time was spent acquiring the baseline in this sort of experiment, which severely limited the range of systems amenable to study. The Nobel prize–winning development of pulsed Fourier transform (FT) NMR (Ernst and Anderson, 1966) enabled the simultaneous excitation of all resonant frequencies in the sample. In FT NMR, a short, intense burst of tuned rf photons is applied to a solenoid that holds the sample, which is at equilibrium in a magnetic field. The current in the solenoid gives rise to an oscillating magnetic field perpendicular to the main magnetic field, and this field tips the direction of the sample's magnetization from parallel to the magnetic field to an orientation where the weak signal from the nuclear spins can be measured. The sample's magnetization precesses about the main magnetic field once the rf pulse is turned off, with individual nuclei precessing at different frequencies depending on their physical and chemical environments. The precessing magnetization of the sample induces an oscillating voltage in the coil that typically behaves like a damped cosine wave, decaying over a time ranging from microseconds to seconds, depending on the sample being studied. This is the time-domain NMR spectrum, known as the "free induction decay" (FID), which is then Fourier transformed into the more understandable frequency-domain spectrum. (Fourier transformation is a mathematical procedure that analyzes the FID to obtain the proportions of the various spectral frequencies present.)

In addition to the information available from FT NMR spectroscopy, one may gain considerable insight into molecular interactions and motion within a material by studying NMR relaxation, either spin–spin relaxation, where nuclei exchange spin states and thus dephase, or spin–lattice relaxation, where excited nuclei lose energy to the bulk sample reservoir surrounding them. Those readers interested in a more detailed introduction to NMR are referred to Farrar and Becker (1971) or to the comprehensive texts of Slichter (1990) and Abragam (1961).

Wide-Line vs. "High-Resolution" NMR

The standard analytical NMR measurement is typically performed on samples that have been dissolved in a suitable solvent. The resulting spectrum consists of sharp lines of varying intensity and frequency from which it is possible to deduce the chemical structure of the solvated molecule. Sharp lines appear because the dissolved substance undergoes isotropic reorientation (sampling all angles with respect to the magnetic field with equal probability) in a time that is short compared to the characteristic NMR measurement time (typically on the order of 10^{-5} to 10^{-4} sec). Each nuclear spin's angularly dependent interactions with its surroundings are completely averaged, and thus only this average resonance, typically a very narrow line with a width on the order of hertz (Hz), is observed. The positions of these narrow lines are determined primarily by the immediate chemical environments of the resonant nuclei and are characterized in terms of "chemical shift." The chemical shift is a spectral line's frequency shift (in Hz) from a known standard divided by the Larmor frequency (in MHz) of the nucleus in the particular magnet, and is thus a unitless number of "ppm" (parts per million).

NMR studies of solid and semisolid systems differ intrinsically from the standard measurement just described. In these systems the angularly dependent, or anisotropic, interactions between the nuclear spins and their surroundings are *not* completely averaged and the resulting frequency spectra are broadened considerably, with widths on the order of kilohertz. Examples of these angularly dependent interactions include the dipole–dipole interaction between protons, the quadrupolar interaction between an electric field gradient and a deuteron's nuclear spin (see the second subsection in Section I.C for an introduction to ^{2}H NMR of membranes) and the chemical shift anisotropy observed in ^{31}P NMR. While these broad, relatively featureless spectra may look dull to the researcher who is more familiar with high-resolution NMR, they actually contain more information. For example, the average width of the spectrum can be correlated with the degree of mobility of the labeled site. Especially in anisotropic systems such as membranes, considerable insight into molecular motion can be gained from a careful NMR study of spectral parameters such as spin–spin or spin–lattice relaxation as a function of the orientation of the label with respect to the magnetic field. Broad-line NMR spectra can often be converted into high-resolution spectra using the technique of magic angle spinning, in which the sample is rotated rapidly about the so-called "magic" angle ($\theta = 54.7°$, where $3\cos^2\theta - 1 = 0$). Magic angle spinning merely averages out the orientation-dependent information in the broad-line spectrum in much the same way as molecular tumbling of molecules in solution averages the orientation-dependent information in standard high-resolution NMR.

^{2}H NMR Primer

The deuterium nucleus ($I = 1$) has a quadrupole moment that results from its nonspherically symmetric distribution of nuclear charge. The interaction dominating deuterium NMR spectroscopy is that between the nuclear quadrupole moment and the electric field gradient at the deuterium nucleus. This "quadrupolar interaction" modifies the separation of the Zeeman nuclear energy levels (Fig. 1) so that the transition from spin up to spin "sideways" ($m = 1 \rightarrow 0$) occurs at a lower energy, and hence lower frequency, than the transition from spin "sideways" to spin down ($m = 0 \rightarrow -1$), resulting in a doublet spectrum. The modulation of the Zeeman energy levels, whose frequencies are on the order of MHz, by the quadrupolar interaction energy (tens of kHz, typically) has been vastly exaggerated in Fig. 1—drawn to scale, the changes in energy levels would be invisible.

When the field gradient is parallel to the magnetic field, the combined Zeeman and quadrupolar energy as a function of spin state m for a deuteron is given by $E_m = -\gamma hBm/2\pi + (e^2qQ/4)(3m^2 - 2)$, where e is the charge on an electron, eq is the field gradient, and Q is the nuclear quadrupole moment. The frequency separation, in hertz, of the two spectral lines in the doublet is calculated from the equation $\Delta\nu = [(E_{-1} - E_0) - (E_0 - E_1)]/h = (3/2)(e^2qQ/h)$.

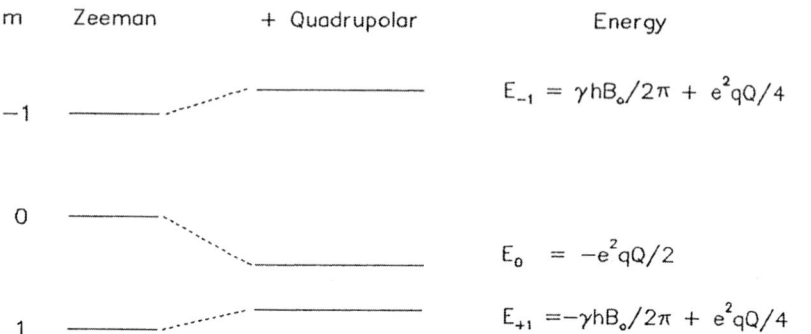

Figure 1   Sketch of the Zeeman and quadrupolar energy levels for a nucleus having spin $I = 1$. The effect of the quadrupolar interaction is to destroy the degeneracy between the two pairs of energy levels, so the NMR spectrum, which is a single line at the Larmor frequency for the Zeeman interaction alone, becomes a doublet centered on the Larmor frequency.

The quantity e^2qQ/h, termed the "quadrupolar coupling constant," is a function of the chemical environment of the deuteron. For example, in hexane e^2qQ/h = 168 kHz (Burnett and Müller, 1971). Note that this quantity is independent of the magnetic field strength. ^{2}H NMR doublets are centered about the Larmor frequency, but in practice this frequency is subtracted away, so spectra are generally shown plotted as a function of frequency, centered on zero. The minimum observed frequency is $\nu_{min} = -3/4(e^2qQ/h)$, and the maximum is ν_{max} = $3/4(e^2qQ/h)$. (A very readable quantitative introduction to NMR studies of nuclei having quadrupole moments is given by Cohen and Reif, 1957).

In our studies we have only examined compounds labeled with deuterons directly bonded to carbon. In these molecules the quadrupolar interaction depends strongly on the angle θ between the C—D bond and the magnetic field, thus causing the resonant frequencies to vary as a function of the orientation of the labeled molecule in the magnet. A single crystal containing a C—D bond will display an NMR spectrum consisting of a doublet whose frequency separation $(\Delta\nu)$ changes according to the function $\Delta\nu \propto (3\cos^2\theta - 1)/2$ (Fig. 2, top). This function can assume values from –0.5 to 1, so for a given C—D bond orientation the observed $\Delta\nu$ is generally smaller than the maximum value occurring at $\theta = 0°$ of $\Delta\nu_{max} = \Delta\nu_Q = 3/2(e^2qQ/h)$. (For the purposes of this chapter, we can assume that the local electric field gradient will always be axially symmetric and will lie along the carbon–deuteron bond axis so that the "asymmetry parameter," η, which complicates the description of the variation of the splitting with orientation, is negligibly small.)

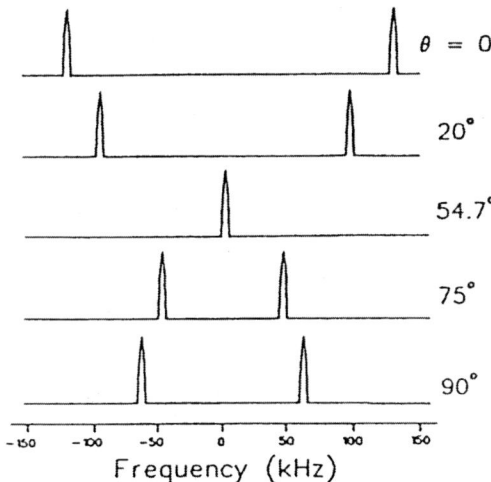

Frequency (kHz)

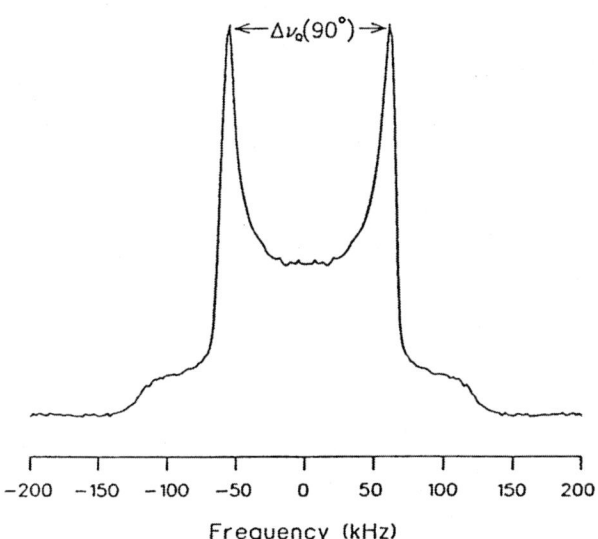

Frequency (kHz)

Figure 2 *Top*: The variation of the doublet splitting as a function of the angle θ between a given C—D bond in a single crystal and the magnetic field. *Bottom*: The "Pake doublet." A powdered crystal will display this characteristic spectrum, which is the superposition of all the component doublets from C—D bonds, which are randomly oriented.

If the single crystal is now pulverized so that all C—D bond orientations are equally probable, the powder will display the well-known "Pake doublet" lineshape (Fig. 2, bottom), which is the sum of all the individual doublet spectra. The separation of the two sharp peaks, for which $\theta = 90°$, characterizes the width of the spectrum: $\Delta v = 3/4(e^2 qQ/h)$. This quantity is known as the quadrupolar splitting. The functional form of the Pake doublet arises from a combination of two factors. First, the relative number of C—D bonds oriented at a given angle with respect to the magnetic field varies as $\sin \theta$. Second, the transformation from angular to frequency terms of the function $3(\cos^2 \theta - 1)/2$ yields $f_1(v) \propto (v_{max} - 2v)^{-1/2}$ for $v_{min} \leq v < v_{max}/2$ and $f_2(v) \propto (v_{max} + 2v)^{-1/2}$ for $v_{min}/2 < v \leq v_{max}$. The observed Pake doublet is the sum of $f_1(v)$ and $f_2(v)$, with the "rough edges" at $\pm v_{max}/2$, where the functions approach infinity, smoothed out by the intrinsic finite line width of the spectral components.

In this section we have attempted to introduce the reader to the salient features of ^{2}H NMR spectroscopy: nuclear spin $I = 1$, doublets whose splittings depend on the quadrupolar interaction at the position of the deuteron, and single crystal vs. powder spectra. We have not as yet addressed the pertinent question: What about molecular motion? How do the rates and classes of molecular motion affect ^{2}H NMR spectra? The second subsection of Section C will discuss some features of ^{2}H NMR that make it a useful technique for probing molecular motions in membranes.

C. Understanding the Physical Properties of Membranes: Information from NMR

Molecular Motions in Membranes

Most biological membranes are complex entities whose foundation is the lipid bilayer, a thin (≈ 5 nm) sheet composed of two layers of amphipathic lipids (e.g., phosphoglycerolipids, sphingolipids, cholesterol) having their hydrophilic "headgroups" facing the aqueous environment on either side of the membrane and their hydrophobic "tails" extending to the bilayer core (to get an idea of some physicists' recent thoughts on lipid membranes, see Bloom, Evans and Mouritsen, 1991). Within this foundation reside membrane proteins, which may serve both structural and functional roles in maintaining cell integrity. Lipid bilayers are usually thought of as liquid crystals: crystalline in that phospho- and sphingolipid molecules only very rarely (times on the order of minutes to hours) flip from one side of the bilayer to the other, but liquid in that within each layer molecules may diffuse freely (lateral diffusion coefficients in the neighborhood of 10^{-12} m^2 sec). In addition, individual lipids within such fluid membranes undergo considerable motion (Gennis, 1989), including axial rotation (in times on the order of a nanosecond) about the lipid long axis, trans-gauche isomerizations (in times on the order of a picosecond) in the hydrocarbon tails, and nodding and shaking of the headgroups (in times on the order of nanoseconds). Further, lipids in fluid bilayers display collective motions—for example, surface undulations having characteristic wavelengths from the size of a few molecules to the cell circumference (microns) are possible (Bloom and Evans, 1991).

Membrane lipids in aqueous environments display a rich selection of phases. Besides the common "fluid bilayer" phase described earlier, other possibilities include "solid," "gel," inverted hexagonal "H_{II}" "cubic," and "micellar" lipid packing. These are not normally of direct interest to those studying biological membranes but, as we will discuss later, may be so in the case of SC intercellular membranes. The solid bilayer phase of a simple membrane (made of dipalmitoylphosphatidylcholine (DPPC), a saturated 16-carbon chained lipid, for example) is one in which the lipid hydrocarbon chains pack in an orthorhombic crystalline array and are fixed in position (Ruocco and Shipley, 1982a,b). This phase, where all lipid chain motion with the exception of methyl group reorientation is suppressed, can be induced by low temperature, low water content, or high pressure. The gel phase is intermediate between solid and fluid bilayers: lateral diffusion is absent, but individual molecules exhibit considerable motion on the microsecond time scale, notably trans-gauche isomerizations and restricted axial wobbles. Chain packing becomes hexagonal, with individual chains no longer locked in place with respect to their neighbors. The remaining three examples of lipid polymorphism, inverted hexagonal (H_{II}), cubic, and micellar, are nonbilayer phases. The H_{II} phase consists of long cylinders of lipid (tails pointing away from the cylinder center) surrounding aqueous cores roughly 5 nm in diameter. These cylinders are packed in hexagonal arrays. Lipid motion in this phase is much like that in fluid bilayers. Cubic phases can take many forms, one example being that the lipid/water cylinders of the H_{II} phase can be interwoven such that the cylinder cross sections form a cubic array. Micelles, usually formed from single-chained lipids, are like small golf balls, hydrocarbon tails forming the interior and headgroups packed around the outside. Being very small, micelles tumble rapidly in aqueous solution due to Brownian motion.

^2H NMR as a Probe of Lipid-Phase States

As we have just described, different membrane phases are distinguished both by their molecular packing arrangements and by the types and rates of molecular motion characteristic of a particular phase. In the introduction to ^{2}H NMR (second subsection of Section I.B) we completely neglected the effects of molecular motion on the shape of the NMR spectrum. ^{2}H NMR is intrinsically a local probe, intramolecular in nature, measuring the quadrupolar interaction at the position of the deuteron for a given C—D bond orientation. If the C—D bond orientation fluctuates, the quadrupolar interaction becomes averaged over the range of the fluctuations. Depending on the rate of a given type of molecular motion as well as its symmetry, such averaging yields a variety of spectral "signatures" that can allow the identification of the phase of the lipid membrane. Often, however, it is necessary to combine the results of techniques such as x-ray scattering and neutron scattering, which are sensitive to long-range (e.g., intermolecular or interlayer) packing to obtain an unambiguous picture of the membrane's molecular organization. It is important to note that such long-range orders must exist for these methods to be successful; this may not always be the case in tissue.

In order to get a feeling for the rates of motion to which ^{2}H NMR spectroscopy is sensitive, it is necessary to introduce the concept of the "NMR time scale" (Bloom and Thewalt, 1995). For a Pake doublet, the NMR time scale may be approximated as simply the inverse of the quadrupolar splitting, so a deuterium-labeled methylene group in a sample of solid hexane, for which $\Delta\nu = 126$ kHz, would have a corresponding time scale of ≈ 1 μsec. As we shall see, ^{2}H NMR splittings are often narrowed due to motion, which increases the relevant time scale accordingly. Lipid molecular motions can be subdivided into three regimes: those slow on the NMR time scale, to which the NMR spectrum is insensitive; those comparable to the characteristic NMR time, which typically cause gross deviations from classic Pake doublet lineshapes; and those fast on the NMR time scale, whereupon only the average quadrupolar splitting is evident in the spectrum.

Figure 3 catalogs five different ^{2}H NMR spectral shapes obtainable from lipid phases. We first discuss the solid phase: in a solid, a lipid deuterated at one or more acyl chain methylene positions will have a ^{2}H NMR spectrum consisting of a single Pake doublet, whose splitting is 126 kHz (see the third subsection of Section I.B). The lipid is essentially motionless on the NMR time scale, and nothing whatsoever can be ascertained about the molecular packing of the lipids in this phase using straightforward ^{2}H NMR spectroscopy. More sophisticated techniques (Bloom et al., 1992), such as T_1 and T_2 relaxation time measurements or two-dimensional NMR, can give some idea of how slow these motions may be, however. For example, a measurement of the rate at which the sample magnetization returns to equilibrium with the external field

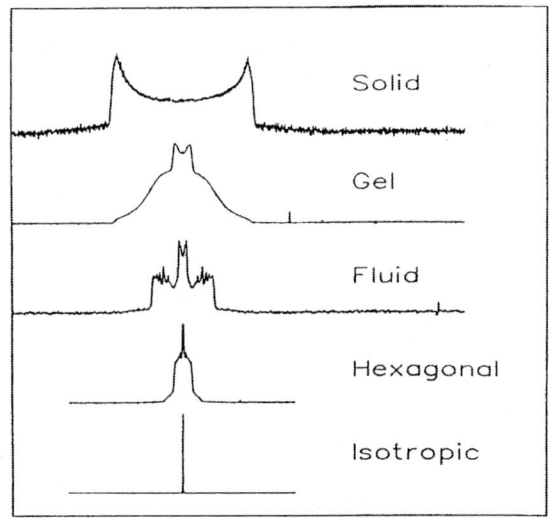

Figure 3 The ^{2}H NMR spectrum of a perdeuterated fatty acid chain in five distinct membrane-phase states.

following an rf pulse, $1/T_{1z}$, can be made in several ways, some of which are insensitive to motions such as lateral diffusion, and one of which is sensitive to diffusion, and thereby measures a relaxation rate $1/T^*_{1z} \geq 1/T_{1z}$. The former techniques, which measure the "true" T_1, include: inversion recovery, where the magnetization is first inverted using a 180° pulse and then measured at a variety of subsequent times—the spectrum starts "upside-down," goes through zero, and at long times is indistinguishable from the equilibrium spectrum; or saturation recovery, where the intensity of the spectrum is measured as a function of the time separating the rf pulses used to tip the magnetization from equilibrium—for regular spectroscopy this time is kept long compared to T_1, but for the saturation recovery technique the times needed are short compared to T_1, which give a low-intensity spectrum due to the fact that the higher-energy nuclear spin states are partially saturated. Relaxation influenced by diffusion, $1/T^*_{1z}$, is measured using a "stimulated echo" technique (Bloom et al., 1992), where the equilibrium magnetization is inverted in two 90° steps, with an intervening time long enough to allow the FID to vanish due to destructive interference of the various precession frequencies in the sample. At a variable time τ_2 later, the magnetization is measured and its decay rate calculated. This decay rate is now a function of normal T_1 relaxation and also has contributions from the loss of signal due to the diffusion during τ_2 of individual molecules into locations having different orientations with respect to the magnetic field. Thus, a ^{2}H NMR T_1 study of "solid" membranes can in fact put limits on the rates of diffusion in the system.

If there is some molecular motion with characteristic times on the order of 10^{-6} sec, the ^{2}H NMR spectrum will no longer have the Pake doublet lineshape discussed earlier. For example, in gel-phase bilayers a perdeuterated lipid acyl chain will have a broad, relatively featureless spectrum, as shown in Fig. 3. These spectra do not lend themselves to easy analysis: The molecular motion in the membrane is not rapid enough to be axially symmetric (see the description of the fluid bilayer below) on the NMR time scale but is fast enough to influence the average value of the quadrupolar interaction and thus the splittings of the individual labels.

The most common physical state of biological membranes is known as the "liquid crystalline" or "fluid" bilayer phase. In these types of membranes, ^{2}H NMR has proven to be especially useful (for reviews see, e.g., Seelig, 1977 or Davis, 1983) in that when performed using chain-deuterated lipids it allows the environment within the bilayers to be examined in considerable detail. Both the degree of chain conformational order and the thickness of the hydrophobic region (given certain assumptions) can be ascertained (Ipsen, Mouritsen and Bloom, 1990). On the NMR time scale, molecular motion in liquid crystalline bilayers is axially symmetric about the lipid long axis, which is on average perpendicular to the plane of the membrane. The effect of this motion on the ^{2}H NMR spectrum is that the quadrupolar splitting of an individual deuteron is no longer dependent on the orientation of the C—D bond with respect to the magnetic field; instead, the splitting varies as a function of the orientation β of the axis of symmetry of the motion with respect to the magnetic field. The functional form of the spectrum is now given by: $\Delta v(\beta) = \Delta v_Q | S_{CD} (3 \cos^2\beta - 1)/2 |$, where the order parameter $S_{CD} = \langle 3 \cos^2_{\beta' - 1} \rangle / 2$ is a measure of the time-averaged orientation (the instantaneous value of which is characterized by β') of a particular C—D bond with respect to the bilayer normal. For liquid crystalline membranes the Pake doublet ^{2}H NMR lineshape (as seen with the pulverized solid crystal) is preserved, but the axially symmetric rotation of the lipids about their long axes causes the maximum obtainable splitting to be only half that observed in the solid phase. The geometry of the labeled acyl chain dictates that the angle β' between the C—D bond and the lipid long axis is 90° in the absence of fluctuations; therefore this maximum splitting occurs for the hypothetical case where the lipids have rigid chains with no conformational kinks, i.e.,

$S_{CD} = -1/2$. In this case the splitting observed for a deuterated acyl chain methylene group is $\Delta v(\beta = 90°) = 3/4(e^2qQ/h)| S_{CD}| = 63$ kHz. (Note that there are some instances where β' is not 90°, due to hydrogen-bonding-induced kinks in the molecule near the aqueous interface, for example, or due to the geometry of the attachment between acyl chain and backbone.) Trans-gauche isomerizations along the lipid acyl chains cause the range of β' values accessed to be broad, an effect that is magnified toward the methyl group at the end of the chain. The result of this conformational disorder is that the magnitude of S_{CD} is reduced from its maximum value of 0.5. Pioneering ^{2}H NMR studies of lipid chain order in membranes (Seelig and Seelig, 1974) labeled individual acyl chain groups and constructed an "order parameter profile" by plotting S_{CD} as a function of carbon number. For a simple membrane dispersion composed of DPPC, a saturated diacylphosphatidylcholine having 16 carbon atoms per chain—for example, the order parameter profile of the *sn*-1 chain—contains a region of approximately 7–9 carbons, depending on temperature, with similar splittings corresponding to $| S_{CD} | \cong 0.2$ and known as the "plateau" region. These carbons are denoted C2–C10, numbered from the chain's ester linkage (C1) with the glycerol backbone. The splittings of C11–C15 progressively decrease, indicating enhanced floppiness toward the chain's end, and the C16 splitting is further narrowed by a factor of 3 due to the extra motional averaging of the methyl rotor. The fluid bilayer spectrum illustrated in Fig. 3 is a superposition of Pake doublets arising from each deuteron in a perdeuterated hydrocarbon chain (in this case palmitic acid).

The spectrum of lipids in the H_{II} phase is also a superposition of Pake doublets. In this phase, however, the individual lipids experience axially symmetric motion on the NMR time scale about two different axes. First, as in the fluid bilayer phase discussed earlier, there is the rapid rotation of the lipid about its long axis. Second, the hexagonally packed cylinders are small enough that lipids can diffuse right around the cylinder in a time short compared to microseconds. The result of these two perpendicular axially symmetric motions is that there is an additional halving of the quadrupolar splitting in the H_{II} phase in comparison with the fluid bilayer splitting (Cullis and de Kruijff, 1979). The Pake doublet arises from the random distribution of cylinder axis orientations with respect to the magnetic field; information as to the precise location of a lipid on a particular cylinder is not obtained. For a given deuterated methylene group, the observed splitting will in fact be less than half that in the fluid bilayer phase (Lafleur et al., 1990). This is due to the enhanced conformational freedom of the chains: They each have a conical space to fill in the H_{II} phase as opposed to a cylindrical space. The order parameter profile constructed from lipid chains in the H_{II} phase typically has a very limited plateau region, which gives the spectrum its characteristic appearance: closely spaced doublets superimposed so that the spectral intensity slopes upward towards the methyl peaks.

An isotropic line implies that the deuterated molecule being studied is experiencing motion on the NMR time scale that completely averages the function characterizing the orientation dependence of the quadrupolar interaction, $(3 \cos^2 \theta - 1)/2$, so the splitting collapses and the spectrum is a single resonance at the Larmor frequency. Examples of lipid phases that yield isotropic ^2H NMR spectra include: micelles, whose tumbling in solution means that the label samples all orientations with respect to the magnetic field; cubic phases, whose geometry means that a diffusing deuterated label will sample all of the tetrahedral lattice coordinates; and melts, where the labels move randomly within oily droplets.

Comparison of NMR with Other Methods

Every biophysical technique is intrinsically biased. It is crucial to understand the biases inherent in each particular measurement in order that the experimental results obtained from a variety of techniques may be compared critically and understood analytically.

One distinguishing characteristic of different types of measurements is the time scale to which they are sensitive (Bloom and Thewalt, 1994). Standard techniques can be classified broadly into those providing essentially an instantaneous "snapshot" of the sample, such as IR spectroscopy, those whose longer inherent time scales allow molecular motion to be reflected in the spectrum, such as NMR or ESR spectroscopy, and those that report the average behavior of the whole sample, such as calorimetry. The snapshot techniques (which include both x-ray and neutron diffraction) give no direct information on molecular motion in membranes (although such information can sometimes be inferred), because the motions are orders of magnitude slower than the technique's time scale, and hence the lipids appear frozen. As already discussed, NMR's time scale is useful in classifying lipid motions in membranes—the same is true for electron spin resonance (ESR) spectroscopy, although the ESR time scale is three orders of magnitude shorter: 10^{-9} sec rather than 10^{-6} sec.

Techniques can also be divided into those that provide local information about the environment of a particular probe and those that provide long-range information on the arrangement of molecules in the sample. Spectroscopy—

whether NMR, ESR, fluorescence, IR, or Raman—usually falls into the former category. Although the probe in all these techniques reports its own view of the membrane, if the time scale of the spectroscopy is long enough that a motion such as axial rotation or lateral diffusion occurs, the probe will report its average environment, which will contain some information on larger-scale membrane properties. In addition, NMR relaxation measurements can be used to probe lipid motions whose characteristic rates vary over many orders of magnitude (Gennis, 1989). X-ray diffraction and neutron scattering techniques allow long-range membrane structure to be determined. For example, small-angle x-ray diffraction gives bilayer repeat spacings in multilamellar systems, while wide-angle x-ray diffraction yields the chain-packing geometry in membranes. These scattering techniques are being refined and now also have the capability to measure lipid motions in certain instances. As well, light-scattering techniques are being developed that can probe membrane dynamics on the submicron distance scale.

Finally, techniques can be categorized on the basis of their sensitivity. NMR is intrinsically rather insensitive, since the population difference between ground state and excited nuclear spins is typically only one part in 10^5. ESR and fluorescent probes are much more sensitive, although the chemical structure of these probes is in general more dissimilar to the lipid membrane components than is an isotopically labeled lipid NMR probe. With the exception of the quenching of fluorescence due to high probe concentrations, spectroscopic techniques have the fundamental quality of being able to "see" all the probes in the sample. This can make them very useful in studying samples containing coexisting phases, since the proportions of the given phases can, under favorable circumstances, be determined. However, no information whatsoever as to the large-scale bilayer or other membrane structure can be unambiguously obtained from these techniques without corroboration from, for example, x-ray or neutron scattering. To be fruitful, however, scattering techniques require that there be enough coherent structure in the sample to give clear diffraction peaks, so if the sample is amorphous or contains microscopic regions of phase coexistence, the information obtained will be incomplete. Note that neutron scattering is intrinsically more sensitive than x-ray for membrane structure determination, since the relative scattering cross sections (i.e., nuclear sizes) of protons and deuterons are very different, so the combination of ^2H NMR and neutron scattering is a very powerful one. X-ray scattering works best with elements of high atomic weight, but with the large photon fluxes available from modern synchrotron sources this is no longer a problem.

II. APPLICATION OF ^{2}H NMR TO MODELS OF SC LIPID

A. Introduction

Model Membrane Experiments

As has been extensively discussed elsewhere (Schurer and Elias, 1991; Wertz, Kremer, and Squier, 1992; Gray et al., 1982), the lipids of the stratum corneum intercellular spaces are unusual in mammalian biology, in that ceramides make up a substantial mole fraction of the total. Furthermore, the final lipid composition of the stratum corneum intercellular membranes is considerably different from that found in the intracellular organelles in which these lipids are first synthesized (Squier et al., 1991b; Grayson et al., 1985; Wertz et al., 1984), and extensive lipid modifications occur during epidermal differentiation.

An obvious hypothesis is that this unusual membrane lipid composition is related directly to membrane function in some way. Within the restricted area of lipid bilayers, lipid composition is known to be an important determinant of physical properties. There are several prominent examples. First, the temperature at which the hydrocarbon chains "melt" when assembled in bilayers (the "gel-to-liquid-crystalline transition temperature," T_c) marks an abrupt change in many of the physical properties of such bilayer systems; for example, water permeability through such bilayers increases by several orders of magnitude above the transition. Second, the presence of cholesterol within bilayers composed of amphipathic lipids has a profound effect on lipid motion, mechanical properties (such as resistance to shear), and permeability to water.

With this background in mind, it can easily be appreciated that the unusual lipid composition of *stratum corneum* intercellular membranes may result in equally unusual physical properties. The most obvious example of this is the nature of the hydrophilic headgroups. A feature of SC intercellular membrane lipid structure is that in comparison with other more conventional mammalian membranes, the headgroups are very small: carboxyl groups in the case of free fatty acids, and hydroxyl groups for ceramides. Furthermore, a low pH (< 6) may render the free fatty acid effective headgroup "size" even smaller due to protonation (Cullis, Hope and Tilcock, 1986). As mentioned earlier, epidermal differentiation is marked by enzyme activity that has the effect of removing the headgroups from precursor lipids (during the formation of the SC intercellular domains), and the effect of this wholesale change on membrane physical properties begs investigation.

Because of the complexity of lipid compositions in these and other membranes, the "model membrane" approach has been adopted in many laboratories. This allows creation of lipid/water systems of defined composition, and the effect of these compositions on selected physical properties can be determined. Several studies have been made of systems modeled on the SC intercellular membranes, and examples from these will be given shortly.

Modeling the Dispersing Media

In model membrane studies, the dispersing aqueous medium also plays an important role in determining the behavior of the entire system, and attention must therefore be paid to the composition of this medium as it is to the composition of the lipid phase. Investigation of "lipid polymorphism" in lipid/water dispersions has found that factors such as pH, ionic strength, and water concentration may all have an effect on the phases manifested (Cullis, Hope and Tilcock, 1986). Consideration of this aspect of the model must therefore not be neglected, although any line of investigation is clearly made more complicated by varying such factors.

Careful control of the aqueous phase may be particularly important in models of SC intercellular membranes. In comparison of biological membranes that exist in the internal milieu, the SC membranes would seem to exist in a more extreme position. Not only are they removed from their blood supply by the distance of an entire epithelium, but they do themselves form a permeability barrier, thus insulating themselves from physiological buffering capacities. Furthermore, these membranes are very close to the body's external surface, a very hostile biological environment that is normally a gas. Evaporation of water from stratum corneum is, of course, a fact, and it seems logical that this would also affect the aqueous interspaces of SC intercellular membranes. Not only is water concentration in these regions likely to be low (relative to "excess water"), but ion concentration may well be relatively high.

To our knowledge, there are no detailed studies of the physical properties of the aqueous regions of SC intercellular spaces, and these indeed would be difficult to carry out. However, there is evidence in the literature that bears on this question. It is well established that the surface pH of skin in humans is less than 6 (Treffel et al., 1994). This suggests that a "neutral" pH is unlikely to occur in SC, and one in the range 5–6 is more probable. Similarly, Elias and co-workers have demonstrated the presence of calcium ions in SC intercellular spaces (Lee et al., 1992); others (Lindberg et al., 1992; Warner et al., 1988) have shown by x-ray microanalysis that there is a relatively high ion concentration within the stratum corneum.

In the absence of more definitive studies on this question, the major point to be made is that the nature of the aqueous compartment of the SC intercellular regions may well play an important role in determining the phase behavior of the lipids that make up the associated intercellular membranes, and this must not be forgotten in model membrane studies.

The "Complete" Phase Diagram

The terms *phase diagram* and *phase behavior* recur in this field, and they deserve some consideration. In physical chemistry, a phase diagram may be constructed for any system that is not homogeneous as applied conditions (such as temperature and composition) are varied. In this context, a *phase* is defined as a particular arrangement of molecules having intermolecular interactions that govern the assembly's physical properties. For a defined system (where the composition of all elements is known), a phase diagram will describe the reproducible behavior of this system under defined conditions. A commonly studied example of a phase diagram is that of water, where as temperature and pressure are varied, ice, liquid water, and water vapor are all observed.

The determination of phase diagrams has a long history in the study of lipid/water systems, most noticeably in the study of soaps and related classes of lipids, but also in the area of lipid bilayers. As discussed in the first subsection of Section I.C, lipid bilayers may have a number of phases (liquid crystalline, gel, solid, etc.) and phase diagrams have been constructed for some lipid mixtures (e.g., for phosphatidylcholine/cholesterol membranes in excess water: Vist and Davis, 1990; Thewalt and Bloom, 1992). Several points should be made. First, the greater the number of components in the system, the more complex is the phase diagram, and it is intuitively obvious that a complex mixture of lipids (e.g., ceramide, cholesterol, free fatty acids), together with a complex dispersing medium (e.g., water concentration, ionic strength, pH), will result in an extremely complex phase diagram. Second, even the phase diagrams of "simple" lipid mixtures (e.g., DPPC, cholesterol, and water) prove to be quite complex, and they have been under continuing investigation for many years. The prospect of constructing such a diagram for the complex mixture known to exist in the SC intercellular spaces is daunting and would require considerable resources in time, money, and skilled manpower. For these reasons, we believe that the construction of a "complete" phase diagram for SC lipids is an unralistic objective for the moment and that efforts would be better directed to discerning the important features of the phase behavior of these unusual mixtures and to relating these to other physical properties (such as water permeability) as early as possible.

B. Epidermal Ceramide Models

Mammalian stratum corneum (SC) consists of highly cornified cells embedded in a matrix of lipid bilayers (Matoltsy, 1976). These extracellular lipids are arranged in the form of multiple lamellae that are believed to constitute the major barrier to percutaneous penetration (Michaels et al., 1975; Elias, 1983). As discussed, the SC lipid membranes are made up predominantly of ceramides, cholesterol, free fatty acids, cholesteryl sulfate, and small amounts of some less well-defined nonpolar components (Gray et al., 1982; Yardley and Summerly, 1981). Six groups of ceramides have been characterized in porcine SC, as shown in Fig. 4 (Wertz et al., 1983). This classification was based on the polarity of the ceramides, with ceramide 1 being the least polar.

An understanding of the phase behavior of the SC lipids and of the structure/function relationship of these heterogeneous class of lipids is crucial to the understanding of the epidermal barrier function on a molecular level. But there has been relatively little work in this area, presumably because: (a) the detailed lipid composition of SC was not known even as recently as 10 years ago; (b) the methods used to isolate these nonphospholipids from

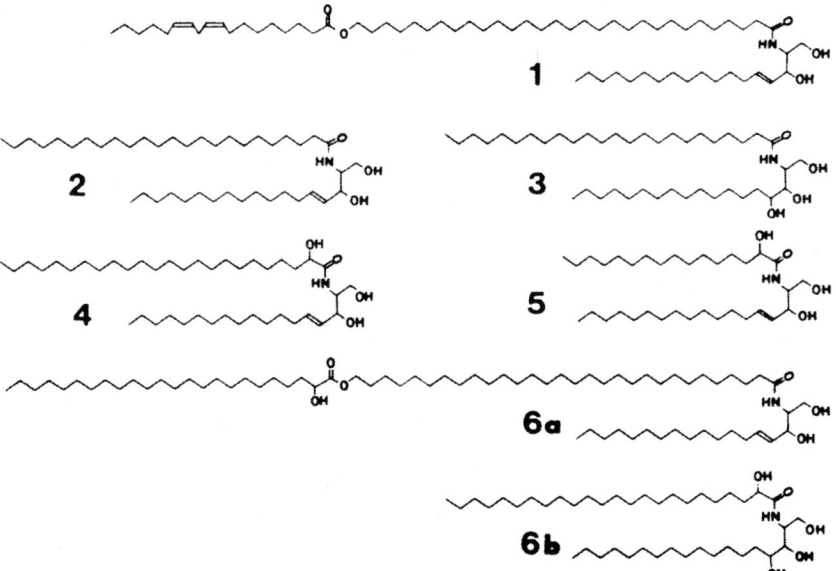

Figure 4 Representative structures of the six groups of ceramides found in mammalian stratum corneum. (Courtesy of Dr. D. T. Downing, University of Iowa.)

epidermis are laborious; and (c) there is a lack of awareness of the problem among membrane scientists. However, with the realization of transdermal drug delivery as an important controlled delivery method, there is increased interest in the epidermal barrier function, and various methods have been used to study SC membrane structure in tissue and tissue preparations (Golden et al., 1987; Knutson et al., 1985; Rehfeld et al., 1988; White et al., 1988; Madison et al., 1987). However, as previously discussed, the use of model systems with isolated lipid mixtures offers the advantage of known composition and enables one to alter the composition to study the effects of different components. While the model system containing SC ceramides resembles SC in its lipid composition, the phase behavior reported in such investigations can only be taken as an approximation of the phase behavior of lipids in native SC. Furthermore, the SC is made of corneocytes that are embedded in a matrix of extracellular lipid lamellae (Matolsty, 1976). The corneocyte cell envelope consists of a monolayer of lipids that has been suggested to serve as a template in the assembly of the multilamellar structures in SC (Swartzendruber et al., 1987; Abraham and Downing, 1990). The effect of the corneocyte lipid envelope on these lipid bilayers was not considered in these in vitro studies. However, due to the difficulty in incorporating deuterated lipids into native SC and due to the low sensitivity of the NMR technique, the model systems offer a good first approximation to the SC tissue. As part of an effort to understand the structure–function relationship of the SC lipids, such an investigation of the SC lipids using solid-state ^{2}H NMR spectroscopy (Abraham and Downing, 1991, 1992) has been undertaken. In these studies, model systems made up of SC ceramides, cholesterol, cholesteryl sulfate, and palmitic acid deuterated at specific positions were used.

The lipid composition of the model systems used in ^{2}H NMR investigations is shown in Table 1. Mixture 1, containing 38 mole % each of ceramides, and cholesterol and 19% palmitic acid, and 5% cholesteryl sulfate, was taken as a close approximation to the in situ lipid composition of SC. Figure 5 shows the ^{2}H NMR spectra of α-deuterated palmitic acid in the ceramide—and in the DPPC-containing mixtures from Table 1. Because there is only one source of deuterium in these samples, the spectral assignment is fairly straightforward. The spectra at 25°C showed symmetric powder patterns for all the mixtures except mixture 3, suggesting that the lipids in these mixtures were in a bilayer configuration. Ceramide or DPPC-containing mixtures with the largest amount of cholesterol (1 and 4) were more fluid than other mixtures, as seen from the smaller Δv_q and S_{CD} values in Table 2. The rigid ring structure of cholesterol interferes with the close packing of the acyl chains in the gel phase and hence with the mobility of the chains. It should be noted that the S_{CD} for the α-CD$_2$

Table 1 Lipid Composition of Model Systems Used in ^{2}H NMR Investigations

		Mole percent of*:			
Mixture	Ceramides	Cholesterol	Palmitic acid	Cholesteryl sulfate	DPPC
1	38	38	19	5	—
2	57	19	19	5	—
3	76	—	19	5	—
4	—	38	19	5	38
5	—	19	19	5	57
6	—	—	19	5	76

*The final mixtures were 50% by weight of lipid water. α-CD$_2$ PA and ω-CD$_3$ PA were used in separate experiments.

palmitic acid in mixtures 1–6 is in the range 0.27–0.32. This value is in excellent agreement with the $S_{CD} = 0.25$ observed at 50°C for the C-2 position of perdeuterated palmitic acid in equimolar mixtures of bovine brain ceramide, cholesterol, and palmitic acid (Fenske et al., 1994). Based on our observed S_{CD}, our results suggest that the SC lipid mixtures exhibit considerable fluidity near the headgroup regions, even at 25°C, and are not in the rigid crystalline state. A rigid crystalline state would give rise to an order parameter of 1, such as that seen for hydrated palmitic acid, as shown in Table 2. There was gradual loss of symmetry as the amount of cholesterol in these mixtures was decreased and the amount of ceramides or DPPC was increased concomitantly. This was more pronounced in the ceramide-containing mixtures; e.g., the spectrum from mixture 3 was highly anisotropic. This was interpreted in terms of nonaxially symmetric averaging of the quadrupole splittings corresponding to the different orientations of the C—D bond in these bilayers, presumably resulting from an extended network of lateral hydrogen-bonding between the palmitic acid and the ceramide headgroup. This is consistent with the observations made by Pascher (1976) in monolayer studies using ceramides. Such H-bonding could be an important factor modulating the barrier property of the bilayers in the SC.

As the temperature was raised from 25°C to 80°C, there was a gradual decrease in the Δv_q until 70°C in the spectrum from mixture 1. At 70°C, there is a second pair of quadrupolar peaks with reduced Δv_q. The appearance of the inner quadrupolar peaks suggested the formation of a new phase. This new phase is more mobile than the lamellar phase, most probably a hexagonal (H_{II}) phase. The quadrupolar peaks with reduced Δv_q appeared at 60°C in mixtures

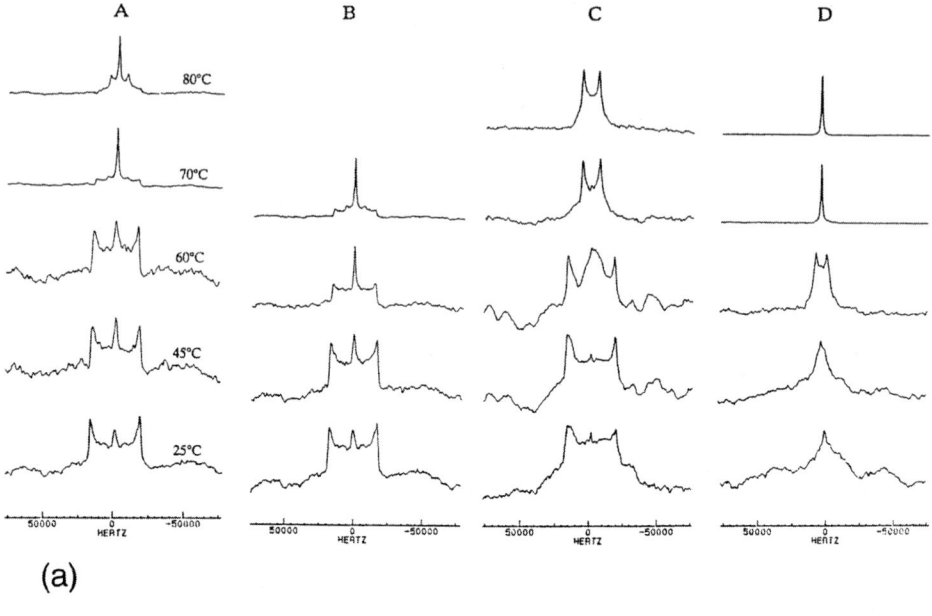

(a)

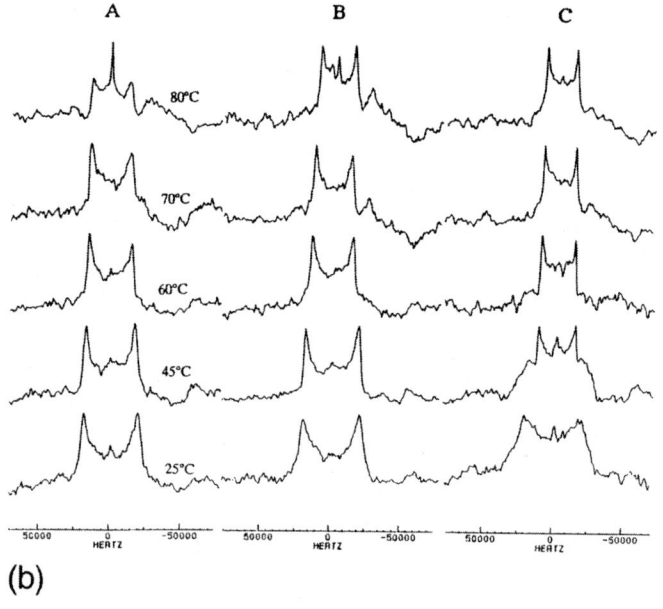

(b)

Figure 5 (a) ^{2}H NMR spectra of α-CD$_2$ palmitic acid intercalated in bilayers made from the ceramide-containing mixtures shown in Table 1. A: Mixture 1. The spectra

Table 2 Deuterium quadrupolar splitting (Δv_q) for the α-CD_2 palmitic acid in the different lipid mixtures

Mixture	Quadrupolar splitting, Δv_q (kHz)	Order parameter, S_{CD}
1	35.2	0.276
2	35.7	0.280
3	—	—
4	38.6	0.303
5	40.5	0.318
6	41.0	0.322
Palmitic acid	116.7	0.915

2 and 3. Freeze-fracture electron microscopic investigation of these mixtures at temperatures above 70°C confirmed the more mobile phase to be the H_{II} phase (Abraham and Downing, 1991). In the control samples containing DPPC instead of the SC ceramides, the lipids remained in the bilayer configuration throughout the temperature range 25°C–80°C.

The results from the lipid mixtures containing the ω-CD_3 palmitic acid also indicated that the ceramide-containing mixtures formed the H_{II} phase at temperatures above 70°C, while the DPPC-containing control samples remained in the bilayer configuration at all temperatures. Figure 6 shows the ^2H NMR spectra from the ω-CD_2 palmitic acid in the ceramide-containing mixtures. The results from the mixtures containing ω-CD_3 palmitic acid provide some insight into the fluidity of the hydrocarbon interior of these bilayers. The Δv_q in mixture 1, which approximates the in situ SC lipid composition, is slightly lower than the corresponding DPPC-containing mixture (mixture 4), indicating that the SC lipids have considerable fluidity in the hydrocarbon region, even at 25°C. Also, the Δv_q for mixtures 1 and 4 was lower than that for other mixtures containing less or no cholesterol. However, as the temper-

---

were obtained after heating the sample to the desired temperature. B: Spectra from mixture 1, obtained after cooling the sample to the given temperature. C: Mixture 2. D: Mixture 3. (Reproduced from Abraham and Downing, 1991). (b) ^2H NMR spectra of α-CD_2 palmitic acid intercalated in bilayers made from the DPPC-containing mixtures shown in Table 1. The Δv_q decreased gradually from 38–41 kHz to 20 kHz as the temperature was increased from 25°C to 80°C, and there was no indication of a hexagonal phase with a smaller Δv_q. A: Mixture 4. B: Mixture 5. C: Mixture 6. (Reproduced from Abraham and Downing, 1991).

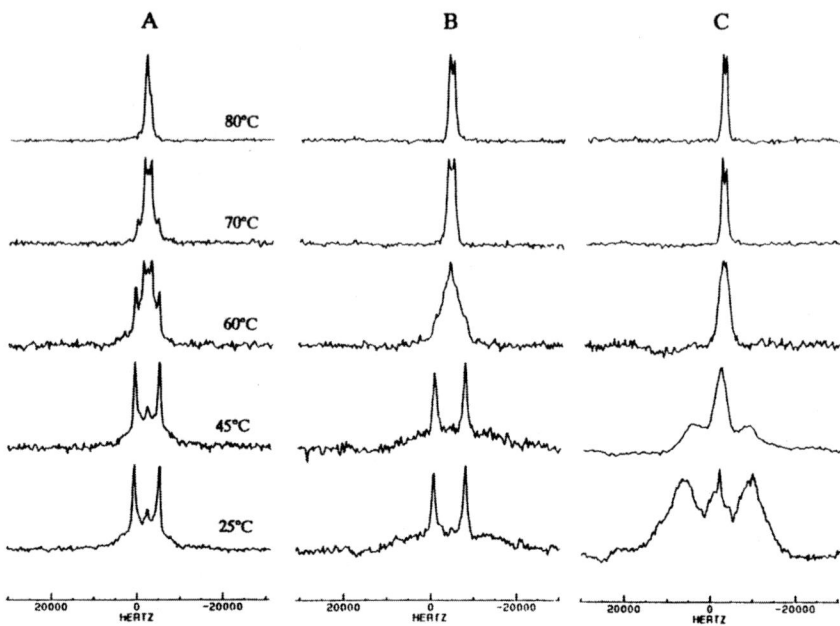

Figure 6 ^{2}H NMR spectra of ω-CD$_3$ palmitic acid intercalated in bilayers made from the ceramide-containing mixtures shown in Table 1. The inner pair of quadrupolar peaks with Δv_q of 0.9–1.7 kHz correspond to the hexagonal phase. A: Mixture 1. B: Mixture 2. C: Mixture 3.

ature was increased, the order parameter of the bilayers declined with decreasing amount of cholesterol. This is illustrated in Fig. 7, where the values cross over, as the amount of cholesterol was lowered, as a function of temperature. This is in accordance with the dual ability of cholesterol to disorder the rigid bilayers and to condense, or order, the fluid bilayers (Stockton and Smith, 1976). The formation of the hexagonal phase by the SC ceramide-containing mixtures suggests that the SC lipid mixture could, under proper impetus, form nonbilayer structures.

Recognition of polymorphism in SC lipids is significant to understanding the membrane function in SC. The SC lipids originate from the lamellar granules formed in the viable layers of epidermis. During the final stages of epidermal differentiation, these granules discharge their lipid contents in the form of membranous disks, which then rearrange to form the extracellular lipid sheets (Lavkar, 1976). This reassembly has been suggested to involve a membrane fusion process wherein the membranous disks fuse edge to edge (Landmann, 1986). Although this has not been conclusively shown, such membrane fusion processes would logically involve the formation of transient nonlamellar structures by the lipids at the site of fusion. Hexagonal structure formation also involves the formation of nonbilayer structures such as inverted micelles. Thus the observation that the SC lipids could form hexagonal structures supports a possible pathway for membrane assembly via the formation of transient nonbilayer structures, during the final stages of epidermal differentiation. Physiological conditions, such as decreased headgroup size and ionization, that result from the changes in the lipid composition, along with decreased water content during the final stages of differentiation, are some of the factors that could promote the formation of transient nonlamellar structures.

The extraordinarily effective barrier property of the SC has been attributed to the highly ordered arrangement of the intercellular lipids in bilayer configuration. This poses a serious challenge to the delivery of drugs through skin at therapeutic levels. Molecules such as Azone, ethanol, and oleic acid are being used to fluidize the SC lipid bilayers with the aim of enhancing the penetration of drug molecules through SC. If the SC lipid mixtures could be induced to form hexagonal or other nonbilayer structures by the addition of molecules of suitable geometry, or by the use of any external stimulus, one could enhance the percutaneous penetration of drugs severalfold.

C. Bovine Brain Ceramide Models

Bovine brain ceramides are prepared commercially from sphingomyelin derived from the same source. The obvious disadvantage is that these are not derived from epidermis, and their specific composition of sphingosine bases and associated acyl chains differs from epidermal ceramides. In particular, the unusual "Type I" epidermal ceramide is not present (see Section II.B), and bovine brain mixtures appear in general to be less complex. The immediate advantage of using bovine brain ceramides is that they are readily available in sufficient quantities to perform broad-line NMR experiments (e.g., Blume et al., 1993), and they can be compared with the sphingomyelin from which they are derived. The relation between model membrane experiments using bovine brain ceramide and lipid-phase behavior in mammalian SC in vivo is unknown, and the interpretation of such model membrane experiments must obviously be placed in the context of available information derived from tissue.

We have selected several results that we believe are pertinent to the

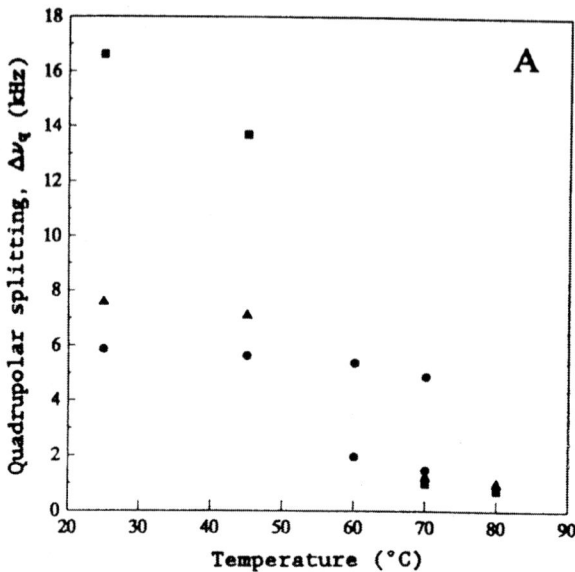

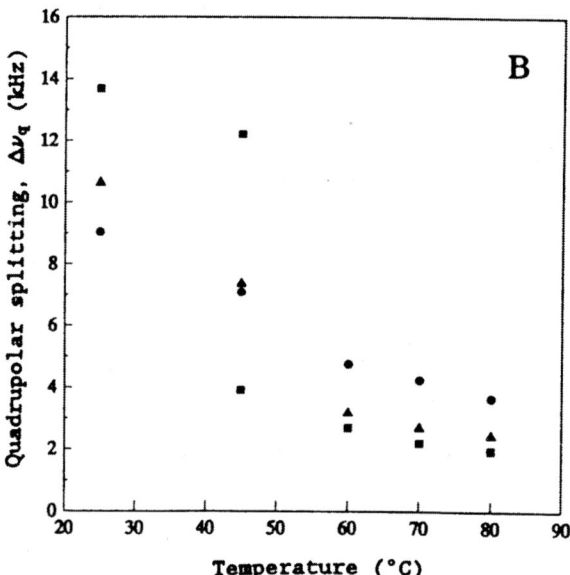

Figure 7 Quadrupolar splitting ($\Delta\nu_q$) of ω-CD_2 palmitic acid in bilayers as a function of temperature. (A) Ceramide-containing mixtures, mixture 1 (circles), mixture 2

problem at hand. In Fig. 8 are temperature-dependent spectra derived from an equimolar mixture of bovine brain sphingomyelin, cholesterol, and per-deuterated palmitic acid (PA-d$_{31}$) dispersed in buffer at pH 5.2. Over this temperature range, the spectrum is typical of that found for liquid crystalline lipid bilayers containing a lot of cholesterol, and it exhibits a maximum order parameter of $S_{CD} \approx 0.4$. With increasing temperature the spectrum narrows very slightly and the individual peaks sharpen—this is also found for spectra derived from conventional phospholipid/cholesterol bilayers (Vist and Davis, 1990; Thewalt and Bloom, 1992). However, when bovine brain ceramide is substituted for sphingomyelin (Fig. 9), the spectra vary considerably with temperature. Furthermore, at all temperatures the spectra show evidence for *coexisting* lipid environments. Even at 75°C, where the spectrum consists mainly of an isotropic line, there is still a small amount ($\approx 6\%$) of the fluid bilayer spectrum present. This is discussed in detail elsewhere (Kitson et al., 1994), but an interesting finding is that at temperatures below about 42°C, there is a significant "solid" lipid environment in which the lipid motion is more restricted than found in a conventional gel-phase bilayer. The potential significance of this for passive diffusion of various solutes across the epidermal permeability barrier is that if similar immobilized lipid domains were to exist in SC extracellular membranes, they would severely limit such diffusion.

In Fig. 10 the change in phase behavior of these ceramide models can be appreciated as a function of temperature and pH. The first moment of the distribution ("M_1") is shown on the y-axis and corresponds to the relative amounts of deuterated lipid probe (in this case PA-d$_{31}$) present in the various coexisting lipid phases. Thus at pH 5.2 and 6.2 we observe a plateau of M_1 values at temperatures less than about 42°C that corresponds to a spectrum having about 80% of the palmitic acid reporter present as a "solid." In analogous experiments using proton NMR (not shown), we have found that much of the ceramide present must also exist in such an immobilized phase (Thewalt et al., 1992), and more recently the use of deuterated cholesterol

---

(triangles), mixture 3 (squares). (B) DPPC-containing mixtures, mixture 4 (circles), mixture 5 (triangles), mixture 6 (squares). In both the ceramide- and the DPPC-containing mixtures, the high-cholesterol-containing mixtures (1 and 4) have smaller Δv_q at 25°C (gel phase) and larger Δv_q at 80°C (liquid crystalline phase) than the other mixtures. The crossover of the Δv_q values occurs around the transition temperature for these mixtures (60–70°C for the ceramide-containing mixtures and ≈ 45°C for the DPPC-containing mixtures).

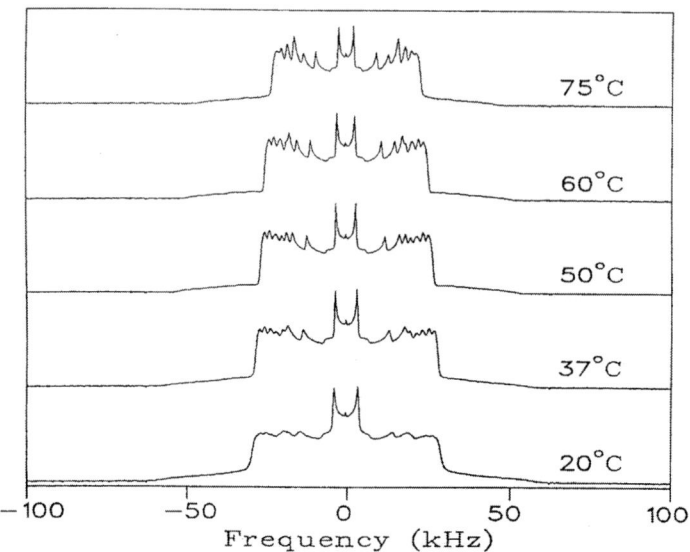

Figure 8 The temperature dependence of the ^{2}H NMR spectrum of an equimolar mixture of sphingomyelin, cholesterol, and PA-d$_{31}$ dispersed at pH 5.2. ^{2}H NMR spectra were acquired at 46 MHz using the quadrupolar echo technique with a pulse spacing of 40 vsec and a 90° pulse length of 40 vsec. Repetition time = 0.3 sec.

(Fig. 11) has shown that this species is similarly solid in the same temperature range (Fenske et al., 1994). Thus we have reason to believe that the entire lipid dispersion is involved in the formation of this very immobilized phase.

III. SUMMARY AND FUTURE PROSPECTS

In the model membrane studies discussed here, results from experiments using bovine brain ceramides differed from those using epidermal ceramides in the presence of a "solid phase" in the former, i.e. a lipid organization in which molecular motion is less than in a gel, and similar to that observed in an anhydrous powder. Model membranes composed of epidermal ceramides are clearly an advantage in studying the behavior of SC intercellular membranes, and appropriate NMR studies to detect such a phase will resolve this issue. One possible explanation is found by considering the kinetics of the formation of the solid phase: In the bovine brain ceramide mixtures it was very slow to form, on the order of days to weeks, and was even more sluggish at pH 7.4

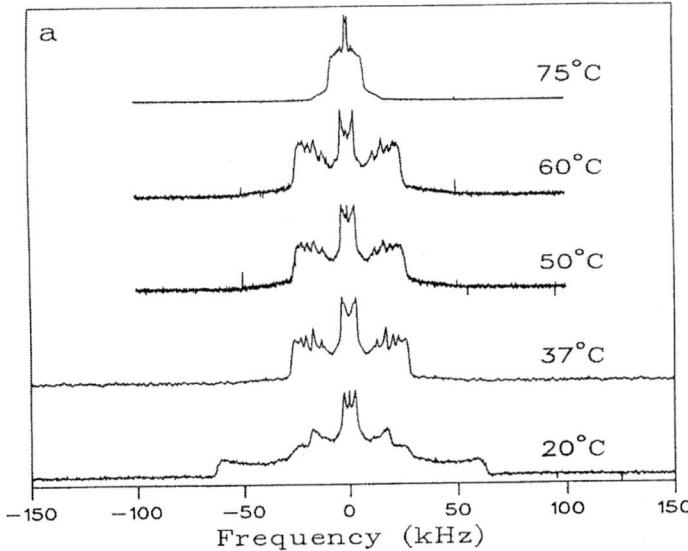

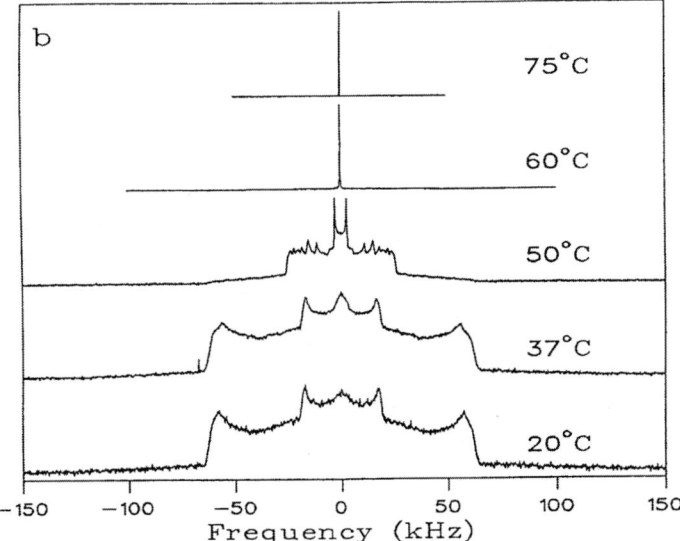

Figure 9 The temperature dependencies of ^{2}H NMR spectra of equimolar dispersions of bovine brain ceramide, cholesterol, and PA-d$_{31}$ at (a) pH 7.4 and (b) pH 5.2. Repetition time = 50 sec at temperatures $\leq 50°$C, 1 sec at 60 and 75°C.

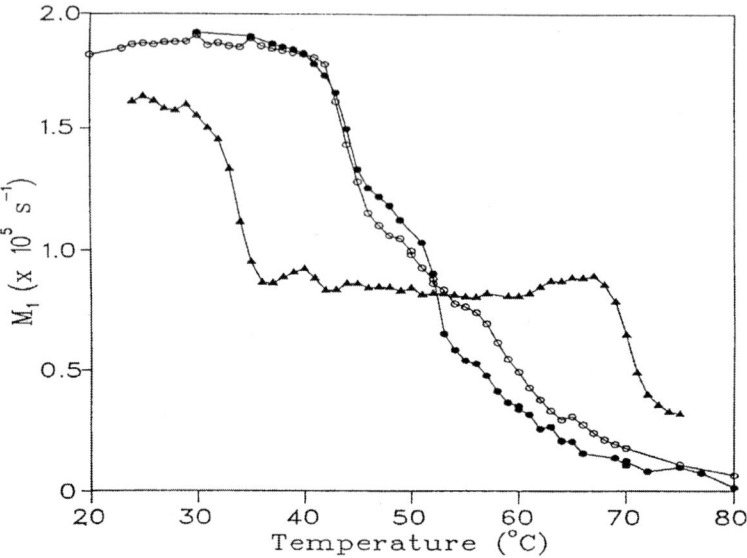

Figure 10 The average width of the ^{2}H NMR spectrum (M_1) as a function of temperature and pH. Closed circles: pH 5.2; open circles: pH 6.2; closed triangles: pH 7.4. Repetition time: 50 sec at all temperatures where the sample contained some solid component, then 1 sec at higher temperatures. (In practice, the quadrupolar echo intensity was checked every few degrees at the 1-sec repetition time toward the completion of the solid-to-fluid transition, and when the echo intensity differed by ≤ 1% between the short and long repetition times, a 1-sec repetition time was used for all higher temperatures.)

than at the lower pH values. ^{2}H NMR measurements made prior to the completion of equilibration showed far less solid signal; indeed, the spectrum looked very similar to the ordered liquid crystalline bilayer spectrum observed at higher temperatures. We can speculate that this solid phase is a tightly packed network of lipids where inter- and intralipid hydrogen bonds (Boggs, 1987) have squeezed out much of the water. Such tight packing has been observed in some phospholipids, e.g., dilauroylphosphatidylethanolamine (Seddon et al., 1983), and slow kinetics are characteristic of the formation of such a phase. For in vivo SC intercellular membranes, the gradual appearance of a solid phase might be crucial in that the lamellae would have enough time to form at the base of the SC while they are still in a mobile state. The significance of such a solid phase is that it is likely to present an obstacle to diffusion in any membrane. This has been shown to be the case in model

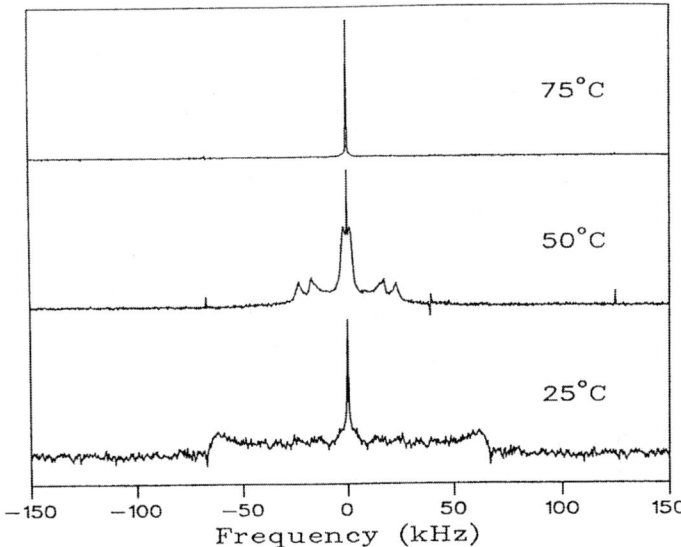

Figure 11 The temperature dependence of ^{2}H NMR spectra of an equimolar dispersion of bovine brain ceramide, cholesterol-d$_5$, and PA at pH 5.2.

membranes when diffusion is both lateral (i.e., within the plane of the bilayer) (Saxton, 1989) or across the bilayer (Haines, 1994). An interesting corollary speculation is that the much decreased epidermal turnover time found in psoriasis would work against the development of such a solid phase, even if lamellar body formation and extrusion were normal. If the solid phase is significant in determining epidermal permeability, one would predict a corresponding increase in permeability in the lesions of psoriasis.

Another issue of considerable interest is the effect of pH on the phase behavior of models containing epidermal ceramides, since such a strong effect was noted on the bovine brain ceramide models. The studies are in agreement in demonstrating the presence of the inverted hexagonal (H$_{II}$) phase at higher temperatures (e.g., > 60°C), although in work with bovine brain ceramide this occurred only at pH > 7. In our view, the practical significance of such studies is not necessarily related only to the normal physiology of the stratum corneum, but also to possible therapeutic applications. The complex phase behavior of these lipid mixtures in vitro suggests that these or other phase transitions might be produced by therapeutic intervention, with important changes in epidermal permeability as the result. Thus, the application of technology to "promote" the H_{II} phase, or to reduce the extent of a "solid" phase, might have significant impact on the transdermal flux of applied compounds.

A major limitation of ^2H NMR (in comparison to other physical techniques) in these studies is achieving the appropriate signal-to-noise ratios, since tens of milligrams of epidermal ceramides are required for individual experiments. However, we believe that the systematic investigation of such models should yield considerable insight into the physical basis of the permeability barrier and, as a practical benefit, contribute to the construction of models predicting epidermal permeability. As reviewed here, an important *advantage* of broad-line ^2H NMR is that components in complex mixtures can be studied separately, and these results are therefore complementary to those achieved using scattering methods, such as x-ray diffraction, and other spectroscopic techniques, such as FTIR and ESR.

Once such systems are better understood, ^2H NMR may be useful in experimental perturbation of the model. For example, the addition of deuterated "penetration enhancers" would allow study of the various environments experienced by such molecules; and for the same system, phase behavior can be monitored by similar or other means (e.g., x-ray diffraction, FTIR, DSC). As illustrated by the studies in this volume, a combination of physical methods is likely to lead to a rigorous understanding of the basis of the epidermal permeability barrier and thus to rational therapeutic intervention.

ACKNOWLEDGMENTS

^2H NMR investigations of SC lipids were performed at the High-Field NMR facility at the University of Iowa and were supported in part by a grant from the United States Public Health Service (AR 32374). Other studies were supported by the Natural Sciences and Engineering Research Council of Canada, the Canadian Dermatology Foundation, and the British Columbia Health Research Foundation. J. T. acknowledges lively discussions with Prof. M. Zuckermann.

REFERENCES

Abragam, A. (1961). *The Principles of Nuclear Magnetism.* Oxford University Press, London and New York.
Abraham, W. and Downing, D. T. (1990). Interaction between corneocytes and stratum corneum lipid liposomes in vitro. *Biochim. Biophys. Acta 1021*:119.

Abraham, W. and Downing, D. T. (1991). Deuterium NMR investigation of polymorphism in stratum corneum lipids. *Biochim. Biophys. Acta 1068*:189.

Abraham, W. and Downing, D. T. (1992). Lamellar structures formed by stratum corneum lipids in vitro: A deuterium NMR study. *Pharm. Res. 9*:1415.

Bloom, M. and Evans, E. (1991). Observation of surface undulations on the mesoscopic length scale by NMR. In: L. Peliti, ed. *Biologically Inspired Physics*. Plenum Press, New York, p. 137.

Bloom, M. and Thewalt, J. (1994). Spectroscopic determination of lipid dynamics in membranes. *Chem. Phys. Lipids 73*:27.

Bloom, M. and Thewalt, J. L. (1995). Time and distance scales of membrane domain organization. *Molecular Membrane Biology 12*:9.

Bloom, M., Evans, E. and Mouritsen, O. G. (1991). Physical properties of the fluid lipid-bilayer component of cell membranes: A perspective. *Quart. Rev. Biophys. 24*:293.

Bloom, M., Morrison, C., Sternin, E. and Thewalt, J. (1992). Spin echoes and the dynamic properties of membranes. In: D. M. S. Bagguley, ed. *Pulsed Magnetic Resonance: NMR, ESR, and Optics*. Oxford University Press, London, p. 274.

Blume, A., Jansen, M., Ghyczy, M. and Gareiss, J. (1993). Interaction of phospholipid liposomes with lipid model mixtures for stratum corneum lipids. *Int. J. Pharm. 99*:219.

Boggs, J. (1987). Lipid intermolecular hydrogen bonding: Influence on structural organization and membrane function. *Biochim. Biophys. Acta 906*:353.

Burnett, L. J. and Müller, B. H. (1971). Deuteron quadrupole coupling constants in three solid deuterated paraffin hydrocarbons: C_2D_6, C_4D_{10}, C_6D_{14}. *J. Chem. Phys. 55*:5829.

Cohen, M. H. and Reif, F. (1957). Quadrupole effects in nuclear magnetic resonance studies of solids. In: F. Seitz and D. Turnbull, eds. *Solid State Physics*. Academic Press, New York, p. 321.

Cullis, P. R. and de Kruijff, B. (1979). Lipid polymorphism and the functional roles of lipids in biological membranes. *Biochim Biophys. Acta 559*:399.

Cullis, P. R., Hope, M. J. and Tilcock, C. P. (1986). Lipid polymorphism and the roles of lipids in membranes. *Chem. Phys. Lipids 40*:127.

Davis, J. H. (1983). The description of membrane lipid conformation, order and dynamics by ^2H NMR. *Biochim. Biophys. Acta 737*:117.

Downing, D. T., Stewart, M. E., Wertz, P. W., Colton, S. W., Abraham, W. and Strauss, J. S. (1987). Skin lipids: An update. *J. Invest. Dermatol. 88*:2s.

Elias, P. M. (1983). Epidermal lipids, barrier function, and desquamation. *J. Invest. Dermatol. 80*(suppl):44s.

Elias, P. M. and Menon, G. K. (1991). Structural and lipid biochemical correlates of the epidermal permeability barrier. *Adv. Lipid Res. 24*:1.

Ernst, R. R. and Anderson, W. A. (1966). Applications of Fourier transform spectroscopy to magnetic resonance. *Rev. Sci. Instrum. 37*:93.

Farrar, T. C. and Becker, E. D. (1971). *Pulse and Fourier Transform NMR*. Academic Press, New York and London.

Fenske, D. B., Thewalt, J. L., Bloom, M. and Kitson, N. (1994). Models of *stratum corneum* intercellular membranes: ^{2}H NMR of macroscopically oriented multilayers. *Biophys. J. 67*:1562.

Gennis, R. B. (1989). *Biomembranes*. Springer-Verlag, New York.

Golden, G. M., Guzek, D. B., Kennedy, A. H., McKie, J. E. and Potts, R. O. (1987). Stratum corneum lipid phase transition and water barrier properties. *Biochemistry 26*:2382.

Gray, G. M. and White, R. J. (1978). Glycosphingolipids and ceramides in human and pig epidermis. *J. Invest. Dermatol. 70*:336.

Gray, G. M. and Yardley, H. J. (1975a). Lipid compositions of cells isolated from pig, human, and rat epidermis. *J. Lipid Res. 16*:434.

Gray, G. M. and Yardley, H. J. (1975b). Different populations of pig epidermal cells: Isolation and lipid composition. *J. Lipid Res. 16*:441.

Gray, G. M., White, R. J., William, R. H. and Yardley, H. J. (1982). Lipid composition of the superficial stratum corneum cells of the pig epidermis. *Br. J. Dermatol 106*:59.

Grayson, S., Johnson-Winegar, A. G., Wintroub, B. U., Isseroff, R. R., Epstein, E. H., Jr. and Elias, P. M. (1985). Lamellar body-enriched fractions from neonatal mice: Preparative techniques and partial characterization. *J. Invest. Dermatol. 85*:289.

Haines, T. H. (1994). Water transport across biological membranes. *FEBS Lett. 346*:115.

Ipsen, J. H., Mouritsen, O. G. and Bloom, M. (1990). Relationships between lipid membrane area, hydrophobic thickness and acyl-chain orientational order. The effects of cholesterol. *Biophys. J. 57*:405.

Kitson, N., Thewalt, J., Lafleur, M. and Bloom, M. (1994). A model membrane approach to the epidermal permeability barrier. *Biochemistry 33*:6707.

Knutson, K., Potts, R. O., Guzek, D. B., Golden, G. M., McKie, J. E., Lambert, W. J. and Higuchi, W. I. (1985). Macro- and molecular-physical considerations in understanding drug transport in the stratum corneum. *J. Controlled Release 2*:67.

Lafleur, M., Cullis, P. R., Fine, B. and Bloom, M. (1990). Comparison of the orientational order of lipid acyl chains in the L_α and the H_{II} phases. *Biochemistry 29*:8325.

Lampe, M. A., Burlingame, A. L., Whitney, J., Williams, M. L., Brown, B. E., Roitman, E. and Elias, P. M. (1983a). Human stratum corneum lipids: Characterization and regional variations. *J. Lipid Res. 24*:120.

Lampe, M. A., Williams, M. L. and Elias, P. M. (1983b). Human epidermal lipids: Characterization and modulations during differentiation. *J. Lipid Res. 24*:131.

Landmann, L. (1986). Epidermal permeability barrier: Transformation of lamellar granule-disks into intercellular sheets by a membrane-fusion process, a freeze-fracture study. *J. Invest. Dermatol. 87*:202.

Lavkar, R. M. (1976). Membrane coating granules: The fate of the discharged lamellae. *J. Ultrastruct. Res. 55*:79.

Lee, S. H., Elias, P. M., Proksch, E., Menon, G. K., Mao-Quiang, M. and Feingold, K. R. (1992). Calcium and potassium are important regulators of barrier homeostasis in murine epidermis. *J. Clin. Invest.* *89*:530.

Lindberg, M., Forslind, B., Sagström, S. and Roomans, G. M. (1982). Elemental changes in guinea pig epidermis at repeated exposure to sodium lauryl sulfate. *Acta Derm. Venereol.* *72*:428.

Madison, K. C., Swartzendruber, D. C., Wertz, P. W. and Downing, D. T. (1987). Presence of intact intercellular lipid lamellae in the upper layers of stratum corneum. *J. Invest. Dermatol.* *88*:714.

Matoltsy, A. G. (1976). Keratinization. *J. Invest. Dermatol.* *67*:20.

Michaels, A. S., Chandrasekaran, S. K. and Shaw, J. E. (1975). Drug permeation through human skin. Theory and in vitro experimental measurement. *Am. Inst. Chem. Eng. J.* *21*:985.

Pascher, I. (1976). Molecular arrangements in sphingolipids. Conformation and hydrogen bonding of ceramides and their implication on membrane stability and permeability. *Biochim. Biophys. Acta* *455*:433.

Potts, R. O. and Guy, R. H. (1992). Predicting skin permeability. *Pharm. Res.* *9*:663.

Rehfeld, S. J., Plachy, W. Z., Williams, M. L. and Elias, P. M. (1988). Calorimetric and electron spin resonance examination of lipid phase transitions in human stratum corneum: Molecular basis for normal cohesion and abnormal desquamation in recessive X-linked ichthyosis. *J. Invest. Dermatol.* *91*:499.

Ruocco, M. J. and Shipley, G. G. (1982a). Characterization of the subtransition of hydrated dipalmitoylphosphatidylcholine bilayers: X-ray diffraction study. *Biochim. Biophys. Acta* *684*:59.

Ruocco, M. J. and Shipley, G. G. (1982b). Characterization of the subtransition of hydrated dipalmitoylphosphatidylcholine bilayers: Kinetic, hydration and structural study. *Biochim. Biophys. Acta* *691*:309.

Saxton, M. J. (1989). Lateral diffusion in an archipelago. Distance dependence of the diffusion coefficient. *Biophys. J.* *56*:615.

Schurer, N. Y. and Elias, P. M. (1991). The biochemistry and function of stratum corneum lipids. *Adv. Lipid Res.* *24*:27.

Seddon, J. M., Harlos, K. and Marsh, D. (1983). Metastability and polymorphism in the gel and fluid bilayer phases of dilauroylphosphatidylethanolamine. *J. Biol. Chem.* *258*:3850.

Seelig, J. (1977). Deuterium magnetic resonance: Theory and application to lipid membranes. *Quart. Rev. Biophys.* *10*:353.

Seelig, A. and Seelig, J. (1974). The dynamic structure of fatty acyl chains in a phospholipid bilayer measured by deuterium magnetic resonance. *Biochemistry* *13*:4839.

Slichter, C. P. (1990). *Principles of Magnetic Resonance*. Springer-Verlag, Heidelberg.

Squier, C. A., Cox, P. and Wertz, P. W. (1991a). Lipid content and water permeability of skin and oral mucosa. *J. Invest. Dermatol.* *96*:123.

Squier, C. A., Wertz, P. W. and Cox, P. (1991b). Thin-layer chromatographic analyses of lipids in different layers of porcine epidermis and oral epithelium. *Arch. Oral Biol. 36*:647.

Stockton, G. W. and Smith, I. C. P. (1976). A deuterium NMR study of the condensing effect of cholesterol on egg phosphatidylcholine bilayer membranes. I. Perdeuterated fatty acid probes. *Chem. Phys. Lipids 17*:251.

Swartzendruber, D. C., Wertz, P. W., Madison, K. C. and Downing, D. T. (1987). Evidence that the corneocyte has a chemically bound envelope. *J. Invest. Dermatol. 88*:709.

Thewalt, J. and Bloom, M. (1992). Phosphatidylcholine: cholesterol phase diagrams. *Biophys. J. 63*:1176.

Thewalt, J., Kitson, N., Araujo, C., MacKay, A. and Bloom, M. (1992). Models of *stratum corneum* intercellular membranes: The sphingolipid headgroup is a determinant of phase behavior in mixed lipid dispersions. *Biochem. Biophys. Res. Commun. 188*:1247.

Treffel, P., Panisset, F., Faivre, B. and Agache, P. (1994). Hydration, transepidermal water loss, pH and skin surface parameters: Correlations and variations between dominant and non-dominant forearms. *Br. J. Dermatol. 130*:325.

Vist, M. R. and Davis, J. H. (1990). Phase equilibria of cholesterol/dipalmitoyl-phosphatidylcholine mixtures: ^{2}H nuclear magnetic resonance and differential scanning calorimetry. *Biochemistry 29*:451.

Warner, R. R., Myers, M. C. and Taylor, D. A. (1988). Electron probe analysis of human skin: Element concentration profiles. *J. Invest. Dermatol. 90*:78.

Wertz, P. W. and Downing, D. T. (1983). Ceramides of pig epidermis: Structure determination. *J. Lipid Res. 24*:759.

Wertz, P. W., Downing, D. T., Freinkel, R. K. and Traczyk, T. N. (1984). Sphingolipids of the stratum corneum and lamellar granules of fetal rat epidermis. *J. Invest. Dermatol. 83*:193.

Wertz, P. W., Swartzendruber, D. C., Abraham, W., Madison K. C. and Downing, D. T. (1987). Essential fatty acids and epidermal integrity. *Arch. Dermatol. 123*:1381.

Wertz, P. W., Kremer, M. and Squier, C. A. (1992). Comparison of lipids from epidermal and palatal stratum corneum. *J. Invest. Dermatol. 98*:375.

White, S. H., Mirejovsky, D. and King, G. I. (1988). Structure of lipid domains and corneocyte envelopes of murine stratum corneum. An x-ray diffraction study. *Biochemistry 27*:3725.

Yardley, H. J. and Summerly, R. (1981). Lipid composition and metabolism in normal and diseased epidermis. *Pharmacol. Ther. 13*:357.

5

Characterization of Stratum Corneum Barrier Properties Using Fluorescence Spectroscopy

Louk A. R. M. Pechtold
University of Leiden, Leiden, The Netherlands

William Abraham and Russell O. Potts
Cygnus, Inc., Redwood City, California

I. INTRODUCTION

In the past decade a number of physical techniques have been used to evaluate the unique barrier properties of mammalian skin [1]. This chapter deals with the use of another physical technique, fluorescence spectroscopy, to study the barrier properties of the human stratum corneum (SC), specifically with respect to the transport of ions and water. The SC is the outermost layer of the human epidermis and consists of keratinized epithelial cells (corneocytes), physically isolated from one another by extracellular lipids arranged in multiple lamellae [2]. Due to a high diffusive resistance, this extracellular SC lipid matrix is believed to form the major barrier to the transport of ions and water through the human skin [3–5]. The objective of the fluorescence studies described here is to understand how such extraordinary barrier properties are achieved. First the phenomenon of fluorescence is described, followed by an evaluation of the use of anthroyloxy fatty acid fluorescent probes to study the physical properties of solvents and phospholipid membranes. Finally, the technique is applied to the SC to study its diffusional barrier to iodide ions and water.

II. FLUORESCENCE SPECTROSCOPY

A. Introduction

Fluorescence involves the emission of a photon by a fluorophore, which accompanies the transition from the lowest vibrational energy level of the excited electronic state (S_1) to one of the vibrational levels of the ground electronic state (S_0) [6]. The process is preceded by energy absorption during which the fluorescent molecule goes from the ground electronic state (S_0) to a vibrational level in the excited electronic state $(S_n, n = 1, 2, 3, \text{etc.})$. Subsequently, the fluorophore relaxes to the lowest vibrational level of the first excited electronic state (S_1), dissipating the excess absorbed energy in a nonradiative way, also known as *internal conversion*. Finally, the molecule relaxes back to the ground electronic state, emitting the remaining vibrational energy in the form of a fluorescence photon. The characteristics of this photon are a function of the energy level of the fluorophore prior to its emission, and are known to be affected by various processes that reflect interaction of the fluorescent molecule with the surrounding medium.

Upon absorption, the dipole moment of the fluorophore is increased, and surrounding polar solvent molecules rearrange themselves in response to that change. However, the excited fluorescent state is short-lived relative to solvent reorientation, preventing the system from reaching the energetically optimal position. As a result, the fluorophore relaxes to the ground state well before an equilibrium with the dipole moments of neighbor molecules has been established. These reorientation steps result in a loss of vibrational energy, shifting the emission spectrum toward lower energy (i.e., toward longer wavelengths) compared to the absorption spectrum. This shift is known as a *Stokes shift*, which increases with increased solvent polarity. In addition, hydrogen bonding and complexation between the fluorophore and the solvent molecules, as well as conformational changes of the fluorophore in the excited state, can cause Stokes shifts.

The fluorescence spectrum can also be altered by collisional quenching, in which a quenching agent collides with the fluorophore in the excited state, resulting in a nonradiative energy loss. This interaction causes a decrease in the fluorescence intensity and a decrease in the average time the fluorophore spends in the excited state. The latter is also known as the *fluorescence lifetime*. Since quenching involves diffusion of the quencher to the fluorophore during its lifetime, this method reveals information on the accessibility of the fluorophore.

Upon excitation, the fluorophore absorbs only photons whose electric vectors are orientated parallel to its absorption transition dipole. Any angular displacement between absorption and emission can depolarize the resultant fluorescence. For example, rotational diffusion of the fluorophore during its excitation lifetime will result in emission that is no longer parallel to the initial absorption. Anisotropy is a measure of the average angular displacement during the fluorescence lifetime. Since rotational diffusion depends on such properties as the viscosity of the surrounding medium, anisotropy can reveal information on the rigidity or "microviscosity" near the probe.

B. The Use of Anthroyloxy Fatty Acid Probes in Solvents and Membranes

Membranes exhibit a common structure, with lipid molecules arranged in the form of one or more bilayers, or lamellae. Since lipids are generally nonfluorescent, lipid-bound fluorophores are an excellent tool to study this environment. These membrane probes are poorly soluble in water, and hence they partition readily into the hydrophobic regions of the membranes. The derivatives of anthroyloxy fatty acids (AF), with the fluorophore 9-anthroic acid esterfied to the 2, 6, 9, 12, or 16 position along a fatty acid acyl chain (stearic acid or palmitic acid), are frequently used. The structure of an AF probe is shown schematically in Fig. 1

Low molecular weight solvents have been used to study the effects of polarity and hydrogen bonding on a fluorescent probe. For example, Garrison et al. studied the effect of various low molecular weight solvents on AF fluorescence [7]. Their results showed these fluorophores to be very sensitive to solvent polarity, shifting the emission maximum to longer wavelengths as the solvent polarity increased. In other words, as dipole–dipole interactions between solvent molecules and fluorophore increased, a greater Stokes shift was observed. Stokes shifts were even greater in protic solvents like ethanol and chloroform, which can interact with the carbonyl group of the fluorophore by intermolecular hydrogen bonding. Of all AF probes studied, 2-AF was the least sensitive to protic solvents, since intramolecular H-bonding between the fluorophore and the fatty acid carboxyl group prevented interaction with solvent molecules. These results showed that the emission spectra of AF probes are highly sensitive to solvent polarity and hydrogen-bonding ability.

These same AF probes have been widely used to study the bilayer structure in a variety of lipid membranes [8–12]. Since the fluorophore is attached at a known position along a fatty acid acyl chain, AF probes have been used to evaluate bilayer structures as a function of depth. When partitioned into a membrane, the fluorophore is localized deeper in the bilayer as its attachment site to the fatty acid is moved further away from the carboxyl

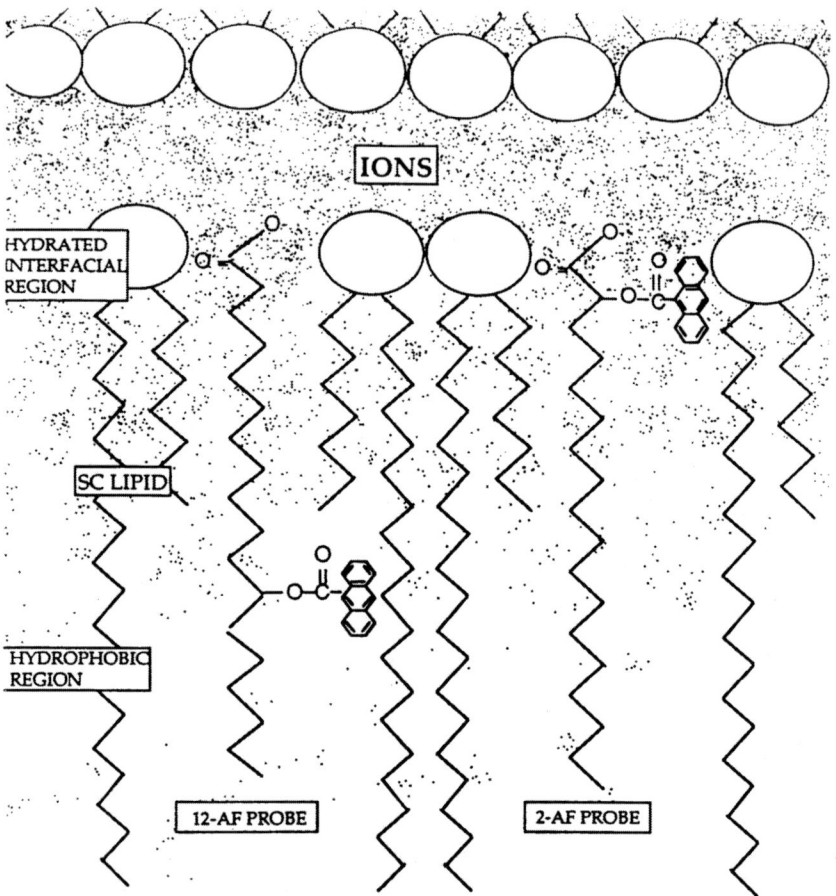

Figure 1 A schematic drawing of the SC extracellular lamellar-lipid domain with incorporated AF probes. The molecular dimensions are not drawn to scale.

group. For example, in 2-AF the probe is located near the bilayer headgroups, while in 16-AF the fluorophore is located nearer the bilayer center. In addition, iodide ions are known to quench the fluorescence associated with AF probes and have been used to study the accessibility of these probes in model and biological membranes [9,10]. The results clearly showed that quenching gradually decreased as the fluorophore was located further away from the lipid–water interface. Similarly, changes in lifetime, anisotropy, and emission spectra of AF probes in phospholipid membranes revealed a decreasing gradient of polarity and viscosity from the surface to the bilayer center [8,11]. These results suggest that the polar headgroup region of these bilayers is ordered and hydrated, while the bilayer interior is less well ordered and more anhydrous.

The AF probes are unusual in that an increase in vibrational energy associated with energy absorption causes a redistribution of electrons, resulting in a conformational change in the excited state [7,11–13]. In the ground state the anthracene and carboxyl group of the fluorophore are perpendicular to each other (known as the *Frank–Condon geometry*), while in the excited state they are co-planar [12]. The co-planar conformation is characterized by a longer lifetime and a lower vibrational energy, shifting the emission spectrum beyond that due to polarity and hydrogen bonding alone. Hindrance of this reorientation, such as that due to high local rigidity, causes a larger population of fluorophores to remain in the Frank–Condon geometry, resulting in a larger Stokes shift and a shorter lifetime. Hence, further information can be obtained on the local rigidity or microviscosity of the bilayer environment from lifetime and Stokes-shift data. In summary, AF probes have been widely used to study the organization of lipid bilayers in a large number of biological and model membrane systems.

III. THE SC BARRIER PROPERTIES TO IONS AND WATER

A. Introduction

The human skin consists of two distinct layers: the dermis and the epidermis. The outermost layer of the human epidermis, the SC, consists of terminally differentiated keratinocytes embedded in a continuous array of extracellular lipid lamellae [2]. These lamellae consist primarily of ceramides, free fatty acids, and cholesterol [4]. Since the polar headgroups of ceramides are known to facilitate lateral hydrogen-bonding with adjacent molecules, and since these lipids have acyl chains more than 24 carbons long, these extracellular lamellae form a rigid structure at physiological temperatures. There is now considerable evidence that SC lipids govern the permeability of water vapor through the SC. For example, lipid removal by solvent extraction leads to a 1000-fold permeability increase [14]. More importantly, SC water permeability seems to be highly correlated with the mobility of the lipid acyl chains [15]. This would suggest that the water barrier properties of SC are associated with the hydrocarbon region of the extracellular lamellae. In this way the hydrocarbon regions of the extracellular lipid lamellae form a continuous barrier to water inside the SC, forcing water and ions to traverse a highly tortuous pathway and so extending the diffusion pathway [5].

On the other hand, water and ion transport may also follow alternative routes. For instance, various skin appendages span the dermis and epidermis, such as sweat glands, sebaceous glands, and hair follicles [16]. Because these appendages extend through the SC, they may act as aqueous shunts to the interior, avoiding transport through the SC lipid matrix. It is believed that these appendages may play a major role in the transdermal transport of ions under passive conditions (e.g., the applications of a chemical gradient). During iontophoresis, when an electrical potential gradient applied across the skin serves as the driving force for ion migration [17], transport through these shunt routes may play an even greater role [18–21]. In addition, it has been proposed that ion transport may also occur through highly conductive pathways not associated with the skin appendages [22]. Since appendages and other highly conductive pathways make up a very small percentage of the total skin surface [23], nonappendageal ion transport (involving the SC lipid lamellar matrix) may still contribute substantially to the net flux through skin under both passive and iontophoretic conditions. In this case, the accessibility of the bilayer interior to these charged species should increase. Consistent with this hypothesis, metal ions [24–26] have been localized within the extracellular spaces following passive diffusion and iontophoresis.

To understand how the extracellular lipid lamellae act as a barrier to the percutaneous transport of water and ions, detailed information on its structure and accessibility is required. The AF fluorescence membrane probes have been used to provide information on the dynamics of SC membranes. The following sections describe the findings obtained using this approach.

B. Characterization of the Microenvironment Within SC Lipid Bilayers

Because the dynamics of phospholipid membranes have been well characterized using AF probes [8–13], fluorescence results obtained with hydrated human SC were compared to aqueous suspensions of unilamellar distearoylphosphatidylcholine (DSPC) vesicles. DSPC was also used because its phase transition temperature (55°C) is close to that of SC lipids (65°C). The microenvironment inside DSPC and SC membranes was studied by measuring fluorescence lifetimes, and shifts in emission maxima were compared to excitation maxima (Stokes shifts), along with quenching of a series of AF probes by iodide. Stokes shifts (Δv) [6] were calculated as:

$$\Delta v = \frac{1}{\lambda_{ab}} - \frac{1}{\lambda_{em}} \qquad (1)$$

where λ_{ab} and λ_{em} are the wavelengths of the absorption and emission maximum, respectively. The fluorescence lifetime (τ) was calculated from a biexponential decay model used to describe the intensity of AF probes in bilayers [7,13].

$$I(t) = \alpha_1 e^{-t/\tau_1} + \alpha_2 e^{-t/\tau_2} \qquad (2)$$

where $I(t)$ is the intensity decay, α_1 and α_2 are the pre-exponential factors, and τ_1 and τ_2 are the individual lifetimes. The fractional contributions (f_i) of each lifetime is given by

$$f_i = \frac{\alpha_i \tau_i}{\sum_{i=1}^{\infty} \alpha_i \tau_i} \qquad (3)$$

Tables 1 and 2 summarize Stokes-shift (Δv) and lifetime data, respectively, for a series of AF probes in DSPC and human SC. Since Stokes-shift data in hexane should reach a minimum value due to the absence of a dipole moment and hydrogen-bonding in this solvent [7], findings with hexane were compared to those of SC and DSPC in Table 1. The data show that while the Δv of 2-AF through 12-AF in DSPC were similar to values obtained in hexane, much smaller values were obtained in fully hydrated SC. Consequently, the

Table 1 Steady-State Emission Maxima (λ_{em}) and Calculated Stokes Shift (Δv) for various *n*-AF Probes in Hexane, DSPC Vesicles, and Human SC at 20°C

	Hexane		DSPC		SC	
Probe	λ_{em} (nm)	Δv^* (cm^{-1})	λ_{em} (nm)	Δv^* (cm^{-1})	λ_{em} (nm)	Δv^* (cm^{-1})
2-AF	446	3420	445	3370	433	2750
6-AF	442	3220	—	—	429	2530
9-AF	442	3220	444	3320	430	2580
12-AF	442	3220	444	3320	431	2640
16-AF	443	3270	453	3770	441	3160

$*\Delta v = \dfrac{1}{\lambda_{ex}} - \dfrac{1}{\lambda_{em}}$, using 387 nm as λ_{ex}.

Table 2 Lifetimes (τ_1, τ_2, τ_{avg}), Their Fractional Contributions (f_1, f_2), and Stern–Volmer Constants (K_{sv}) of n-AF Probes in DSPC vesicles and human SC at 20°C

Medium and probe	$\tau_1^{*\dagger}$ (ns)	$f_1^{*\dagger}$ (10^{-2})	$\tau_2^{*\dagger}$ (ns)	$f_2^{*\dagger}$ (10^{-2})	$\tau_{avg}^{\ddagger}$ (ns)	$K_{sv}^{\S}$ (10^{-1} M
DSPC						
2-AF	1.80 ± 0.42	14 ± 2	9.80 ± 0.38	86 ± 2	8.69 ± 0.25	$16.7 \pm 1.$
6-AF	1.54 ± 0.35	11 ± 2	10.09 ± 0.54	89 ± 2	9.14 ± 0.35	—
9-AF	2.00 ± 0.32	12 ± 1	11.44 ± 0.15	88 ± 1	10.30 ± 0.06	$23.1 \pm 0.$
12-AF	1.74 ± 0.39	9 ± 2	11.91 ± 0.64	91 ± 2	10.95 ± 0.40	$20.3 \pm 0.$
16-AF	1.80 ± 0.41	5 ± 1	13.74 ± 0.24	95 ± 2	13.12 ± 0.17	$10.0 \pm 1.$
SC						
2-AF	1.14 ± 0.62	27 ± 4	9.30 ± 0.92	73 ± 4	7.07 ± 0.79	$1.2 \pm 0.$
6-AF	0.96 ± 0.63	26 ± 3	8.84 ± 1.07	74 ± 3	6.80 ± 1.03	$0.7 \pm 0.$
9-AF	0.78 ± 0.44	27 ± 3	8.15 ± 0.47	73 ± 3	6.19 ± 0.38	$0.6 \pm 0.$
12-AF	1.03 ± 0.44	25 ± 6	9.09 ± 0.52	75 ± 6	7.10 ± 0.67	$0.5 \pm 0.$
16-AF	1.10 ± 0.59	20 ± 2	11.10 ± 0.62	80 ± 2	9.13 ± 0.57	$0.4 \pm 0.$

[*]Data represent average ± S.D. of four measurements on two different DSPC suspensions or on three differ
pieces of skin.
[†]For DSPC, c^2 ranged from 8 to 3, and for SC from 0.6 to 6.
[‡]Apparent lifetime (τ_{avg}) was calculated as $\tau_{avg} = f_1\tau_1 + f_2\tau_2$.
[§]Data represent average ± S.D. obtained with three different DSPC suspensions or pieces of skin.

$\Delta\nu$ in SC cannot be explained by polarity and hydrogen-bonding of the surrounding medium alone. Rather the results are explained better in terms of hindered fluorophore reorientation in the excited state, similar to results obtained with other lipid systems [7,11–13]. Thus, the unusual Stokes shifts seen with AF probes in SC suggests a rather "rigid" environment in the lipid lamellae, which hinder the fluorophore reorientation.

Lifetime data in Table 2 show two populations of fluorophores, with a short (τ_1) or a long (τ_2) lifetime. From the two lifetimes, an average lifetime (τ_{avg}) was calculated:

$$\tau_{avg} = f_1\tau_1 + f_2\tau_2 \tag{4}$$

which is the summation of the two lifetimes weighted by their fractional contributions. As a function of the location of the fluorophore, lifetimes in DSPC and SC follow the same trend but differ greatly in their absolute value. Namely, lifetime increased as the probe was located further from the carboxyl headgroup, for both DSPC and SC. Compared to DSPC, however, the τ_{avg} values in SC were smaller and with a larger f_1 value, suggesting that in SC a larger population of probes exhibit a shorter lifetime. Taken together with the Δv values shown in Table 1, these lifetime data strongly suggest that in SC a large population of fluorophores experience a hindered reorientation and thus that SC bilayers are significantly more rigid than hexane or DSPC.

C. The SC Barrier to Water and Ions

Passive Conditions

Since iodide is known to act in phospholipid vesicles as a collisional quencher for AF probes [6,9] by a diffusive process, fluorescence quenching was described by the Stern–Volmer relationship [6]:

$$\frac{I_0}{I} - 1 = K_{sv}[Q] \tag{5}$$

where I_0 is the fluorescence intensity of the unquenched fluorophore, I is the intensity at quencher concentration $[Q]$, and K_{sv} is the Stern–Volmer constant, which reflects the quenching efficiency [14]. The quenching results obtained with AF probes in SC (Fig. 2) show that K_{sv} generally decreased as the fluorophore is located further down the acyl chain. Since quenching efficien-

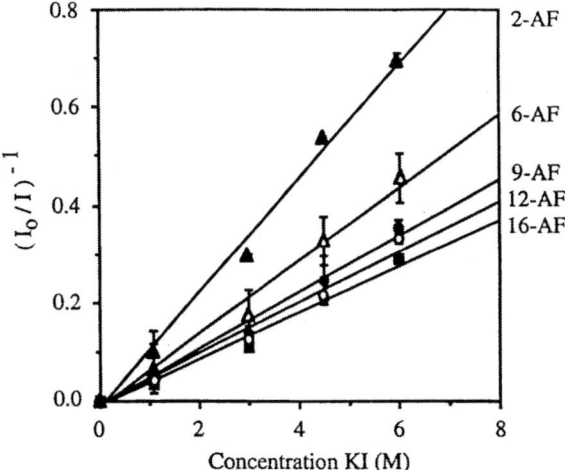

Figure 2 Fluorescence intensity quenching $[(I_0/I) - 1]$ of AF probes in SC as a function of iodide (KI) concentration. Data represents the average $\pm$ S.D. and are obtained from three different pieces of skin. *Symbols*: solid triangles (2-AF); open triangles (6-AF); solid circles (9-AF); open circles (12-AF); solid squares (16-AF).

cies reflects ion accessibility, these results demonstrate that when the fluorophore was located further away from the fatty acid polar headgroup (i.e., deeper within the bilayer), it was less accessible to the quencher. This gradient in accessibility is consistent with results obtained with other lamellar lipid systems [8,10], and suggests that the AF probes were localized in a bilayer structure where more iodide was present near the bilayer headgroup region than near the core. While the trend is the same in SC and DSPC, the K_{sv} values are an order of magnitude smaller in SC [27]. These differences in quenching efficiencies between SC and DSPC could reflect differences in bilayer structure. On the other hand, SC is made up predominantly of proteins such as keratin (approximately 80% w/w of dry SC). Since many proteins bind anions, the concentration of free iodide in the SC bilayer could be reduced due to protein binding, hence reducing the K_{sv}. Regardless of the difference in quenching magnitude between DSPC and SC, these results also show that iodide was found within the lamellar lipid structure of both. Therefore, the combined results strongly suggest that under passive conditions the SC lipid lamellar matrix is accessible to iodide ions.

Iontophoretic Conditions

During iontophoresis, an electric potential gradient applied across the skin serves as the driving force for ion migration through this tissue [17]. Increasing the current at constant resistance will therefore increase ion migration, accompanied by a flow of water. Because iodide quenching of AF probes requires collision of the ion and the fluorophore during the lifetime of the excited state [6], a change in fluorescence intensity serves as an indicator of the close proximity of the ion to the fluorophore within the SC bilayer. Quenching of AF probes in SC was measured before, during, and after iontophoresis. To distinguish the effect of passive from iontophoretically enhanced ion accessibility, current was applied after quenching under passive conditions (see above) had reached steady state. Iodide anions were introduced using a Ag/AgI cathode placed in the donor chamber, which contained 1.1 M KI, while a Ag anode was placed in the receiver chamber containing Hepes. Due to the combination of a Ag/AgI electrode with a KI solution on the cathodal side, iodide is the primary anionic current carrier through the skin. The effect of current density on iodide iontophoresis was evaluated at current densities of 100 and 300 μA/cm^2. During iontophoresis, spectra were recorded every 30 minutes until the fluorescence intensity reached a constant value and, hence, quenching had reached steady state.

The results showed that quenching decreased in proportion to current density, suggesting that as the current increased, more quenching agents (iodide) entered the SC lipid lamellae. Iontophoretically enhanced quenching also decreased as a function of the position of the fluorophore along the fatty acid acyl chain (Fig. 3), qualitatively similar to results obtained under passive conditions (see above). Therefore, these results point to a gradient in accessibility within the SC bilayer, and suggest that the lamellar lipid structure remains relatively unperturbed, even during iontophoresis. On the other hand, additional quenching due to iontophoresis suggests that under an applied electric current SC lipid bilayers were more accessible to iodide.

To ensure that any decrease in intensity during iontophoresis was due only to quenching and not to probe migrating out of the SC, the amount of probe in the SC was determined after iontophoresis at the highest current density studied. In these experiments, 16-AF was used, since its high quantum yield enabled the detection of small amounts of probe. The results showed that the probe-to-lipid mole ratio in SC was unchanged by iontophoresis and that the probe was not found in the remaining skin, electrodes, or donor and receiver solutions. These results demonstrate that AF probes did not migrate

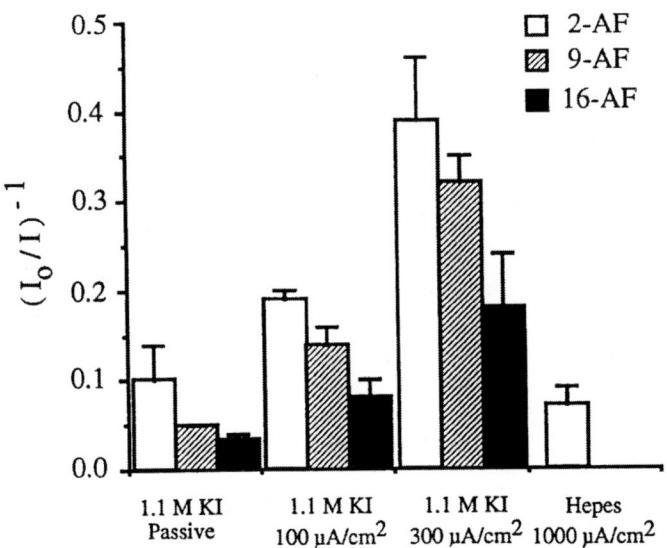

Figure 3 Quenching results, $(I_0/I) - 1$, of 2-, 9-, and 16-AF using KI under passive conditions and iontophoresis at 100 and 300 $\mu A/cm^2$, together with the control involving iontophoresis in Hepes buffer alone at 1000 $\mu A/cm^2$.

out of the SC due to an applied electric field. Any decrease in fluorescence intensity during iontophoresis, therefore, must be due to quenching.

Since water and buffer components could also contribute to the observed quenching, iontophoresis in Hepes served as a control experiment. For these experiments, 2-AF was used, since its fluorophore is the most accessible and hence is the most sensitive to quenching. Iontophoresis with buffer alone at a current density of 1000 $\mu A/cm^2$ resulted in increased quenching (Fig. 4), suggesting that SC lipid bilayer interior became more accessible to water and buffer components. However, since the magnitude of quenching was much smaller than that obtained with iodide iontophoresis at a 30% lower current density, it can be concluded that the contribution of water and buffer components to the quenching was small relative to iodide. The relative quenching efficiencies of water versus iodide are not known. Nevertheless, these results strongly suggest that during an applied electric field, the SC lipid bilayer interior becomes more accessible to water and ions. This would imply that during iontophoresis, ion and water transport through the human skin is associated, at least in part, with the SC lipid matrix.

The increased accessibility of the SC bilayer to water and ions is consistent with iontophoresis causing increased hydration of the SC [3,15]. However, according to x-ray diffraction results [3], increased hydration due to iontophoresis resulted in no significant swelling of the SC bilayers, suggesting that hydration did not alter the lipid lamellar structure. Similar results were obtained with infrared (IR) spectroscopy [28,29], whereby iontophoresis caused an increase in the SC hydration (as measured by oxygen–water absorbance), yet no change in the carbon–hydrogen (C–H) stretching frequencies was observed. Since changes in C–H stretching frequencies correspond to altered SC lipid order [15], these results imply that iontophoresis does not affect the organization of SC bilayers. Together with our results, these IR [28,29] and x-ray [3] data suggest that during iontophoresis, the SC bilayer interior becomes more accessible to water and ions; however, no structural alteration occurs.

The lack of SC lipid bilayer alteration during iontophoresis is contrary to the conclusion drawn from published results involving skin impedance measurements [3]. In these experiments, as current was applied across the skin, the electrical impedance was measured as a function of temperature. At around 65°C, a 100-fold decrease in the electrical resistance was observed, which corresponded to a solid-to-fluid phase change affecting the structure of SC bilayers, as observed using other techniques [13,15,30]. As the current density was increased from 13 to 130 $\mu A/cm^2$, the impedance decrease occurred at a lower temperature, suggesting a current-induced perturbation of the SC bilayer structure. However, the results from differential scanning calorimetry (DSC) studies show that increased hydration shifts the SC lipid-phase transition to lower temperatures due to water-dependent, freezing-point depression [15,30]. Therefore, an alternative explanation could be that the current-induced shift in SC lipid-phase transition temperature results from increased hydration [3,28] and not from a perturbation of the SC bilayer structure, consistent with the results presented.

The results of the present study show that quenching of AF probes is a useful tool to the study of the presence of ions within SC bilayers during iontophoresis. However, since quenching only indicates the presence of the ion in close proximity to the fluorophore, no detailed information is obtained on how the ion migrated into the SC bilayer. In addition, since the probes are located in SC bilayers, there is also no information on how the ion migrated through other structures of the SC (e.g., paracellular, transcellular, or appendageal) and to what extent ions in the SC bilayer contribute to the total ion transport through the SC. Nevertheless, the results show that the interior of the SC lipid bilayer becomes more accessible to ions and water due to an applied electric field. This electrohydration may be essential to enhanced skin transport seen with both electroporation [31–33] and iontophoresis [18,31].

REFERENCES

1. Potts, R. O. Physical characterization of the stratum corneum. In: J. Hadgraft, R. H., Guy, eds. Transdermal Drug Delivery. Marcel Dekker, New York, 1990, pp. 23–58.
2. Elias and D. S. Friend. The permeability barrier in mamalian epidermis. *J. Cell Biol.* 65:180–191 (1975).
3. Craane-van Hinsberg. *Transdermal peptide iontophoresis*, Ph.D. Dissertation, Leiden University, The Netherlands, 1994.
4. Yardley, H. D., and Summerly, R. Lipid composition and metabolism in normal and diseased epidermis. *Pharmacol Ther.* 13:357–383, 1981.
5. Potts and M. L. Francoeur. The influence of stratum corneum morphology on water permeability. *J. Invest. Dermatol.* 96:495–499 (1991).
6. Lackowicz. *Principles of Fluorescence Spectroscopy*, Plenum Press, New York, 1983.
7. Garrison, M. D., Doh, L. M., Potts, R. O., and Abraham, W. Fluorescence spectroscopy of 9-anthroyloxy fatty acids in solvents. *Chem. Phys. Lipids 70*:155–162, 1994.
8. Thulborn and W. H. Sawyer. Properties and the locations of a set of fluorescent

probes sensitive to the fluidity gradient of the lipid bilayer. *Biochim. et Biophys. Acta 511*:125–140 (1978).

9. Langner and S. W. Huie. Iodide penetration into lipid bilayers as a probe of membrane lipid organization. *Chem. and Phys. of Lipids 60*:127–132 (1991).

10. Chalpin and A. M. Kleinfeld. Interaction of fluorescence quenchers with the n-(9-anthroyloxy) fatty acid membrane probes. *Biochim. et Biophys. Acta 731*:465–474 (1983).

11. Thulborn, L. M. Tilley, W. H. Sawyer, and E. Treloar. The use of n-(9-anthroyloxy) fatty acids to determine fluidity and polarity gradients in phospholipid bilayers. *Biochim. et Biophys. Acta 558*:166–178 (1979).

12. Matayosi, E. D. and Kleinfeld, A. M. Emission wavelength-dependent decay of the 9-anthroyloxy-fatty acids membrane probes. *Biophys. J. 35*:215–235, 1981.

13. Garrison, L. M. Doh, L. A. R. M. Pechtold, R. O. Potts, and W. Abraham. Fluorescence spectroscopic evaluation of stratum corneum lipids and related model systems. In K. R. Brain, V. J. James, and K. A. Walters (eds.), *Predictions of Percutaneous Penetration*, I.B.C. Technical Services Ltd., London, 1993, pp. 1–7.

14. Potts, R. O., and Francoeur, M. L. Lipid biophysics of water loss through the skin. *Proc. Natl. Acad. Sci. USA 87*:3871–3873, 1990.

15. Golden, D. B. Guzek, R. R. Harris, J. E. McKie, and R. O. Potts. Lipid thermotropic transitions in human stratum corneum. *J. Invest. Dermatol. 89*:255–259 (1986).

16. Urmacher, C. Histology of normal skin. *Am. J. Surg. Pathol. 14*:671–686 (1990).

17. Schultz. *Basic principles of membrane transport*, Cambridge University Press, New York, 1969.

18. Burnette and D. Marrero. Comparison between iontophoretic and passive transport of thyrotropic releasing hormone across excised nude mouse skin. *J. Pharm. Sci. 75*:738–743 (1986).

19. Abramson, H. A. and Gorin, M. H. Skin reactions. IX: The electrophoretic demonstration of the patent pores in the living human skin; its relation to the change of the skin. *J. Phys. Chem. 44*:1094–1102, 1940.

20. Cullander, C. and R. Guy. Visualisation of iontophoretic pathways with confocal microscopy and the vibrating probe electrode. *Solid State Ionics 53–56*:197–206 (1992).

21. Grimnes. Pathways of ionic flow through human skin in vivo. *Acta Derm. Venerol. 64*:93–98 (1984).

22. Scott, A. I. Laplaza, H. S. White, and J. B. Phipps. Transport of ionic species in skin: Contribution of pores to the overall skin conductance. *Pharm. Res. 10*:1699–1709 (1993).

23. Schaeffer, F. Watts, J. Brod, and B. Illel. Follicular penetration. In R. C. Scott, R. H. Guy, and J. Hadgraft (eds.), *Prediction of Percutaneous Penetration: Methods, Measurements, and Modelling*, IBC Technical Services, London, 1990, pp. 163–173.

24. Boddé, M. A. M. Kruithof, J. Brussee, and H. K. Koerten. Visualisation of normal and enhanced $HgCl_2$ transport through human skin in vitro. *Int. J. Pharm.* 53:13–24 (1989).

25. Sharata, H. and R. R. Burnette. Percutaneous absorption of electron-dense ions across normal and chemically perturbed skin. *J. Pharm. Sci.* 77:27–32 (1989).

26. Monteiro-Riviere, A. O. Inman, and J. E. Riviere. Identification of the pathway of iontophoretic drug delivery: light and ultrastructural studies using mercuric chloride in pigs. *Pharm. Res.* 11:251–256 (1994).

27. Wertz, P. W. and Downing, D. T. Ceramides of pig epidermis: Structure determination. *J. Lipid Res.* 24:759–767, 1983.

28. Green, P. D. and J. Hadgraft. FT-IR investigations into the effect of iontophoresis on the skin. In K. R. Brain, V. J. James, and K. A. Walters (eds.), *Predictions of Percutaneous Penetration*, I.B.C. Technical Services Ltd., London, 1993, pp. 37–43.

29. Clancy, J. Corish, and O. I. Corrigan. A comparison of the effects of electric current and penetration enhancers on the properties of human skin using spectroscopic (FTIR) and calorimetric (DSC) methods. *Int. J. Pharm.* 105:47–56 (1994).

30. Oh, L. Leung, D. Bommannan, R. H. Guy, and R. O. Potts. Effect of current, ionic strength and temperature on the electrical properties of skin. *J. Control. Rel.* 27:115–125 (1993).

31. Bommannan, D., Tamada, J., Leung, L., and Potts, R. O. Effect of electroporation on transdermal iontophoretic delivery of luteinizing hormone release hormone (LHRH) in vitro. Pharm. Res. 11:1809–1814, 1994.

32. Vanbever, R. Lecouturier, N., and V. Préat. Transdermal delivery of metoprolol by electroporation. *Pharm. Res.* 11:1657–1662 (1994).

33. Chizmadzhev, Y. A., Zarnitsin, V. G., Weaver, J. C., and Potts, R. O. Mechanism of electroinduced ionic species transport through a multilamellar lipid system. *Biophys. J.* 68:749–765, 1995.

6
Impedance Spectroscopy: Applications to Human Skin

Ronald R. Burnette
University of Wisconsin, Madison, Wisconsin

John D. DeNuzzio
Becton Dickson and Company, Research Triangle Park, North Carolina

I. INTRODUCTION

Transport properties of biological membranes and tissues are commonly determined through classical flux experiments. However, the experimental setup and analytical procedures involved in such studies are laborious and time-consuming. Furthermore, transient flux responses are difficult to measure accurately. Alternatively, impedance spectroscopy allows rapid experimental determination of the transient and steady-state conduction properties of materials.

Impedance spectroscopy (IS) is a measurement of the conductive and dielectric properties of electroactive systems over a wide range of frequencies. Its popularity and applicability has increased dramatically over the past 25 years with the advent of fast-response potentiostats and frequency response analyzers. Impedance spectroscopy has been applied extensively in electrochemistry, especially in battery and sensor research, and it has been used to study active transport in biological membranes. Skin impedance has also been investigated with IS, but many of these studies attempted to correlate impedance with hydration and provided no insight into the mechanism of charge transport. More recent studies have used IS to elucidate the pathways of ion transport through skin, with special emphasis on understanding the mechanism of transdermal delivery of charged compounds via iontophoresis. The objective of this chapter is to introduce the basic theory and experimental techniques of impedance spectroscopy, and to review the current literature on impedance measurements of skin.

II. THEORY OF IMPEDANCE SPECTROSCOPY

Impedance spectroscopy is a well-established technique in electrochemistry, and it has been the topic of numerous articles and books. It is actually a subset of a broader category of spectroscopy that includes dielectric and conductance responses. All three terms (impedance, conductance, and dielectric response) are intimately related and are grouped under the general heading of *immittance spectroscopy* by MacDonald and Johnson [1]. For further detailed information on the various applications of immittance spectroscopy, the reader is directed to Ref. 1–4.

Impedance is the functional form of resistance that is typically defined by Ohm's law. That is, resistance R is the time-invariant relationship between voltage (V) and current (I):

$$\text{Ohm's law:} \quad R = \frac{V}{I}$$

Impedance, on the other hand, includes the transient response of the system as well as the long-term, steady-state response defined by Ohm's law. The entire time course of impedance is usually captured by transforming the measurement to the frequency domain. This is an inverse transform in which transient responses occur at high frequencies and long-term, steady-state responses are approached at low frequencies.

$$\text{frequency} = \frac{1}{\text{time}}$$

Thus, in its simplest form, impedance (Z) is the function that describes the relationship between voltage and current over a range of frequencies.

An impedance measurement can be made either by applying an electrical potential and monitoring the current response or, conversely, by passing current and monitoring the potential response. Several decades of frequencies can be scanned rapidly and accurately using a frequency response analyzer [4]. An alternative approach applies multiple frequencies simultaneously (white noise) and deconvolutes the response with a lock-in amplifier. The use of an oscillating (a.c.) input function maintains the system near equilibrium during the measurement.

To illustrate the technique, let's consider the case in which the system is stimulated by an applied voltage at a discrete frequency and the response current is measured at the same frequency. At zero frequency, or d.c., impedance is equivalent to resistance as defined by Ohm's law: $R = V/I$. When the impressed voltage is oscillated at a particular frequency, the system responds by passing an oscillating current. If the amplitude of the input voltage is sufficiently small (typically < 10 mV), the system is linear, and the frequency of the response wave (current) matches the frequency of the perturbation (voltage). However, the response current wave may differ from the perturbation in amplitude and phase (Fig. 1). The ratio of the amplitudes of the perturbation to the response waveforms and the phase shift between the signals define the impedance function.

Consider, for example, a test sample of material with a well-defined geometry as shown in Fig. 2. Reversible electrodes are attached to opposite planar faces of the test article, and a sinusoidal electrical potential (V_{ac}) is applied via a waveform generator. The current response is monitored with a frequency response analyzer (FRA), which converts the signal to the frequency domain. The amplitude (A) of the input wave is adjusted to the range in which the system responds linearly, about 10 mV. Thus, the perturbation can be described by the following equation:

input: $V_{ac} = A \sin \omega t$

where ω is the angular frequency and t is time. Likewise, the response current

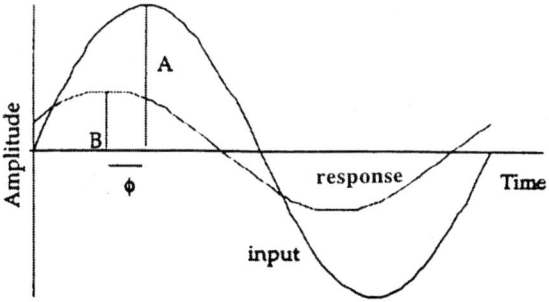

Figure 1 Sinusoidal perturbation and response waveforms illustrating change in amplitude (A and B) and phase shift (ϕ).

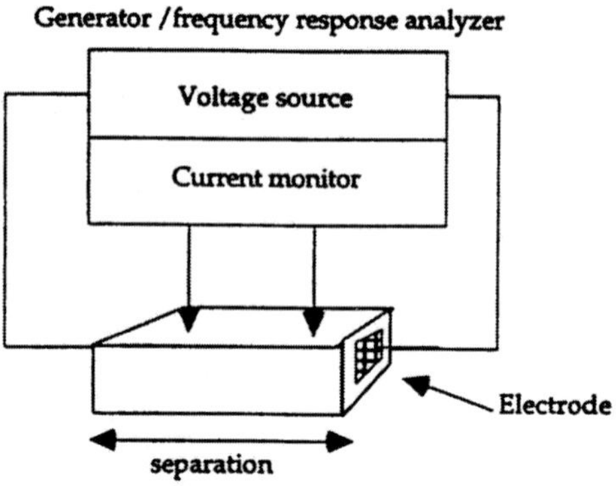

Generator /frequency response analyzer

Figure 2   Experimental setup for impedance measurement.

waveform (I_{ac}) follows the perturbation, but with a different amplitude (B) and shifted in phase by the amount ϕ:

response: $I_{ac} = B \sin (\omega t + \phi)$

The impedance of the system is the function Z:

impedance: $Z = \dfrac{V_{ac}}{I_{ac}} = \dfrac{A \sin \omega t}{B \sin (\omega t + \phi)}$

The mathematics can be simplified by redefining the sine function in terms of real (') and imaginary (") components such that:

input: $V_{ac} = V' + jV''$

response: $I_{ac} = I' + jI''$

impedance: $Z = \dfrac{V' + jV''}{I' + jI''} = Z' + jZ''$

where ($j = \sqrt{-1}$) Thus, the magnitude of the impedance is given by:

magnitude: $|Z| = (Z'^2 + Z''^2)^{1/2}$

and the phase angle is given by:

phase angle: $\phi = \arctan \dfrac{Z''}{Z'}$

The real component (Z') of the impedance function corresponds to the in-phase response, and the imaginary component (Z'') corresponds to the out-of-phase response. In mechanical measurements, these components are also known as "loss" and "storage" moduli. In electrical terms, they correspond to resistive and capacitive portions of the impedance function.

An impedance response can be interpreted graphically as a vector on the complex plane. The imaginary axis is the out-of-phase response (Z''), and the real axis is the in-phase response (Z'). The magnitude of the impedance response $|Z|$ is the length of the vector, and the phase angle ϕ describes its direction (Fig. 3). Each point on the plane defines an impedance response at a particular frequency. Such representations are commonly referred to as *complex plane plots, Nyquist diagrams,* or *Cole–Cole plots.* However, the Cole-Cole plot is actually the complex plane representation of the dielectric response of a material.

Alternatively, an equally powerful visualization of impedance data involves Bode analysis. In this case, the magnitude of the impedance and the phase shift are plotted separately as functions of the frequency of the perturbation. This approach was developed to analyze electric circuits in terms of critical resistive and capacitive elements. A similar approach is taken in impedance spectroscopy, and impedance responses of materials are interpreted in terms of equivalent electric circuits. The individual components of the equivalent circuit are further interpreted in terms of phemonenological responses such as ionic conductivity, dielectric behavior, relaxation times, mobility, and diffusion.

A. Equivalent Analog Circuits

Ideal electric circuit components such as resistors and capacitors have well-defined signatures in the complex plane. The impedance of an ideal resistor Z_R is characterized by a zero phase shift between the input and output

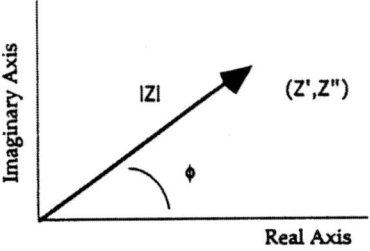

Figure 3 Complex plane representation of impedance vector Z.

waveforms (Fig. 1). This type of impedance response does not vary with frequency, and therefore it has no imaginary component. An ideally resistive impedance response appears as a point on the real axis of the complex plane (Fig. 3).

resistor: $Z_R = Z' + j0$

Conversely, a purely capacitive response is completely out of phase with the perturbation wave. The capacitive impedance Z_C response varies continuously and inversely with frequency and has no real component. In the complex plane, an ideal capacitance (C) appears as a vertical line that does not intercept the real axis.

capacitor: $Z_C = 0 + j \dfrac{-1}{\omega C}$

From these simple expressions of ideal resistance and capacitance, intricate electrical networks can be assembled by applying the rules of series and parallel circuits:

series network: $Z_{\text{series}} = Z_1 + Z_2 + \cdots$

parallel network: $\dfrac{1}{Z_{\text{parallel}}} = \dfrac{1}{Z_1} + \dfrac{1}{Z_2} + \cdots$

One of the most broadly applied equivalent circuits is shown in Figure 4. It consists of a parallel R_pC network in with a resistor R_s. This particular network is a simple representation of an electrochemical cell. R_s represents the

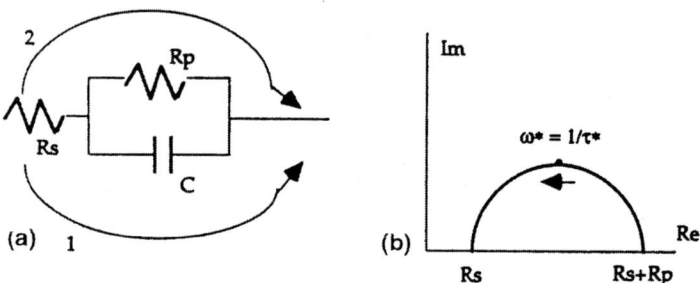

Figure 4   (a) *R-RC* equivalent analog circuit diagram, showing conduction paths 1 and 2. (b) Impedance response of *R-RC* circuit on the complex plane. The arrow indicates the direction of increasing frequency. The frequency at the apex of the arc (ω^*) is related to the time constant (t^*) of the circuit.

bulk resistance of the electrolyte, and the parallel RC models the electrode–electrolyte interface. Current may pass through a combination of two distinct paths. Pathway 1 illustrates the capacitive charging of the system. In an electrochemical cell, this might be nonfaradaic charging of the electrode. Alternatively, this pathway might illustrate reorientation of proteins in a membrane in response to an electric field. Capacitive elements dominate the transient part of the impedance response, and in the frequency domain those transient events transform to high frequency responses. Once the capacitor is charged, the bulk of the current follows pathway 2. This path is totally resistive and is described by the sum $R_s + R_p$. In a real experimental system, this second pathway might correspond to the bulk resistance of the electrolyte and kinetics of the electrode process.

The impedance response of the R-RC circuit in Figure 4a is illustrated on a complex plane plot in Figure 4b. At low frequencies, the data approach the real axis at $R_s + R_p$ (pathway 2), and the capacitive response is illustrated by the arc in the data. The frequency at the apex of the arc (ω^*) corresponds to the characteristic relaxation time (t^*) of the circuit:

$$\text{relaxation time:} \quad t^* = \frac{1}{\omega^*} = \frac{1}{RC}$$

At high frequencies (ω approaches infinity), the capacitive impedance ($Z_c = -j/\omega C$) tends to zero, and the impedance response of the circuit approaches the real axis at R_s.

The complexity of the conduction process in a particular material is reflected in its impedance response and ultimately in its equivalent circuit. Multiple impedance arcs correspond to distinct conduction pathways and separate RC elements in the circuit model. However, the true challenge of impedance spectroscopy is to interpret response functions in terms of the simplest meaningful circuit analogs and to use the electrical analogs as mere guides to the interpretation of the real physical events. The individual components of equivalent circuits should represent specific physical processes in the real system. For example, resistance describes the facility of charge transport through a medium, and capacitance describes space-charge phenomena and dielectric properties such as dipole reorientation. Ideally, each conductive pathway within a system has a unique relaxation time (t^*), which, in turn, is related to the magnitudes of its resistive and capacitive components ($t^* = 1/RC$) of the equivalent circuit. Since these relaxation events are evident at particular frequencies, it is possible to observe many different conduction processes in a system by measuring its impedance response over a wide range of frequencies. In reality, impedance responses are not ideal, and results are sometimes difficult to interpret. Furthermore, equivalent circuits are not unique. Seemingly different network combinations can have identical impedance responses. Therefore, it is usually best to construct the simplest equivalent circuit based on common sense and reasonable estimations of the actual physical processes.

In many cases, the use of ideal equivalent circuits is convenient but not always appropriate. Nonideal behavior might arise from interactions of species, resulting in frequency-dependent capacitances [$C(\omega)$]. Under these conditions, the physical process is more accurately described by a range of relaxation time constants instead of a unique value. Such distributed relaxation events are usually manifested as semicircles depressed below the real axis in the complex plane, and the angle of depression is related to the degree of nonideality. Various distribution functions and constant phase elements have been employed to describe such events. These nonidealities are especially evident in biological systems.

In addition to the complexity of nonideal system responses, IS is limited in that it cannot distinguish chemical composition. Other analytical techniques should complement impedance spectroscopy to determine the actual species involved in the electrochemical processes. Despite these limitations, IS is a powerful and valuable technique for measuring the conduction properties of electroactive systems. It is especially well suited for investigating the transport properties of biological tissues because: (a) small pertubation signals are employed, maintaining the system near equilibrium throughout measurement; and (b) a variety of capacitive and resistive properties of the test material can be determined in a single, brief experiment by analyzing the response over a wide frequency range. In the following sections, the current literature on impedance responses of skin is reviewed.

III. CURRENT LITERATURE ON IMPEDANCE RESPONSES OF SKIN

A. Inferences About Human Skin Determined Through the Use of Impedance Spectroscopy

By observing that the skin's electrical resistance substantially decreased as layers were sequentially removed by tape stripping, Yamamoto and Yamamoto [5] demonstrated that the stratum corneum layer is the primary contributor to the skin's electrical resistance. However, Rosell et al. [6] have shown that even the slightest abrasion to the skin markedly decreases the skin's resistance. In addition, in Leveque and De Rigal's review [7], it is mentioned that stripping can produce a "cracked" skin surface, resulting in a defective contact between the electrode used to determine the skin's impedance and the skin. Therefore, one is led to conclude that although tape stripping is removing the stratum corneum, it could also be causing small abrasions all the way down to the viable epidermal layer, even after the first stripping. This may result in an inappropriate quantitation of the resistance characteristics of the stratum corneum. Nonetheless, several investigators [6,8–10] have confirmed that the stratum corneum represents the skin's primary resistive barrier.

Yamamoto and Yamamoto [5] also showed that the resistance of the stratum corneum was not homogeneous, being higher in the uppermost layers and then becoming smaller in the lowermost layers. In fact, with sequential tape stripping, Yamamoto and Yamamoto found that the skin's impedance became a very low constant value after approximately 15 strippings. This suggests that the deep tissues below the stratum corneum do not act as a barrier to electric current. Yamamoto [11] suggested that the constant impedance observed for the deeper tissue results from the body's homeostatic nature. In addition, Yamamoto's analysis of the skin's impedance showed that the stratum corneum did not obey a Cole–Cole circular arc (as illustrated in Fig. 4b), whereas the skin remaining after complete stripping did [5]. This is a result of the stratum corneum's heterogeneous structure [5]. As was mentioned in the background section, this heterogeneity produces frequency-dependent capacitances that require a range of relaxation constants to characterize the system more fully.

The impedance of the skin has been generally modeled by using a parallel resistance/capacitor equivalent circuit (Fig. 4a). The skin's capacitance is mainly attributed to the dielectric properties of the lipid-protein components of the human epidermis [5,8,9,12]. The resistance is associated primarily with the skin's stratum corneum layer [5,8,9,12]. Several extensions to the basic parallel resistor/capacitor circuit model have appeared in the literature [5,8,9,13]. Most involve two modified parallel resistor/capacitor combinations connected in series [5,8,9]. The interpretation of this series combination is that the first parallel resistor/capacitor circuit represents the stratum corneum and the second resistor/capacitor parallel combination represents the deeper tissues [5,8,9]. The modification generally employed is to add another resistance, either in series and/or in parallel with the original parallel resistor/capacitor combination [8,9]. Realize that because all of these circuits contain a capacitance, they will all exhibit a decrease in impedance as the frequency is increased. This is actually what is observed in all impedance measurements of the skin [5,6,8–15]. In addition, note that the capacitance associated with the skin is 10 times less than that calculated for a biological membrane [12]. This may be because of the presence of water in the skin, which could markedly influence the skin's dielectric constant [12].

Yamamoto and Yamamoto [8,9] showed that not only is the skin's impedance profile quite complex, but, in addition, it was demonstrated that the skin's impedance changes in a very complex manner. In particular, the skin's impedance depends on the season, the time of day at which the impedance is determined, the state of the subject studied, the site at which the impedance is measured, and the electrode paste used to make the impedance measurements. Other investigators have confirmed and amplified on these observations [10–12,14,15,17]. For example: DeNuzzio and Berner [12] demonstrated the important influence that the type of electrolyte present around the electrodes have on the skin's impedance; Clar et al. [10] showed that the time variation occurred not only during the day but from day to day; and Panescu et al. [14] demonstrated that the average impedance of the forearm was less than that for the palm.

Since hydration of the skin has been shown to be the primary variable influencing the skin's impedance [7,10,11,18], one can speculate that the time variation in the skin's impedance may be a strong function of the time variation of the skin's hydration. The reason for the skin's profound dependence on hydration results from the skin's hydroscopic nature [15] coupled with water's significant impact on the skin's dielectric constant [12]. The skin's hydroscopic characteristic is speculated to be in part due to the presence of amino acids in the skin [15]. Hydration probably influences the skin's dielectric constant because the following components are sensitive to an electric field [7]: (a) The keratin protein chains contained in the stratum corneum have a dipole moment. Thus, as the stratum corneum becomes more hydrated, the keratin becomes more flexible and responsive to an applied electric field. (b) As the stratum corneum becomes more hydrated, the ions in the stratum corneum become freer to move and thus more responsive to an applied electric field.

The profound variability in the skin's impedance is one of the primary problems in the application of impedance spectroscopy to the study of the skin. It is thus necessary to control or remove as many factors as possible that lead to the variability in skin impedance before useful information can be obtained from impedance measurements [9]. Several methods have been proposed that can be implemented to decrease the variability of impedance measurements. Such methods include the following:

1. The use of bilateral impedance measurements (e.g., impedance measurements using the right and left forearms) [10].

2. Control of the humidity coupled with sufficient time for equilibration of the subject's skin with moisture in the environment [9].
3. Since the temperature coefficient of electrical conductance is about 2% per degree centigrade, temperature control is important [14,17].
4. Use of an electrode contact fluid whose composition should be balanced according to the relative humidity of the environment such that water exchange between the skin and the environment is not altered [10,15].
5. Because at the millimeter scale different regions of the skin have very different electrical characteristics [14,19–22], electrode dimensions should be on the order of 1 cm^2. For human skin in vivo, this is due in part to the presence of sweat glands, which can represent low-impedance pathways when activated [17].
6. Prevention of electrolyte spread from gel electrodes. If this is not minimized, the impedance can decrease markedly with time. This is because the effective area of the electrode is increased as the electrolyte spreads. The increase in effective contact area then results in a decrease in impedance [6,23].
7. The electrolyte beneath the electrode can penetrate into the skin. If this occurs, the measured impedance will decrease with time [23]. Since electrolyte penetration is to a certain extent unavoidable and its effect depends on the type of electrolyte [11,12]. Yamamoto [11] has recommended using a frequency higher than 10 kHz when performing impedance measurements. At frequencies higher than 10 kHz, Yamamoto demonstrated that the impedance measurement was less dependent on the electrolyte composition. Operating at a higher frequency has the added advantage of minimizing the artifact produced by electrode polarization [7].
8. Electrolysis at the electrodes needs to be minimized, since this will alter electrolyte composition. Partly for this reason, impedance measurements should be made at current densities on the order of 1 $\mu A/cm^2$ or less [17]. Making impedance measurements at 1 $\mu A/cm^2$ or less has the added advantage of minimizing iontophoresis and electroosmosis, which can decrease the skin's impedance with time [16,17].

Even when all of these procedures are implemented, the variability is still great enough that one can generally only use relative impedance measurements for analysis purposes [7].

B. Inferences About the Effect of Cosmetics, Disease, and Permeability Enhancers on Skin Through the Use of Impedance Spectroscopy

Cosmetics influence primarily the stratum corneum's hydration state and therefore have a marked influence on the skin's impedance [7,10]. Despite the problems associated with making accurate impedance measurements, impedance spectroscopy represents the simplest way to get a relative measurement of hydration [7]. By restricting the range of frequencies to 5 Hz to 1 kHz, the measured skin impedance will be due primarily to the stratum corneum [10]. Thus, the skin-moisturizing capabilities of various cosmetics can be assessed. In particular, it has been found that at a frequency of 25 Hz, the measured impedance provides a good indicator of the short- and long-term effects of hydrating agents [10]. Studies have revealed that skin emollients do indeed have water-supplying ability [15].

When an agent such as formaldehyde or urea is applied to the skin, changes in the skin's impedance are observed [18]. It is believed that formaldehyde increases the ratio of unbound to bound water, thus possibly explaining why formaldehyde lowers the skin's resistance [18]. In contrast, urea is observed to increase the skin's resistance. It is speculated that this results because urea increases the amount of bound water in the skin [18]. Also, it appears that the most hydrophilic material does not necessarily produce the greatest effect on the skin's impedance [7]. For example, glycerol decreases the skin's impedance to greater extent than does pyrrolidone carboxylic acid. In addition, it was observed that petrolatum has an occlusive property [15].

Since irritants also influence the hydration state and the integrity of the skin, impedance spectroscopy provides a useful method for the quantification of skin irritant effects. The chief irritant studied has been sodium lauryl sulfate (SLS) [24–26]. Studies show that as the dose of SLS was increased, the amount of decrease in impedance was also increased [26]. By following the skin's impedance after the application of SLS, changes in the skin's conductivity showed up well before any visual signs of skin irritation were detectable [24]. In addition, it was demonstrated that exposure to SLS resulted in a gradual loss in the skin's barrier properties [24]. Finally, skin lotions have been shown to decrease the damage (as assessed by the degree the skin's impedance has decreased) caused to the skin by SLS.

Penetration enhancers such as azone and dodecyl N, N-dimethylaminoacetate appear to increase the skin's impedance [13]. The authors speculate that this may be related to the fact that these enhancers increase the skin's heterogeneity (as assessed, in part, by an observed increase in the skin's fractal dimension) [13]. The authors also speculate that in the case of azone the increase in impedance may also be the result of the formation of an isolating layer.

Impedance spectroscopy has been used in the assessment of skin diseases such as eczema and psoriasis [7]. However, these studies suffer in that these diseases exhibit cracking of the skin. This cracking implies that defective electrode contact is probably made during impedance measurement [7].

C. Inferences About the Effect of Iontophoresis on the Skin Through the Use of Impedance Spectroscopy

The skin's impedance decreases markedly during iontophoresis and then after the cessation of the iontophoresis recovers. After iontophoresis, the impedance recovery is asymptotic, approaching a final value that is less than was observed before iontophoresis began [16]. The rate of decrease in skin resistance is strongly dependent on the applied potential drop across the skin [27]. The greater the potential drop, the more rapid the decrease in resistance [27]. The recovery times for the skin's resistance were found to be dependent on both the duration and the magnitude of the applied electric field [27]. The authors note that these results parallel those found in the electrical breakdown and recovery of bilayer membranes (electroporation [27]. This, they suggest, implies that iontophoresis at a voltage of 2 V using wet electrodes can induce pore formation in the human epidermal membrane and that these pores explain the associated changes in permeability that are observed [27]. However, other authors apparently disagree with this electroporation explanation [14,17]. Both Grimnes [17] and Panescu et al. [14] state that rapid skin breakdown occurred only when dry electrodes were used and at voltages that were much greater than 2 V. Part of the apparent discrepancy may be because Grimnes' [17] and Panescu et al.'s [14] studies were conducted on human volunteers, whereas Inada's studies [27] were carried out on immersed excised human skin.

The passive flux of sodium ions was shown to be highly correlated ($r^2 = 0.98$) to the inverse of the skin's impedance [16]. Note that since this impedance was measured at 0.2 Hz, it represents mainly the skin's electrical resistance. A weaker correlation was obtained for the passive flux of tritiated water [19]. This was found to be true both before and after the application of iontophoresis [16]. Since iontophoresis decreases the skin's impedance, the passive flux was greater after iontophoresis than before iontophoresis [16]. Inada et al. [27] have also demonstrated for tetraethylammonium ion and mannitol that their passive and iontophoretic fluxes are related to the reciprocal of the skin's resistance. In addition, Inada et al. [27] showed that the higher the applied voltage, the greater the drop in skin resistance, which resulted in a higher flux being obtained.

Impedance measurements have been carried out on skin that has been exposed to direct current (DC) iontophoresis and to pulsed depolarization (PD) iontophoresis [28]. Both DC (0.1 mA) and PD (3.0 mA) iontophoresis treated skin did not show any invasion of neutrophiles or any acute inflammation. This histological assessment of skin damage suggested that neither the DC nor the PD iontophoresis caused any skin damage. However, DC iontophoresis did decrease the skin's impedance more than was observed in the case of PD iontophoresis. These results suggest that the DC iontophoretically treated skin sustained slightly more damage than the PD iontophoretically treated skin. Upon application of iontophoresis, the authors suggest that the observed decrease in skin resistance was due to both hydration and damage to the skin.

IV. SUMMARY

Impedance spectroscopy is a remarkably versatile technique for investigating conductive and dielectric properties of electrically active systems. As summarized in this work, it has been applied in numerous studies to evaluate the physical/chemical nature of skin and to understand the transport of ions through human skin.

It is generally accepted that the stratum corneum represents the primary electrical barrier in skin. Though impedance results vary from subject to subject and from site to site on the same individual, the electrical response of skin can be modeled as a simple *RC* network. Nonideal behavior is associated with environmental conditions, the hydration of the skin, and the integrity of the stratum corneum.

REFERENCES

1. MacDonald, J. R. and Johnson, W. B. Fundamentals of impedance spectroscopy. In: J. R. MacDonald, ed. *Impedance Spectroscopy.* New York, Wiley and Sons, 1987, pp. 1–26.
2. Edelberg, R. Electrical properties of skin. In: *Biophysical Properties of Skin.* Harry Elden, ed. New York, Wiley-Interscience, 1971, pp. 513–549.
3. Archer, W., Kohli, R., Roberts, J. and Spencer, T. Skin Impedance Measurement. In: R. Rietschel and T. Spencer, eds. *Methods for Cutaneous Investigation.* New York, Dekker,

4. Gabrielli, C. *Use and Applications of Electrochemical Impedance Techniques.* Solartron Instruments, Schlumberger Technologies, England, Technical Report 12860013, 1990.

5. Yamamoto, T. and Yamamoto, Y. Electrical properties of the epidermal stratum corneum. *Med. Biol. Eng. ??? 151, 1976.*

6. Rosell, J., Colominas, J., Riu, P., Pallas-Areny, R. and Webster, J. G. Skin impedance from 1 Hz to 1 MHz. *IEEE Trans. Biomed. Eng. 35*:649, 1988.

7. Leveque, J. L. and De Rigal, J. Impedance methods for studying skin moisturization. *J. Soc. Cosmet. Chem. 34*:419, 1983.

8. Yamamoto, T. and Yamamoto, Y. Analysis for the change of skin impedance. *Med. & Biol. Eng. & Comput. 15*:219, 1977.

9. Yamamoto, T. and Yamamoto, Y. The measurement principle for evaluating the performance of drugs and cosmetics by skin impedance. *Med. & Biol. Eng. & Comput. 16*:623, 1978.

10. Clar, E. J., Her, C. P. and Sturelle, C. G. Skin impedance and moisturization. *J. Soc. Cosmet. Chem. 26*:337, 1975.

11. Yamamoto, Y. Measurement and analysis of skin electrical impedance. *Acta Derm. Venereol. (Stockh) Suppl. 185*:34, 1994.

12. DeNuzzio, J. D. and Berner, B. Electrochemical and iontophoretic studies of human skin. *J. Controlled Release 11*:105, 1990.

13. Kontturi, K., Murtomaki, L., Hirvonen, J., Paronen, P. and Urtti, A. Electrochemical characterization of human skin by impedance spectroscopy: The effect of penetration enhancers. *Pharm. Res. 10*:381, 1993.

14. Panescu, D., Cohen, K. P., Webster, J. G. and Statbucker, R. A. The mosaic electrical characteristics of the skin. *40*:434, 1993.

15. Tagami, H., Ohi, M., Iwatsuki, K., Kanamaru, Y., Yamada, M. and Ichijo, B. Evaluation of the skin surface hydration in vivo by electrical measurement. *J. Invest. Dermatol. 75*:500, 1980.

16. Burnette, R. R. and Bagniefski, T. M. Influence of constant current iontophoresis on impedance and passive permeability of excised nude mouse skin. *J. Pharm. Sci. 77*:492, 1988.

17. Grimnes, S. Skin impedance and electro-osmosis in human epidermis. *Med. Biol. Eng. Comput. 21*:739, 1983.

18. Campbell, S. D., Kraning, K. K., Schibli, E. G. and Momii, T. Hydration characteristics and electrical resistivity of stratum corneum using a noninvasive four-point microelectrode method. *J. Invest. Dermatol. 69*:290, 1977.

19. Burnette, R. R. and Ongpipattanakul, B. Characterization of the pore transport properties and tissue alteration of excised human skin during iontophoresis. *J. Pharm. Sci. 77*:132, 1988.

20. Cullander, C. and Guy, R. H. Visualization of iontophoretic pathways with confocal microscopy and the vibrating probe electrode. *Solid State Ionics 53–56*:197, 1992.

21. Cullander, C. and Guy, R. H. Sites of iontophoretic current flow into the skin:

Identification and characterization with the vibrating probe electrode. *J. Invest. Dermatol.* *97*:55, 1993.

22. Grimnes, S. Pathways of ionic flow through human skin in vivo. *Acta Derm. Venenreol. (Stockh.)* *64*:93, 1984.

23. Grimnes, S. Impedance measurement of individual skin surface electrodes. *Med. Biol. Eng. Comput.* *21*:750, 1983.

24. Serban, G. P., Henry, S. M. and Cotty, V. F. In vivo evaluation of skin lotions by electrical capacitance: I. The effect of several lotions on the progression of damage and healing after repeated insult with sodium lauryl sulfate. *J. Soc. Cosmet. Chem.* *32*:407, 1981.

25. Ollmar, S. and Emtestam, L. Electrical impedance index in human skin: Measurements after occlusion, in five anatomical regions and in mild irritant contact dermatitis. *Contact Dermatitis* *28*:104, 1993.

26. Ollmar, S., Nyren, M., Nicander, I. and Emtestam, L. Electrical impedance compared with other non-invasive bioengineering techniques and visual scoring for detection of irritation in human skin. *Br. J. Dermatol.* *130*:29, 1994.

27. Inada, H., Ghanem, A. and Higuchi, W. I. Studies on the effects of applied voltage and duration on human epidermal membrane alteration/recovery and the resultant effects upon iontophoresis. *Pharm. Res.* *11*:687, 1994.

28. Numajiri, S., Sakurai, H., Sugibayashi, K., Morimoto, Y., Omiya, H., Takenaka, H. and Akiyama, N. Comparison of depolarizing and direct current systems on iontophoretic enhancement of transport of sodium benzoate through human and hairless rat skin. *J. Pharm. Pharmacol.* *45*:610, 1993.

7

Neutrons, Surfaces, and Skin

Adam C. Watkinson
An-eX Analytical Services, Ltd., Cardiff, Wales

Jonathan Hadgraft and Paul R. Street
University of Wales College of Cardiff, Cardiff, Wales

Randal W. Richards
University of Durham, Durham, England

I. INTRODUCTION

In order to optimize formulations that are to be placed on the skin for local or transdermal drug delivery, it is important to know the mechanisms by which the drug penetrates the skin. The barrier function of the skin may be modified by the absorption of formulation excipients or penetration enhancers that have been deliberately incorporated into the device. It is therefore relevant to consider how these act. The precise mechanism by which drugs penetrate the skin is still a matter of debate, but it is generally thought that many materials diffuse through the stratum corneum through a tortuous pathway around the dead keratinocytes. The matrix that makes up the "cement" that is present in the intercellular channels is a complex array of lipids. The approximate composition is 50% ceramides (predominantly ceramide 6), 25% cholesterol, 15% free fatty acids, and 5% cholesterol sulfate. The important feature of these lipids is that they structure themselves into fairly solid, ordered bilayer arrays. A diffusing molecule therefore has to cross a sequence of bilayers before it encounters either the viable tissue, where is required to act locally, or the blood supply if it is to act systemically. It is the nature of these bilayers that makes the skin a very impermeable membrane.

It is therefore of importance to determine how diffusing molecules and potential penetration enhancers interact with the structured lipids. This can be achieved using a number of spectroscopic techniques, which is the subject of other chapters in this book. Here the use of monolayers and neutron scattering is considered as techniques that can probe the molecular features of ordered lipids and how the ordering may be affected by the presence of enhancers.

One of the problems in dealing with skin is the large biological variability encountered. This is possibly due to the heterogeneous nature of the lipids. In this chapter we have chosen to concentrate on simple lipid structures to provide some insight into molecular interactions that probably occur in the skin. The work demonstrates the power of the techniques and potential pitfalls that can be encountered when using complex membranes such as the skin.

Model membranes have been used, such as multilamellar vesicles composed of dipalmitoyl phosphatidylcholine. It is appreciated that there are no phospholipids in the skin, but the types of interactions expected are similar, and interpretation of the results is much easier, when the lipid is pure. In order to simplify interpretation further, experiments with monolayers have been conducted and the results interpreted in light of published information.

II. MONOMOLECULAR FILMS

One of the most useful and more accessible experimental techniques allowing the behavior of molecules within membranes to be modeled is the study of monolayers. The easiest type of experiments to undertake in this field is the measurement of simple area/pressure isotherms using a Langmuir film balance.

A Langmuir film consists of a monomolecular layer of amphiphiles spread onto a liquid subphase (usually water) via deposition from a volatile solvent. The solvent is allowed to evaporate, leaving the molecules free to orient themselves in the two-dimensional environment at the interface (with their hydrophilic headgroups in the water and their hydrophobic tails in the atmosphere above the water surface). The molecules dissolve or evaporate only to a very limited extent, due to the insolubility of the hydrocarbon chains and the strong headgroup interaction with the water, respectively.

The characteristics of a monolayer are studied by measuring the changes in surface pressure upon compressing and/or expanding the monolayer. These changes are usually measured by means of a Wilhelmy plate hung from a microbalance that dips into the subphase surface. The plot of surface pressure against area per molecule is known as a "pressure-area isotherm" (because compression takes place at a constant temperature). When the monolayer is in the two-dimensional solid or fully condensed phase, the molecules are closely packed enough for quantitative information regarding molecular cross-sectional area to be ascertained by extrapolation of the isotherm to zero pressure. These measurements have been shown to agree with those values obtained by computer modeling.

The use of this simple technique has shed light on the mechanisms by which Azone® and oleic acid may exert their well-documented enhancing effects. The study of mixed monolayers of dipalmitoylphosphatidylcholine (DPPC) and Azone or oleic acid (Lewis and Hadgraft, 1990) has revealed, in some detail, possible differences in the way in which these compounds may act as enhancers. Monolayer experiments have also been used to examine the behavior of a complex mixture of lipids (representing those in the stratum corneum) and the way in which these are affected by the presence of Azone (Schuckler and Lee, 1991). Although there are many interesting results in the literature arising from such experiments, it is perhaps these that are the most relevant. Therefore, it is on these results that this section will primarily concentrate.

Studies using the phospholipid DPPC as a model for the stratum corneum lipids are very much simpler to conduct than those involving complex lipid mixtures and are thus more often employed. Figure 1 depicts a typical compression isotherm for a DPPC monolayer with its clearly visible liquid-expanded/liquid-condensed (LE/LC) transition region. This situation is directly analogous (Blume, 1979) to that observed by light-scattering techniques (e.g., Beastall et al., 1988) on heating liposomes of DPPC through their phase-transition temperature.

The phase change seen when heating DPPC liposomes involves a decrease in turbidity of the liposomal suspension due to a decrease in their refractive index. This decrease in light scattering occurs because the chains of the lipid are no longer in an ordered trans configuration but contain significantly more gauche conformers, making the refraction of light less efficient. In a monolayer experiment, the change seen on compression of a DPPC film in the pressure range 0–40 mN N^{-1} is from a less ordered system, at low pressure, to a more ordered system at high pressure. The difference between the "starting states" of the lipid chains in the liposome and monolayer experiments is explained by the relatively high surface pressure of a liposome (about 30 mN m^{-1}) at which, according to the DPPC pressure–area isotherm, the lipid chains are in an ordered or trans state; i.e., it is the structural restraints within a liposome that create a high internal surface pressure and make the chains adopt a predominantly trans conformation.

Any changes in the position or magnitude of the LC/LE transition of a

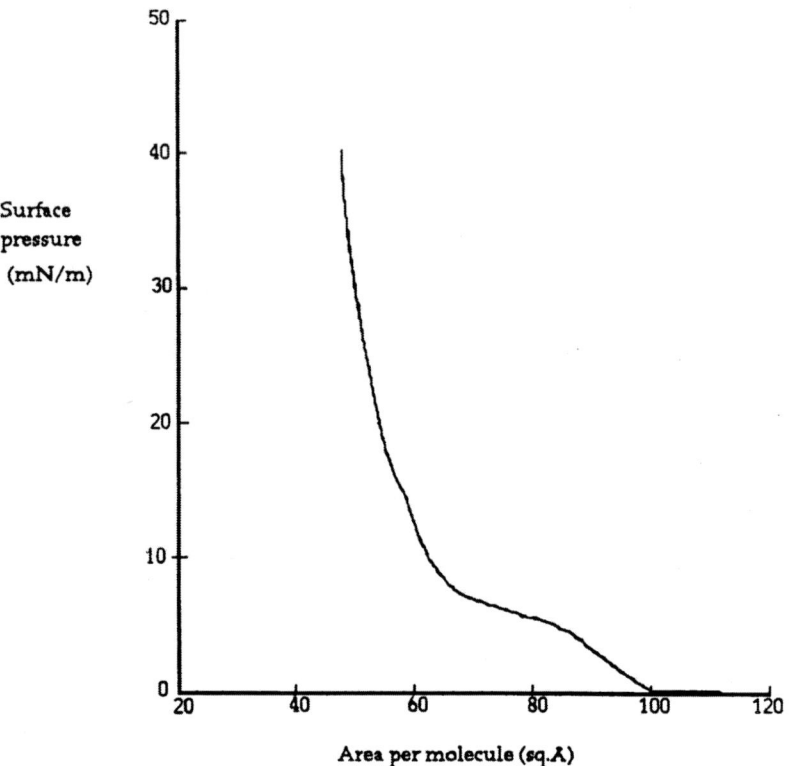

Figure 1 Compression isotherm of pure DPPC monolayer.

DPPC/enhancer mixed monolayer are indicative of a change in the state of the alkyl chains of the lipid in that monolayer.

A.   Oleic Acid/DPPC Monolayers

The effect of the incorporation of a secondary compound such as Azone or oleic acid (OA) into monolayers of DPPC is dramatic. In the case of oleic acid, the LE/LC transition is slowly abolished (at 10% OA, the effect is significant in that the surface pressure at which the transition occurs is raised) on increasing the ratio of enhancer to lipid. It is completely removed at concentrations above 50% enhancer (Lewis and Hadgraft, 1990).

       The effect is thought to arise from destabilization of the LC phase of the phospholipid, with a concurrent increase in chain disorder and consequent disruption of the cooperativity of the LE/LC transition. This type of effect has been inferred from many studies on the effect of unsaturated lipids on membrane structure (Stubbs and Smith, 1984) and is reflected in plots of molecular area against monolayer composition at fixed surface pressures where, on inclusion of OA, there is some positive deviation (Lewis and Hadgraft, 1990; Street and Hadgraft, unpublished data) from ideal mixing in the LC region (measured at 15 mN m^{-1}). Indeed, it has been shown by external reflectance FTIR (Mitchell and Dluhy, 1988) that in the region of the LE/LC transition, a film of DPPC exhibits a biphasic character where there is coexistence of fluid and solid phases of lipid (gauche and trans chain states). The inclusion of OA will presumably shift this equilibrium in favor of the LE phase, resulting in expansion of the monolayer.

Oleic acid, therefore, appears to disrupt lipid packing without producing a great expansion of the monolayer. The reason for this relatively small expansion from ideality has been explained in terms of a reorganization of DPPC packing that allows easier accommodation of the OA. DPPC has a large headgroup cross section (relative to that of the alkyl chains), resulting in a tilted orientation at the interface in both the LE and LC phases (Hauser et al., 1981). It is thought that the OA molecules can therefore be accommodated within the monolayer, to some extent, by "straightening up" the DPPC molecules relative to the interface. This process would allow significant free-volumes to be created, which could then be filled by the much smaller OA molecules. This type of explanation has been used to explain partially the condensing effect of cholesterol on phospholipid monolayers (Presti, 1985).

If, as suggested by FTIR data, the situation here involves two, essentially separate, phases of OA and DPPC, one might expect a two-stage collapse in isotherms of mixed monolayers of these two components. Although it has been concluded that in the gel phase, complete separation of oleic acid and DPPC is unlikely (Lewis and Hadgraft, 1990), there is evidence from biphasic-type collapse pressures of OA/DPPC monolayers that a fair degree of phase separation does occur. It is well established that some degree of phase separation is likely in most biphasic systems, and there are several excellent review articles on this theme (e.g., Jain, 1983).

Mixed monolayers of OA and DPPC do appear to exhibit "squeeze-out" at surface pressures above that of the collapse pressure of oleic acid (about 32 mN m^{-1}), implying the coexistence of two separate phases at these higher pressures (Street et al., unpublished data). The surface pressures at which squeeze-out begins are composition dependent and always greater than the collapse pressure of a pure OA monolayer. The pressure of onset increases as the DPPC/OA ratio increases, possibly implying some increase in the degree of miscibility with this compositional change. This behavior has also been documented for a series of OA esters for which squeeze-out from OA ester/DPPC monolayers begins above the collapse pressure of the pure ester (Street and Hadgraft, 1992). In these studies, squeeze-out of the esters began at lower pressures than that of OA due to the lower equilibrium spreading pressures of the compounds involved. The fact that the onset pressure of squeeze-out is composition dependent suggests perhaps that phase separation occurs only at those pressures approaching that of collapse. If components were phase separated at lower pressures, then the onset pressure of squeeze-out would always be the same, being equal to the collapse pressure of the pure monolayer. The mixing behavior of oleic acid and DPPC has been found to be apparently ideal at pressures above those around the LC region (Lewis and Hadgraft, 1990), implying either complete miscibility or immiscibility at these pressures. This, coupled with the squeeze-out behavior and the expansion from ideality at lower pressures, further enhances the argument that phase separation is a pressure-dependent phenomenon and that in these systems it occurs only at fairly high surface pressures. Even if this is the case, it is still quite possible that separate phases of OA exist in bilayers and indeed in the lamellar lipid sheets of the stratum corneum, because the pressures in these systems may be high enough to induce phase separation.

There are many cases in which other techniques have been applied to biphasic systems in order to establish the nature of mixing. For example, fluorescence microscopy of DPPC monolayers containing 2% of a fluorescent probe have shown the coexistence of solid and fluid phases of DPPC at intermediate pressures (Weis, 1991). Similar results have been achieved with a variety of other phospholipids using the same technique (Vaz et al., 1989). The recent application of laser light scattering to this area (Street et al., unpublished data) has yet to produce any conclusive evidence, but the future for this particular technique is also promising. It also provides information about the viscoelastic properties of the monolayer and how these are affected by the inclusion of penetration enhancers.

B. Azone/DPPC Monolayers

A second and potentially more potent enhancer of percutaneous absorption that has received much attention in recent years is Azone. Compressional investigation of monolayers consisting of Azone and DPPC have revealed much regarding its possible mechanism of action as an enhancer. The effect of Azone on the LC/LE phase transition of DPPC is very much greater than that of OA (the transition being abolished completely on incorporation of 30% Azone), and although Azone has a tendency to dissolve slowly into the subphase, a very considerable expansion from ideality occurs at even the lowest mole fraction investigated (0.1). Indeed, the maximum expansions recorded at low surface pressures are in the region of 33% over what would be expected if the mixing were ideal.

These expansions have been partially accounted for by the application of computer graphics to determine molecular areas of the components of the system. The headgroup cross-sectional area of DPPC has been calculated at 52 $Å^2$, and those of two energetically similar conformers of Azone were calculated as 45 $Å^2$ (end-on projection) and 58 $Å^2$ (ring face projection). Energy calculations revealed that although the linear form of Azone is the global energy minimum, the "bent" conformer is within 10 kcal mol^{-1} of it and thus easily achieved (Lewis and Hadgraft, 1990). In an interfacial region it seems reasonable to expect that the preferential interaction of the amide group with the water subphase might favor the adoption of the latter "bent" conformer and thus increase the area of the Azone headgroup. Under these conditions it is possible for the alkyl chains of the adjacent DPPC molecules to undergo greater freedom of rotation due to the low penetrative nature of the Azone molecule (Azone chain length C_{12}, DPPC chain length C_{16}) compared to the area it occupies in the monolayer. Large expansions from ideality of mixed monolayers of alkyl alcohols have also been accounted for (Shah and Shiao, 1975) by the induction of greater thermal motion in the longer-chain molecules propagating along the molecules toward the headgroup. This necessitates greater molecular areas at the interface to accommodate the flexing moieties.

It seems that a combination of the distorted Azone headgroup and the greater flexibility of lipid alkyl chains may account for the expansions seen. This may also explain why OA does not have as great an expansive effect on the monolayer in that it has a small headgroup and a long alkyl chain that will prevent any significant increase in DPPC chain mobility because of its depth of penetration into the hydrophobic regions of the monolayer. Indeed, further studies (Lewis et al., 1990) have revealed that increasing the length of the alkyl chain of the Azone molecule brings about a marked decrease in the observed deviation from ideality in mixed monolayers with DPPC. An Azone derivative with a C_{16} chain was found to mix seemingly ideally with DPPC, producing no deviation from ideality, whereas a derivative of the intermediate C_{14} chain length was found to induce small positive deviations. This trend is well reflected in the varying ability of Azone-type compounds to enhance percutaneous penetration. It has been found in vitro (with human skin) that the enhancement ratios of Azone analogs of different chain length are optimized at C_{12} (Hoogstraate et al., 1991). SAXS measurements (Bouwstra et al., 1992) have revealed that structural disruption of stratum corneum lamellae occurs on treatment with Azone derivatives and that this effect is greatest when the enhancer has a chain length of C_{10} or longer. These results confirm the suggestion that it is the spatial freedom given to the alkyl chains of the DPPC lipid that is an important factor in determining the mixing characteristics of these compounds.

The possibility of Azone forming a separate phase within the DPPC has been poorly investigated to date, although it can be inferred that, as with OA, it is only likely to occur at high surface pressures (from observations of squeeze-out behavior in mixed monolayers). This would account for the observed expansion from ideality (Lewis and Hadgraft, 1990) at low surface pressures and the composition-dependent nature (Street and Hadgraft, 1992) of the pressure at which squeeze-out begins.

C. Monolayers of Stratum Corneum Lipids

The lipid lamellae within the stratum corneum are thought to consist of a complex mixture of compounds but to contain predominantly cholesteryl sulfate (5%), free fatty acids (15%), cholesterol (25%), and ceramides (50%) (Abraham and Downing, 1990). Unlike DPPC monolayers, those formed from stratum corneum lipids do not undergo any obvious phase transitions during compression); therefore the information available from the resulting isotherms is more limited. The behavior of monolayers consisting of these types of compounds has been investigated in the presence and absence of Azone.

The pressure/area isotherm for a cholesterol monolayer is of a very noncompressible liquid condensed type (Ries, 1976). The compressibility of a cholesterol monolayer is increased only slightly on the introduction of low concentrations of Azone ($X_{Az} = 0.2$); but if the mole fraction of Azone in the film is increased to 0.4 and above, the compressibility increases dramatically and the film can be classed as liquid expanded. Another feature of these higher Azone concentrations is a small kink in the isotherm at approximately 32 mN m^{-1}. This pressure is equal to the collapse pressure of a pure Azone monolayer found by these workers, and the kink in the Azone/cholesterol isotherm may be due to squeeze-out of Azone (Schuckler and Lee, 1991).

A fairly detailed study of the behavior of various (Löfgren and Pascher, 1977) synthetic ceramide monolayers has been conducted in an attempt to ascertain the structural features of these compounds that determine the manner of their packing in bilayer systems. The most important finding in this work was probably that the presence of a 4,5-trans double bond in the lipid chain was generally found to improve the packing ability of these compounds. This result implies that in this case it is the conformational behavior of the chains that dictates the packing and not that of the headgroup.

Monolayers of pure ceramide (with the 4,5-trans double bond) show a slightly greater compressibility and are also more easily expanded by the presence of Azone than those of cholesterol (the change to LE occurring at X_{Az} = 0.15). Azone again appears to be squeezed out of the monolayer at the same pressures as in the cholesterol isotherms (Schuckler and Lee, 1991). Monolayers consisting of a mixture of bovine brain ceramides (BBC) have been shown to expand upon inclusion of Azone above the X_{Az} = 0.2 level (Harrison et al., 1993). In the same work it was found that cholesterol was better able to support Azone in a monolayer than BBC but that the inclusion of cholesterol in a BBC monolayer led to a decrease in its ability to support Azone (seen by an increase in squeeze-out or molecular loss). This was explained by hypothesizing that BBC and cholesterol interact strongly with each other to the exclusion of Azone and hence destabilize its presence in the monolayer.

A mixed monolayer consisting of stearic acid (9.9%), palmitic acid (36.8%), myristic acid (3.8%), oleic acid (33.1%), linoleic acid (12.5%), and palmitoleic acid (3.6%) produces an expanded area/pressure isotherm on which Azone has no apparent effect in terms of either expansion or compressibility (Schuckler and Lee, 1991). Squeeze-out of Azone from such films was not reported, but the surface pressures measured were not high enough for this to occur. The addition of cholesterol (to produce a 50:50 mixture) to this type of fatty acid monolayer results in a reduction of compressibility. However, the addition of ceramide has a much smaller condensing effect on the combined fatty acids (ratio 55:45), and the combination of all three components (free fatty acids/cholesterol/ceramide, 31:31:38) produces a liquid condensed film of moderate compressibility. The condensed nature of this film therefore results primarily from the presence of the membrane-stiffening cholesterol. In the presence of only small quantities of Azone (X_{Az} = 0.025), the mixed film becomes liquid expanded in nature, and there is also evidence of Azone squeeze-out at approximately 32 mN m^{-1}.

In general, these mixed monolayers seem to be destabilized by the presence of Azone, which causes a concentration-dependent transition from solid or liquid condensed behavior to a liquid expanded type of film. There is also substantial evidence that squeeze-out of Azone occurs in all cases and at similar pressures. It is therefore possible that Azone can exist as a separate phase in stratum corneum lipids at a lower pressure than in monolayers of DPPC. In either case it seems likely that Azone may well exist in pools in the stratum corneum.

Attempts at the measurement of permeation through these type of monolayers have also been undertaken. The rate of water loss from the subphase through the films was measured by following weight changes in a sample of adsorbent material (LiCl) suspended above the monolayer, as in the method of Barnes et al. (1980). Although the results gained are not conclusive because of a large scatter of data, it appears that both cholesterol and mixed lipid monolayers were made more permeable to water molecules in the presence of 40% Azone (Schuckler and Lee, 1991). The permeation of acetone through these films was not found to be substantially altered by the presence of Azone. This anomalous result was explained by suggesting that much of the acetone may be solubilized in the monolayer itself.

III. NEUTRON SPECTROSCOPY

To the majority of pharmaceutical and biological scientists, the neutron is simply part of the subatomic makeup of the molecules they study every day. In recent years, however, advances in particle physics have allowed the spectrum of people using neutron facilities, such as those at the Rutherford Appleton Laboratories (RAL), U.K., to broaden considerably. The application of neutron spectroscopy to the field of percutaneous penetration is not yet well established, but it has already produced some interesting results, and it is hoped that these will prompt further utilization of this powerful technique in this and other pharmaceutically oriented areas of research.

As mentioned earlier, the study of model monolayer and bilayer systems has become an integral part of the search for the mechanisms of percutaneous penetration and its enhancement. However, the extremely complex nature of the lipid structures that exist within the stratum corneum has promoted the use of simple mono- or biphasic models in experiments of this nature. Perhaps the most commonly used model for stratum corneum lipids is dipalmitoylphosphatidylcholine (DPPC); and although there are no phospholipids in the stratum corneum lipid matrix, this compound has served as a useful substitute and predictive model for their general behavior. In neutron spectroscopy the examination of multilamellar systems such as liposomes is often carried out using the technique of small-angle neutron scattering (SANS), and the study of monomolecular films is conducted using the method of neutron reflectometry. The following two sections describe these techniques and some of the recent experiments relevant to the field of percutaneous absorption that have been conducted using them.

A. Small-Angle Neutron Scattering (SANS)

Introduction

The basic principle of a SANS experiment is that a beam of neutrons is incident on a sample and the resultant pattern of scattered radiation intensity is examined. Much of the information that can be gained from SANS experiments is similar in nature to that produced by small-angle x-ray scattering studies (see Chapter 2). Indeed, the relationship between scattering vector, $\mathbf{Q}$, and Bragg repeat distance, d, is the same in both cases ($d = 2\pi/\mathbf{Q}$). However, there are several reasons why neutron scattering can often prove a more useful technique than x-ray scattering. Neutrons are principally scattered by atomic nuclei and not electrons (as x-rays are). Hence, because the nucleus is a point scatterer, the scattered intensity does not decrease with increasing scattering vector, $\mathbf{Q}$. (This is a significant advantage in high-resolution studies of structure.) Second, different isotopes of the same element may scatter neutrons differently; thus, using isotopic substitution, the scattering of chemically similar samples can be changed to great advantage. This approach is especially useful in the pharmaceutical sciences, because hydrogen and deuterium have coherent scattering lengths (b_i, the degree to which atoms scatter neutrons) that are opposite in sign, as shown with other examples in Table 1 (data taken from Richards, 1989, and Gray, 1972). The scattering length density of a molecule (ρ, the degree to which it scatters neutrons) is calculated from the coherent scattering lengths of its constituent atoms using Eq. 1,

$$\rho = N_A d \sum \frac{b_i}{M_m} \tag{1}$$

Table 1 Coherent Scattering Lengths, Incoherent Scattering Cross Sections, and Absorption Cross Sections for Some Elements

Element	Coherent scattering length (cm × 10^{12})	Incoherent scattering cross section (cm^2 × 10^{24})	Absorption cross section (cm^2 × 10^{24})
H	−0.374	79.9	0.33
D	0.667	2.00	0.00
C	0.665	0.00	0.00
N	0.936	0.46	1.88
O	0.580	0.00	0.00
P	0.510	—	—

where, b_i = scattering length of nucleus i in the scattering molecule, M_m = relative molecular mass of the scattering molecule, d = density of scattering substance, and N_A = Avogadro's number. That is, the calculation of scattering length density from individual nuclei is equivalent to identifying these nuclei as point scatterers over which the scattered intensity is averaged.

The intensity of the scattered neutron beam is related to numerous parameters, but a full discussion of these is not appropriate here. There are several texts that give a more detailed account of these variables and of SANS in general (e.g., Richards, 1989). However, one of the most important parameters in the determination of the pattern and intensity of scattered radiation is the contrast factor, as defined in Eq. 2,

$$K = (\rho_p - \rho_m)^2 \qquad\qquad\qquad (2)$$

where ρ_p and ρ_m = the scattering length densities of the particle and matrix (or solvent), respectively.

As a consequence of this relationship it is sometimes possible to "match out" the spectrum of a solute or a dispersed particle (reduce its scattering intensity to zero) by dissolving it in a solvent of the same scattering length density, i.e., produce a situation in Eq. 2 where $\rho_p = \rho_m$, making K equal to zero. When an aqueous solvent is required, this is often accomplished by using a mixture of H_2O and D_2O, where the ratio of the two components is adjusted to make the scattering length density of the mixture equal to that of the solute. Once this has been accomplished, other components can be incorporated into the system, and any scattering pattern that appears can be attributed solely to that component.

Simple Experiments Using SANS

There are several published reports on SANS studies carried out on aqueous dispersion of lipid in water. The measurement of interlamellar repeat distances within multilamellar liposomes is probably the most easily accomplished and reported type of experiment. The repeat distance measured is the length of the lipid molecule plus that of the water layer that separates the hydrophobic layers of the liposome (Fig. 2). This distance has been determined using the technique for several different lipid/water multilamellar systems. For example, the interlamellar repeat distance for multilamellar liposomes of DPPC has been measured by several workers as approximately 60 Å (Winter and Pilgrim, 1989; Martel and Ahmed, 1990; Watkinson et al., 1991). Figure 3 depicts typical SANS data for DPPC at different concentrations in D_2O and shows clear Bragg peaks at $\mathbf{Q} \cong 0.1$, corresponding to an interlamellar repeat distance

Repeat distance

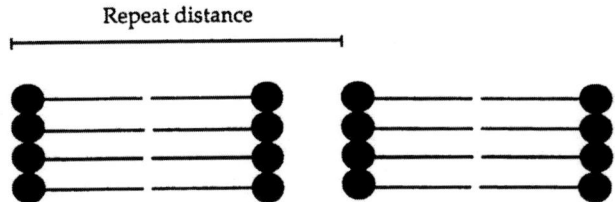

Figure 2   Repeat distance measured in a multilamellar system by SANS.

of 62 Å (data from Watkinson et al., 1991). The effective balance of resolution and intensity is obvious. By recording SANS data over a temperature gradient (22 to 43°C), the liquid-condensed (LC) to liquid-expanded (LE) phase transition of DPPC and the accompanying decrease in interlamellar spacing of approximately 30 Å has been followed using this technique (Winter and Pilgrim, 1989).

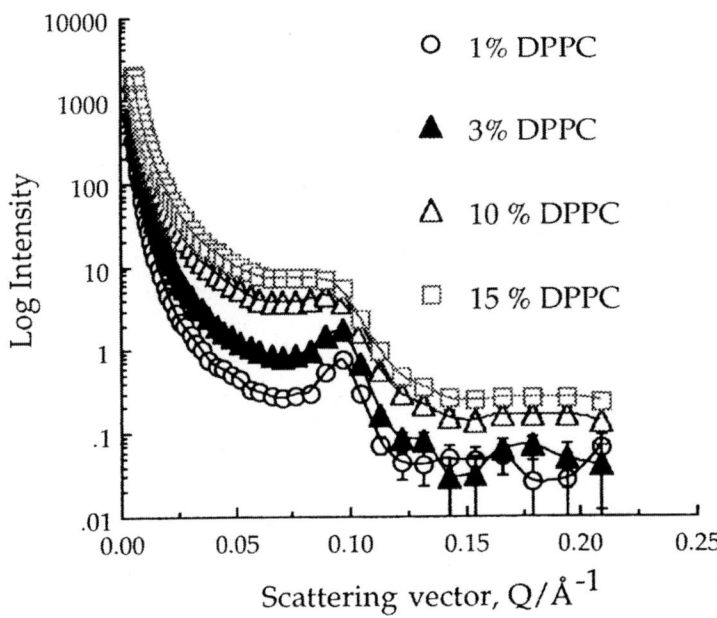

Figure 3   Effect of concentration on the SANS spectrum of DPPC multilamellar systems.

SANS and Percutaneous Penetration

Insight into the way in which oleic acid may act as a penetration enhancer can be gained by using the "matching-out" technique described earlier. As was first suggested by Ongpipattanakul et al. (1991), it may be possible that oleic acid does not distribute itself homogeneously in a lipid bilayer but forms discrete pools or islands in a sea of skin lipids. This type of oleic acid distribution will necessitate the formation of defects where the two species meet, and it has been suggested that it is along these interfacial defects that facilitated permeation occurs.

To investigate this phenomenon using neutron scattering, an experiment was devised (Watkinson et al., 1991) in which perdeuterated oleic acid was incorporated into a liposome of hydrogenous DPPC in a solvent of H_2O/D_2O such that the DPPC produced no spectrum—i.e., the DPPC was "matched out." Therefore, any spectrum produced should be due solely to the incorporated deuterated oleic acid. However, the oleic acid will produce a Bragg peak only if it is distributed within the liposome in a uniform manner. If the oleic acid is not distributed uniformly (which may be interpreted as its forming concentrated regions within the liposome), then no Bragg peak would be expected. The results of this experiment suggested that the oleic acid was not distributed in a regular pattern (there was no Bragg peak from the oleic acid), confirming the theory proposed by Ongpipattanakul et al. It should be pointed out that control experiments do need to be conducted and that this method of experimentation is still in its infancy. For example, it would be most useful to conduct experiments incorporating deuterated Azone into "matched-out" DPPC and look for the absence or presence of a Bragg peak in the neutron-scattering spectrum of such a system.

Unlike x-ray scattering [SAXS on stratum corneum produced a Bragg peak corresponding to the interlamellar repeat distance of the lipid bilayers (Bouwstra et al., 1992)], attempts at investigating the structure of stratum corneum using SANS have been largely unsuccessful. This is probably due to the need for a dense packet of material to be placed in the beam, for which, at present, the facilities are not available. However, several experiments have been attempted (Watkinson et al., 1991), and it is feasible that under the right conditions it would be possible to match out the spectrum of stratum corneum by hydrating it in an atmosphere of D_2O/H_2O (the correct ratio of these two components would have to be determined experimentally). Theoretically it would then be possible to incorporate molecules into stratum corneum and investigate their distribution within the skin. There are obviously many pitfalls associated with such a project, biological variation being possibly the greatest, but nevertheless it is one worth undertaking in the future.

B. Neutron Reflectometry

Introduction

Due to the wave–particle duality of neutrons, they can be reflected and refracted in a manner similar to light. Reflected neutron beams can interfere with each other to produce a reflected beam intensity that is characteristic of the reflecting material (Lekner, 1987). Detailed analysis of the reflectivity is able to able to provide information on the structural organization normal to the surface on which the beam is incident. Neutron reflectometry is particularly useful (vis à vis x-ray reflectometry), since selective isotopic labeling can be used to highlight particular regions of interest in a surface structure. This is especially valuable for monolayers on surfaces.

The Critical Reflection of Neutrons

Consider a beam of neutrons in medium 1 incident on a perfectly smooth surface of a medium 2 at an angle θ. Some of the beam is specularly reflected (angle of reflection = glancing incident angle), and some is refracted into medium 2 with an angle θ_2 (Fig. 4). A neutron refractive index can be defined for medium 2 as

$$n = \frac{k_1}{k_2} = 1 - \left(\frac{\lambda^2}{2\pi}\right)\rho_1 \tag{3}$$

where k_1 and k_2 are the neutron wave vectors in mediums 1 and 2, respec   ly, λ is the neutron wavelength, and ρ_1 is the scattering length density. Total reflection takes place at incident angles less than a critical angle θ_c, and

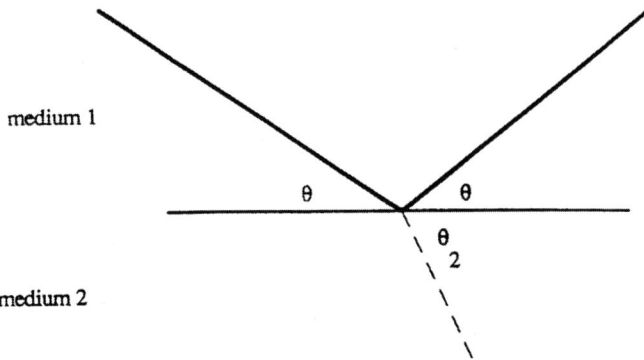

Figure 4 The critical reflection of neutrons.

$$\cos \theta_c = \frac{n_2}{n_1} \tag{4}$$

For small θ_c (generally the case), the cosine can be expanded and we obtain

$$\mathbf{Q}_c = 4\pi^{0.5}(\rho_1 - \rho_2)^{0.5} \tag{5}$$

Fresnel's equations can be used to calculate the dependence of the reflectivity [(reflected beam intensity)/(incident beam intensity)] on the incident angle expressed in terms of the scattering vector $\mathbf{Q}$ (Fig. 5),

$$R(\mathbf{Q}) = \left[\frac{\mathbf{Q} - (\mathbf{Q}^2 - \mathbf{Q}_c^2)^{0.5}}{\mathbf{Q} - (\mathbf{Q}^2 - \mathbf{Q}_c^2)^{0.5}} \right]^2 \tag{6}$$

where $\mathbf{Q}_c$ is the scattering vector corresponding to the critical incident angle θ_c; i.e., $\mathbf{Q}_c = (4\pi/\lambda) \sin \theta_c$.

If an intervening layer is now placed between the two media, the reflectivity will be modified due to interference effects between neutrons reflected from upper and lower interfaces. Apart from the incident angle, factors that determine the reflectivity are the scattering length density of the layer, the layer thickness, and the scattering length densities of the upper medium and the subphase.

The layer is described by an optical matrix, M (Born and Wolf, 1980), where

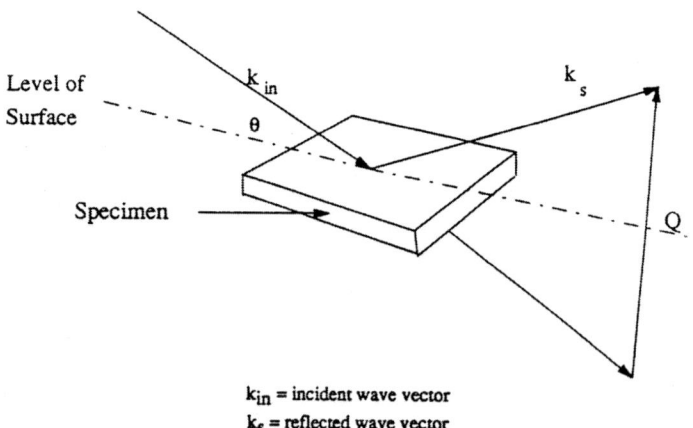

k_{in} = incident wave vector
k_s = reflected wave vector

Figure 5 Schematic of neutron reflection from a plane surface.

$$M = \begin{bmatrix} -\cos\beta & \left(\dfrac{-i}{p_l}\right)\sin\beta \\ -ip_l\sin\beta & \cos\beta \end{bmatrix} \tag{7}$$

This description can be applied to each layer if there are many layers on the subphase, and the relevant optical reflectivity matrix is then the product of all the separate matrices for the n layers.

$$M_r = [M_1][M_2]\cdots[M_n] \tag{8}$$

If the elements of this resultant matrix are indicated as M_{11}, M_{12}, etc., then the reflectivity is given by

$$R(\mathbf{Q}) = \left| \frac{(M_{11} + M_{12}p_2)p_1 - (M_{21} + M_{22})p_2}{(M_{11} + M_{12}p_2)p_1 - (M_{21} + M_{22})p_2} \right|^2 \tag{9}$$

and $\beta = (2\pi/\lambda)n_j d \sin\theta_j$ and $p_j = n_j \sin\theta_j$. Figure 6 shows the reflectivity, in the absence of background scattering, as a function of $\mathbf{Q}$, for a 20-Å-thick layer of scattering length density 3×10^{-6} Å^{-2} on a subphase with scattering length density zero, with air as the upper medium. Note that air has $\rho = 0$, and hence almost all other materials are optically less dense than air for neutrons. Since the scattering length density is determined by the composition of the layer, the

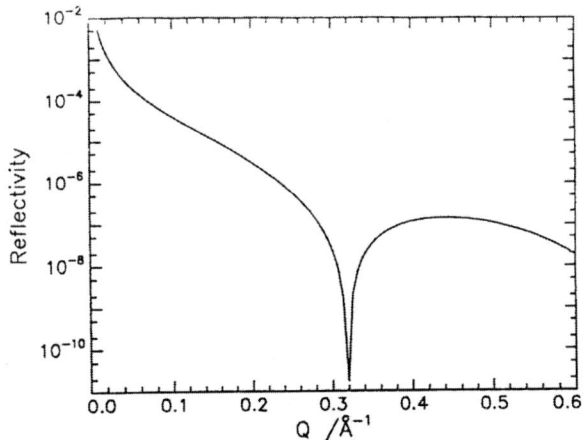

Figure 6 Reflectivity, in the absence of background scattering, as a function of $\mathbf{Q}$, for a 20-Å-thick layer of scattering length density 3×10^{-6} Å^{-2} on a subphase with scattering length density zero, with air as the upper medium.

neutron reflectometry can be used to determine the structure and composition distribution normal to the surface on which the neutron beam is incident, and the essence of a neutron reflectometry experiment is the determination of the intensity of the specular reflected beam as a function of incident angle or $\mathbf{Q}$.

Experimental Considerations

Instruments are now available that have been designed specifically for conducting neutron reflectometry experiments on a wide range of surfaces. One such instrument is the reflectometer CRISP at the ISIS pulsed neutron source, Rutherford Appleton Laboratory (RAL), Didcot, Oxon. (Penfold et al., 1987). CRISP permits a well-collimated neutron beam to impinge on horizontally positioned samples at fixed glancing angles in the range 0.25–1.5°. So-called "time of flight" (TOF) analysis determines the neutron wavelengths and enables CRISP to measure reflectivity profiles simultaneously over a wide range of neutron scattering vector $\mathbf{Q}$ ($= 4\pi \sin \theta/\lambda$). Other reflectometers, such as the D17 spectrometer at Institut Laue-Langevin, Grenoble, France, record reflectivity profiles over a wide range of $\mathbf{Q}$ using a monochromatic neutron beam and measuring reflectivity at a range of angles.

A typical neutron reflectometry experiment records the variation in the intensity of a specularly reflected neutron beam as a function of $\mathbf{Q}$. Often called a *reflectivity profile*, this is determined by the neutron refractive index profile perpendicular to the reflecting surface. The most commonly used method of data analysis relies on the calculation of theoretical reflectivity profiles for a model of the surface using the optical matrix method (e.g., Born and Wolf, 1975). The model of the surface specifies the neutron refractive index profile normal to the surface in terms of a number of discrete elements, and its theoretical reflectivity profile is calculated. This theoretical reflectivity profile is fitted to the experimental data using an automatic regression routine, and the thickness and scattering length density parameters of each layer are adjusted in order to obtain the best possible fit. Reflectometry data for insoluble monolayers are analyzed in terms of one- or two-layer models of the surface layer, and the thickness of the layers d_{fit} can be related directly to the molecular dimensions of the film. The scattering length density ρ_{fit} of a layer is the volume-fraction-weighted sum of all the components present:

$$\rho_{fit} = \sum \alpha_i \rho_{i,\text{theory}} \tag{10}$$

where α_i is the volume fraction of component i and $\rho_{i,\text{theory}}$ is its theoretical scattering length density, calculated from Eq. 2. This allows the volume fraction of water in the headgroup region, or air in the alkyl-chain region, to be calculated.

The most important features of neutron reflectometry experiments are related to the way in which isotopic substitution can be used to highlight specific regions of an interface. Due to the very different scattering lengths of hydrogen and deuterium (discussed earlier), the reflectivity profiles of deuterated materials are markedly different from their protonated equivalents. For example, the scattering length density of H_2O is -0.562×10^{-6} Å^{-2}, whereas that for D_2O is 6.34×10^{-6} Å^{-2}. This important feature is utilized to produce a mixture of H_2O and D_2O that has a scattering length density of zero, the same as air. This mixture gives no specular reflection of neutrons at any angle and is referred to as *air contrast-matched water* (ACMW) or *null-reflecting water*. Therefore a neutron beam incident on a film spread at the air/ACMW interface will be reflected only by the air–monolayer and monolayer–water boundaries. In other words, the neutron beam "sees" surfaces only where there is contrast between the scattering length densities of materials. Moreover, by using selective H/D substitution in the monolayer components, and replacing ACMW by D_2O, it is possible to change the location of the contrast and to highlight different regions of the film. Reflectivity profiles can therefore be obtained for isotopic variations of a system whose physical chemistry is not radically changed by H/D substitution. In analyzing the results of such experiments, the proposed chemical model of the interface must fit all the experimental data.

The Application of Neutron Reflectometry

Neutron reflectometry has been applied to the study of a variety of surfaces, including solid polymeric films, ferromagnetic films, and pure liquid surfaces (Penfold and Thomas, 1990). The technique has also been used in conjunction with Langmuir film balance apparatus to study the adsorption of compounds at the air–water interface, e.g., alkyl trimethylammonium bromide surfactants (Lee et al., 1989), fatty acids (e.g., Grundy et al., 1988), and a variety of polymeric compounds (e.g., Henderson et al., 1991; Henderson, 1993).

Recently, the investigation of monolayer models of biological membranes by neutron reflectometry has received some attention. For example, the changes in the structure of monolayers of dimyristoylphosphatidylglycerol (DMPG) and dimyristoylphosphatidylcholine (DMPC), which accompany the transition from an expanded to a condensed state, were reported by Bayerl et al. (1990). Monolayers composed of a mixture of perdeuterated DMPC and DMPG in the ratio 7:3 were deposited on D_2O and ACMW subphases to provide different points of contrast in the system. Data analysis by the optical matrix method involved one- and two-layer models of the monolayer. The thickness of the monolayer increased, as expected, from 19.5 Å in the expanded state to 22.5 Å in a compressed state. More surprisingly the volume fraction of water in the headgroup region of the expanded monolayer was very large ($\alpha = 0.76$), which indicated that the transition of phospholipids between expanded and condensed phases was associated with considerable changes in the hydration state of the headgroup, possibly due to the dehydration of the glycerol backbone of DMPC molecules. Similar experiments on DPPC monolayers enabled Vaknin et al. (1991) to estimate a variety of structural parameters for condensed DPPC monolayers, such as molecular volume, chain tilt, and the thickness of the lipid headgroups and hydrocarbon chains. From a knowledge of the volume of water molecules, the number associated with the lipid headgroup was estimated. Neutron reflectometry has also been used to study unilamellar phospholipid bilayers adsorbed onto planar solid surfaces submerged in an aqueous phase (Johnson et al., 1991a).

An obvious extension of this work is to study the interaction of compounds on the structure of model membranes using neutron reflectometry. The first study of this kind examined the interaction between the protein spectrin and phospholipid monolayers (Johnson et al., 1991b). Results indicated that spectrin did not significantly alter the thickness of the headgroup of alkyl-chain regions of DMPC monolayers, but the molecular area of the film increased due to penetration of spectrin into the monolayer. This interaction between spectrin and phospholipids is thought to be driven by hydrophobic effects. The volume fraction of spectrin in the headgroup region was estimated to be around 0.09, and a reduction in packing density of lipid acyl chains was observed. Similar studies on monolayers of DMPC/DMPG, in the ratio 7:3, found that the volume fraction of spectrin in the headgroup region increased to 0.22 due to additional electrostatic interaction between the spectrin molecules and the lipid, which carries a net negative charge. The interactions between spectrin and phospholipids have been shown to increase the permeability of membranes toward ionic and polar species, and it has been suggested that these interactions are important in the maintenance of separate gel and liquid-crystalline phases within phospholipid membranes.

Neutron Reflectometry and Skin Penetration Enhancers

The studies just outlined indicate that neutron reflectometry has considerable potential for studying the mode of actions of skin penetration enhancers at a molecular level. Of particular interest in the field of percutaneous absorption is the nature of the interactions between oleic acid (OA) and the structured lipids of the stratum corneum. Phospholipids, although absent from the stratum corneum, are often used to illustrate the general behavior of biological membranes, and, since they are widely available in a variety of deuterated forms, they are ideal for use in neutron reflectometry experiments.

Neutron reflectometry studies on mixed DPPC/oleic acid monolayers have been conducted using the CRISP reflectometer at RAL. First, the structure of DPPC monolayers was determined by measuring reflectivity profiles from three different isotopic forms of the DPPC monolayer system. This was achieved using hydrogenated (h-DPPC) and chain perdeuterated (d-DPPC) phospholipids and two different subphases of D_2O and ACMW. The monolayers were studied at three surface coverages of approximately 50, 60, and 70 $Å^2$/molecule. Examination of the surface pressure-area isotherm reveals that the main LE/LC phase transition for DPPC monolayers occurs over this range of molecular area (Lewis and Hadgraft, 1990).

Reflectivity data were collected for six different isotopic forms of the equimolar DPPC/oleic acid mixed monolayer using either hydrogenated oleic acid (h-OA) or perdeuterated oleic acid (d-OA) in conjunction with h-DPPC or d-DPPC. Additional isotopic variation was provided by using either ACMW or D_2O as the subphase. Again, each monolayer was studied at three surface coverages of approximately 50, 60 and 70 $Å^{-2}$/molecule.

Initial data analysis was conducted using the optical matrix method, with experimental data being fitted to theoretical reflectivity profiles for a uniform one-layer model of interfacial structure. It is possible to determine some structural parameters relating to alkyl-chain structure from the d-DPPC/ACMW, where the hydrogenated phosphatidylcholine headgroup ($\rho = 1.16 \times 10^6$) $Å^{-2}$) contributes little to the overall reflectivity profile, which is determined predominantly by the deuterated chains, $\rho = 7.63 \times 10^6$ $Å^{-2}$ (Fig. 7b). Similarly, the reflectivity profile for the h-DPPC/D_2O system is determined mainly by the D_2O associated with the headgroup; the small scattering length density of hydrogenated alkyl chains ($\rho = 0.46 \times 10^6$ $Å^{-2}$) means that they make a negligible overall contribution (Fig. 7a). The single-layer model of interfacial structure fitted to this data enables structural parameters related to the headgroup region to be estimated independent of the alkyl-chain region.

The thickness of DPPC alkyl chain has been estimated, using the optical matrix method, to be ~ 20 Å at the highest surface coverage (50 $Å^2$/molecule), and this did not appear to change radically during expansion of the monolayer to around 70 $Å^2$/molecule. These results agree well with the theoretical length of 19.15 Å for fully extended C_{16} chains (Tanford, 1972). The estimated

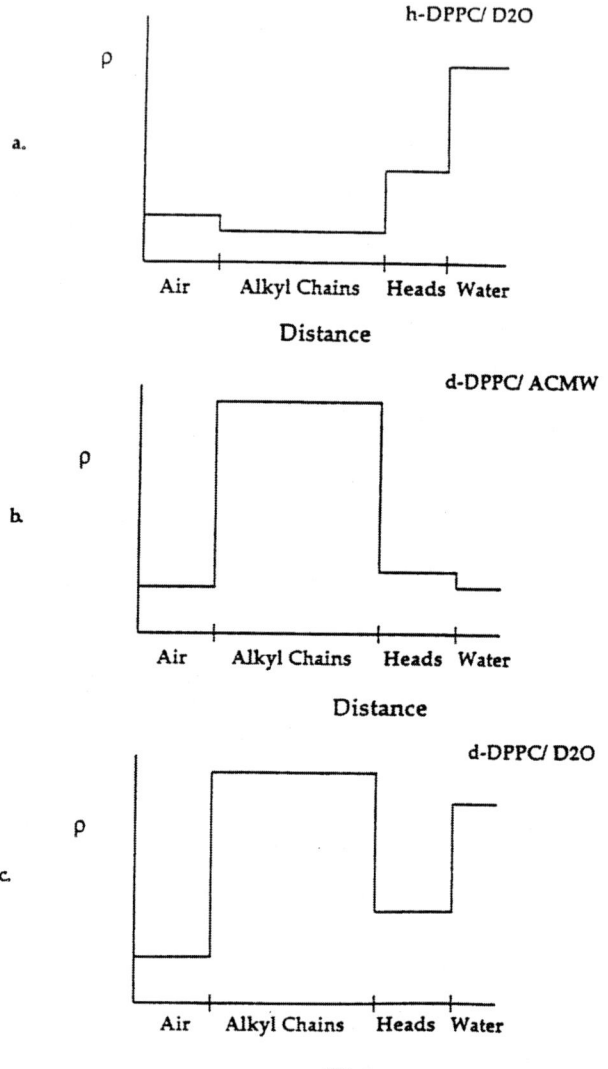

Figure 7   Theoretical scattering length density profiles of different monolayer systems.

thickness of the DPPC headgroup at 50 Å^2/molecule is considerably larger at 14 Å than the theoretical length of a fully extended phosphatidylcholine group, 8 Å (molecular graphics estimates using Chem-X data), which suggests that the close-packing of headgroups is achieved by a staggering of molecules. The close-packing of alkyl trimethylammonium bromide surfactants at the air–water interface is also thought to be associated with staggering of the headgroups (Lee et al., 1989). The staggering of DPPC headgroups appears to remain as the monolayer is expanded, and the thickness of this layer shows a small reduction as it is expanded to 70 Å^2/molecule. Of course, this effect could also be explained by a thick layer of water associated with the headgroup, meaning that the prediction of staggering is debatable.

It is also possible to analyze reflectivity data for DPPC monolayers using a two-layer model of interfacial structure in which the alkyl-chain region is assumed to be well separated from the headgroup region. The fitted values of scattering length density obtained from this method of data analysis can be used to estimate the volume fraction of each component in a given layer. In the alkyl-chain region, the volume fraction of chains is found to decrease from 0.70 to 0.61, as expected, during expansion of the monolayer. The reduction is achieved by incorporation of air into the alkyl-chain region. More important, the fitted scattering length density of this region cannot be accounted for without assuming some penetration of water into the lipid alkyl chains. At the highest surface coverage the volume fraction of water in the alkyl-chain region is estimated to be 0.14, and this reduced to 0.10 with expansion to 60 and 70 Å^2/molecule. The changes in the volume fractions of components in the headgroup region of DPPC monolayers are similar to those already discussed for DMPC monolayers. The reduction in the volume fraction of the DPPC headgroup is accompanied by an increase in the water content of this region, possibly due to the hydration of the glycerol backbone of the phosphatidylcholine group (Bayerl et al., 1990) in expanded monolayers.

It was also possible to analyze data from the DPPC/OA monolayers using the optical matrix method. A one-layer model represents an oversimplification of the complex structure of this monolayer, and the quality of the fits to experimental data is generally poorer than for the DPPC monolayer. Despite these problems it has been possible to estimate the relative volume fraction of DPPC, OA, and water in these mixed monolayers. It is apparent at all surface coverages that the volume fraction of DPPC is approximately twice that of OA, as expected, and that the volume fraction of water in the monolayer increased steadily as the monolayer was expanded to 70 Å^2/molecule.

Kinematic Approximation—Theory

Instead of using the optical matrix method of analysis, a more direct insight into the structure of the spread monolayer can be obtained using the kinematic approximation (Simister et al., 1992; Lu et al., 1992). The kinematic approximation is valid for $\mathbf{Q} \gg \mathbf{Q}_c$ and for low values of reflectivity $[R(\mathbf{Q}) < 10^{-2}]$, and in these cases the specular reflectivity can be written as

$$R(\mathbf{Q}) = \frac{16\pi}{\mathbf{Q}^2} \left| \rho(\mathbf{Q}) \right|^2 \tag{11}$$

where $\rho(\mathbf{Q})$ is the Fourier transform of the scattering length density distribution normal to the surface, $\rho(z)$:

$$\rho(\mathbf{Q}) = \int_{-\infty}^{\infty} \exp(-i\,\mathbf{Q}z)r(z)dz \tag{12}$$

For a surface layer that contains two species i and j then,

$$\rho(z) = n_i(z)b_i + n_j(z)b_j \tag{13}$$

where $n_i(z)$ and $n_j(z)$ are the number density distributions of species i and j that have coherent scattering lengths b_i and b_j. The number of density distributions mentioned here are merely the number of molecules per unit volume as a function of the distance normal (hence $n_i(z)$, the z-axis) to the interface. This is just a way of describing how the molecular configuration of the monolayer changes in this direction. Fourier-transforming Eq. 13 and replacing into Eq. 11 gives

$$R(\mathbf{Q}) = \frac{16\pi^2}{\mathbf{Q}^2} \sum b_i b_j h_{ij}(\mathbf{Q}) \tag{14}$$

where $h_{ij}(\mathbf{Q})$ is known as the partial structure factor and

$$h_{ii}(\mathbf{Q}) = |\, n_i(\mathbf{Q})|^2 \tag{15}$$

$$h_{ij}(\mathbf{Q}) = R_e[n_i(\mathbf{Q})n_j(\mathbf{Q})] \tag{16}$$

and $n_i(\mathbf{Q})$ and $n_j(\mathbf{Q})$ are the Fourier transforms of $n_i(z)$ and $n_j(z)$.

For DPPC monolayers spread on water there are two species in the system, producing three terms in Eq. 17 (two self-terms, h_{DD} and h_{ww}, and one cross-term, h_{Dw}),

$$R(\mathbf{Q}) = \frac{16\pi^2}{\mathbf{Q}^2} \left\{ b_D^2 h_{DD}(\mathbf{Q}) + b_w^2 h_{ww}(\mathbf{Q}) + 2b_D b_w h_{Dw}(\mathbf{Q}) \right\} \tag{17}$$

where D and w refer to DPPC and water, respectively. The terms $h_{ii}(\mathbf{Q})$ and $h_{ij}(\mathbf{Q})$ are the self and cross partial structure factors. Self-terms contain information regarding the thickness and composition of the relevant layer [via the number densities, i.e., the number of molecules per unit volume, $n_i(\mathbf{Q})$, of the component i in the layer]. Cross-terms contain information on the separation of the centers of the distributions of the i and j components of the layer (in this case DPPC and water).

Under some experimental circumstances, equations of the form of Eq. 17 can be simplified to gain information more easily (see later). For example, if null reflecting water is used as the subphase, then in Eq. 17 we have $b_w = 0$, and hence for the DPPC monolayers we have

$$R(\mathbf{Q}) = \frac{16\pi^2}{\mathbf{Q}^2} b_D^2 h_{DD}(\mathbf{Q}) \tag{18}$$

If the monolayer is uniform (Fig. 8), then $n_D(z) = n_{D1}$ for $-d/2 \le Z \le d/2$, where d is the layer thickness and (Champeny, 1973)

$$n_D(\mathbf{Q}) = \frac{2n_{D1}}{\mathbf{Q}} \sin \frac{\mathbf{Q}d}{2} \tag{19}$$

$$\mathbf{Q}^2 h_{DD}(\mathbf{Q}) = 4n_{D1}^2 \sin^2 \frac{\mathbf{Q}d}{2} \tag{20}$$

Similarly if the subphase (in this case water) forms a uniform layer associated with the monolayer that differs from the bulk phase, then

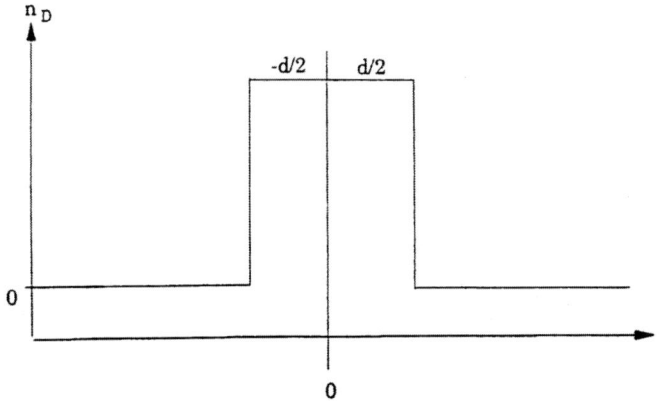

Figure 8 Number density distribution in a monolayer of uniform thickness.

$$Q^2 h_{WW}(Q) = n_{bulk}^2 + 4n_{layer}(n_{layer} - n_{bulk}) \sin^2 \frac{Q\sigma}{2} \qquad (21)$$

where n_{bulk} is the bulk number density of the subphase water, n_{layer} is the density of water associated with or in the monolayer, and σ is the water layer thickness. A value for n_{bulk} can be calculated from the physical density of the subphase (e.g., for pure water, which has a density of 1g cm^{-3} and an RMM of 18, the value of n_{bulk} is 3.3×10^{-2} Å^{-3}, taking Avogadro's number to be 6.023×10^{23}).

Equation 22 describes the cross-term for DPPC and water (containing information about the separation of different monolayer components), where δ_{DW} is the separation distance of the two species:

$$h_{DW} = \pm (h_{DD} h_{WW})^{0.5} \sin Q\delta_{DW} \qquad (22)$$

In order to evaluate the three partial structure factors for the DPPC monolayers it is necessary to measure the reflectivity profiles $R(Q)$ for three different isotopic forms of the DPPC/water system, which sets up three simultaneous equations of the form of Eq. 17. These systems are d-DPPC on ACMW (to give $b_w = 0$, as explained earlier), h-DPPC on D$_2$O (to give $b_D \cong 0$ when compared to b_w), and finally d-DPPC on D$_2$O (to yield the cross-term h_{Dw}).

As already mentioned, the self partial structure factors can be used to determine the thickness and number density (molecules per Å^3) of each component adsorbed at the air–water interface. The number density of the water in the bulk phase (n_{bulk}) and the thickness (σ) and number density of the layer of water associated with the monolayer (n_{layer}) can be determined from the term h_{WW} (as described in Eq. 21). The cross partial structure factors contain information about the spatial relationship between components, which enables the mean distance of separation between two components to be calculated.

The results of partial structure factors analysis of reflectivity data relating to DPPC monolayers on a water subphase are shown in Tables 2 through 4. Table 2 summarizes the results gained from fitting experimental data to Eq. 10 pertaining to the DPPC alkyl-chain region of the monolayer. It is apparent that on expansion of the monolayer, both the expected reductions in thickness and the number density of the DPPC chains occur (Table 2). The decrease in thickness (from 20 Å to 18 Å) is explained by the increased number of gauche conformers introduced into the chains on expansion. The decrease in number density is a function of area per molecule and allows this quantity to be calculated ($1/A_i = n_i/\tau$). On comparison of these values in Table 2 it can

Table 2 DPPC Parameters Calculated from Self-Term h_{DD} for a DPPC Monolayer on a Water Subphase

Nominal area per molecule ($Å^2$)	Number density ($\times 10^4 \ Å^{-3}$)	Thickness ($Å$)	Calculated area per molecule ($Å^2$)
50	8.5 ± 0.2	20 ± 0.5	59
60	8.5 ± 0.2	19 ± 0.6	62
70	7.7 ± 0.2	18 ± 0.5	72

be seen that the calculated value of the monolayer at nominally 50 $Å^2$ is closer to 60 $Å^2$, highlighting an error in the experimental work.

The partial structure factor h_{WW} allows the structure of water in the monolayer to be determined independent of the rest of the monolayer, and this reveals that the thickness of the water layer is approximately 16 $Å$ and does not alter significantly during expansion to higher molecular areas (Table 3).

Analysis of the cross partial structure factors h_{DW} enables the separation of the DPPC and water distributions to be determined. If there were no overlap between water and lipid, the mean distance of separation between the two would be the average of the thickness of the water layer (σ) and lipid layer (τ) in each case (Figs. 9a and 9b). That is, for no penetration of water into the DPPC layer,

$$\delta_{DW} = \frac{\tau + \sigma}{2} \tag{23}$$

The difference between the theoretical separation of water and DPPC and that observed therefore represents the depth to which water is able to penetrate into

Table 3 Water Parameters Calculated from Self-term h_{WW} for a DPPC Monolayer on a Water Subphase

Nominal area per molecule ($Å^2$)	Number density of bulk phase* ($\times 10^2 \ Å^{-3}$)	Number density of associated layer ($\times 10^2 \ Å^{-3}$)	Thickness ($Å$)
50	3.3	0.85 ± 0.08	17.6 ± 0.7
60	3.3	0.8 ± 0.09	15.5 ± 0.7
70	3.3	0.74 ± 0.09	16.0 ± 0.9

*Fixed

Table 4 DPPC–Water Parameters Calculated from Cross-Term h_{DW} for a DPPC Monolayer on a Water Subphase

Nominal area per molecule (Å^2)	$\dfrac{\dfrac{\tau_D}{2} + \tau_W}{2}$ (Å)	δ_{DW} (Å)	Depth of water penetration into alkyl-chain region (Å)
50	18.8 ± 0.6	14.5 ± 0.6	4.3 ± 1.2
60	17.3 ± 0.7	11.8 ± 0.3	5.5 ± 1.0
70	17.0 ± 0.7	10.8 ± 0.4	6.2 ± 1.1

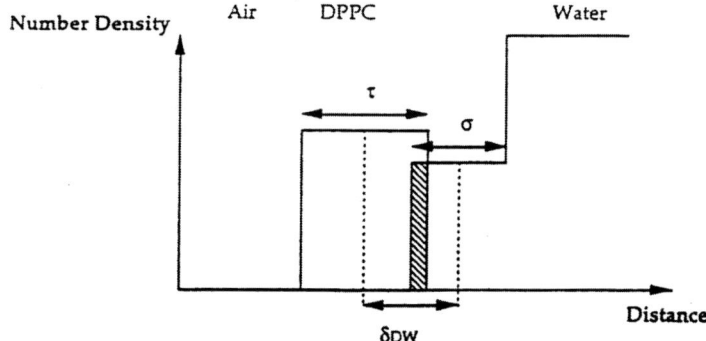

τ	Thickness of DPPC alkyl chains
σ	Thickness of water layer associated with monolayer
$\delta\,\text{DW}$	Distance between the center of DPPC and water distributions
....	Line representing the centre of distribution of water ($\sigma/2$) and DPPC chains ($\tau/2$)
▨	Region of penetration of water molecules into DPPC chains Depth of penetration = $(\tau/2 + \sigma/2) - \delta\,\text{DW}$

(a)

Figure 9 Structural parameter determined by partial structure factor analysis for (a) DPPC and (b) DPPC/OA monolayers.

the DPPC layer (Fig. 9a). At all surface coverages there appears to be considerable penetration of water into the alkyl chains of DPPC, which increases on expansion of the monolayer presumably as the DPPC glycerol backbone hydration levels increase (Table 4).

The equation analogous to Eq. 17 for the DPPC/OA mixed monolayer system is shown as Eq. 24:

$$R(\mathbf{Q}) = \frac{16\pi^2}{\mathbf{Q}^2(b_D^2 h_{DD} + b_O^2 h_{OO} + b_W^2 h_{WW} + 2b_D b_W h_{DW} + 2b_D b_O h_{DO} + 2b_O b_W h_{OW})} \quad (24)$$

The subscripts D, O, and W refer to DPPC, OA, and water, respectively. For DPPC/OA monolayers there are six partial structure factors that need to be evaluated, necessitating reflectivity data from six isotopic variations of the same monolayer.

For the DPPC/OA systems, the equations used to rationalize the partial

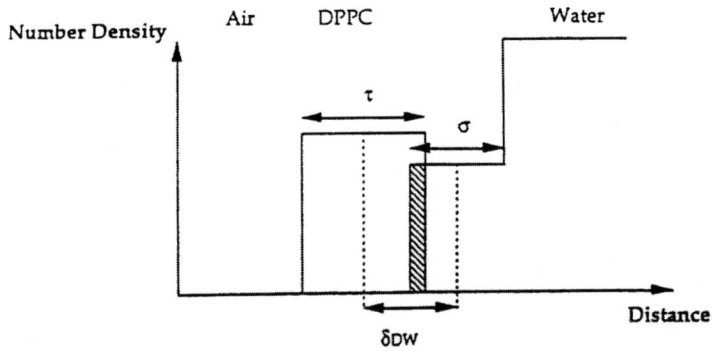

τ Thickness of DPPC alkyl chains

σ Thickness of water layer associated with monolayer

δ_{DW} Distance between the center of DPPC and water distributions

....   Line representing the centre of distribution of water ($\sigma/2$) and DPPC chains ($\tau/2$)

▨   Region of penetration of water molecules into DPPC chains
Depth of penetration = ($\tau/2 + \sigma/2$) - δ_{DW}

(b)

structure factors are identical to those used for the DPPC monolayer except for that describing the cross-term for DPPC and OA (Eq. 25):

$$h_{DO} = \pm (h_{DD}h_{OO})^{0.5} \cos \mathbf{Q}\delta_{DO} \tag{25}$$

Tables 5 and 6 show data derived from the fitting of the two self-terms, h_{DD} and h_{OO}, to Eq. 20 configured for DPPC and OA. Again, there is a reduction in number density on expansion for both monolayer components, and it can also be seen how the OA chain length is greater than that of DPPC at high pressures and, more interestingly, does not change much on expansion. This factor demonstrates that the changes in interfacial structure that occur in DPPC on expansion do not happen for OA, probably because of its more fluid nature at high pressures. This inherent fluidity of OA in proposed phase-separated regions within biological membranes has been used as an explanation for its efficacy as an enhancer (Ongpipattanakul et al., 1991).

The number density of DPPC molecules in OA/DPPC monolayers reflects the packing of lipid alkyl chains. It would be expected that if DPPC chains were packed similarly in the DPPC and DPPC/OA monolayers, then the number densities of the chains, after being corrected for the mole fraction of DPPC present, would be the same. However, it is apparent that at all surface coverages the number density of DPPC chains in the mixed monolayer is less than 50% of its value in the absence of OA. This indicates that there is increased free volume induced in the DPPC alkyl chains by OA.

Calculation of the cross-term partial structure factor fits using Eq. 25 yields values of $h_{DO}/(h_{DD}h_{OO})^{0.5}$ of the order of ± 1.2, which is clearly not possible, since the maximum modulus value of the cosine function is unity. This result implies that there is little separation between the centers of the OA and DPPC distributions.

Attempts to gain an idea of the depth of penetration of water into the mixed monolayers (and compared with the values found for the DPPC) were

Table 5 DPPC Parameters Calculated from the Term h_{DD} for a DPPC/OA Monolayer on a Water Subphase

Nominal area per molecule (Å^2)	Number density ($\times 10^4 \, \text{Å}^{-3}$)	Thickness (Å)	Calculated area per molecule (Å^2)
50	4.7 ± 0.2	17.8 ± 1.0	120
60	4.5 ± 0.2	17.6 ± 0.9	126
70	3.2 ± 0.2	22.3 ± 1.4	140

Table 6 Oleic Acid Parameters Calculated from the Term h_{OO} for a DPPC/OA Monolayer on a Water Subphase

Nominal area per molecule (Å^2)	Number density ($\times 10^4 \text{ Å}^{-3}$)	Thickness (Å)	Calculated area per molecule (Å^2)
50	6.8 ± 0.3	21.5 ± 1.0	68
60	5.7 ± 0.2	21.8 ± 0.9	80
70	5.3 ± 0.2	21.6 ± 1.4	87

somewhat hampered because of the very weak nature of the signal obtained from the d-OA/d-DPPC/ACMW system (in this system, the scattering from the subphase is negligible). To gain the relevant data, the experiment must be repeated using a system of all hydrogenous lipid on D_2O.

The preliminary results just reported for DPPC/OA monolayers illustrate the way in which neutron reflectometry can be used to study the interaction of components in model membrane systems. In particular, the technique has been shown to be useful in the study of the water associated with lipid headgroups. Data analysis by the partial structure factor method offers the potential to study complex multicomponent membrane systems, which have more relevance to the behavior of biological membranes *in vivo*.

IV. CONCLUSION

It is likely that one of the major mechanistic requirements for a good enhancer is the ability to induce some sort of motional freedom in the alkyl-chain region of lipid bilayers. Azone appears to be capable of this. These lipid-chain molecular motions may lead to the easier formation of gauche conformers and thus create a greater number of lipid free volumes. Creation of such free volumes has already been associated with greater skin permeability (Potts et al., 1991), and the positive relationship between molecular size of penetrant and rate of permeation is well established. The action of OA may occur in a similar manner but, because of its longer chain, which impedes adjacent lipid chain motion, to a lesser extent. It is likely that the large kink in the OA molecule created by its cis double bond is an important structural feature in its ability to act in this manner (stearic acid seems to condense DPPC monolayers).

There is now fairly convincing evidence that both of these enhancers are capable of forming discrete islands or pools within lipid bilayers and that facilitated transport may occur along the edges of structural anomalies in the liquid crystal due to the less effective packing of molecules in that region. Comparison of results from skin lipid monolayers with those from DPPC monolayers indicate that the latter films, although much more expanded in nature, are still a useful predictive model for the general behavior of the more complex systems that exist in the stratum corneum.

ACKNOWLEDGMENT

We gratefully acknowledge the assistance of the following members of staff at RAL: Dr. J. Penfold (CRISP), Dr. S. King, and Dr. R. Heenan (LOQ). We thank SERC for financial support, Pfizer (U.S.) for the provision of per-deuterated oleic acid, and Whitby Research for samples of Azone.

REFERENCES

Abraham, W. and Downing, D. T. (1990). Factors affecting the formation, morphology and permeability of stratum corneum lipid bilayers *in vitro*. In: Scott, R. C., Guy, R. H. and Hadgraft, J., eds. *Prediction of Percutaneous penetration*. IBC Technical Services, London, pp. 110–122.

Barnes, G. T., Costin, I. S., Hunter, D. S., and Saylor, J. E. (1980). On the measurement of the evaporation resistance of monolayers. *J. Colloid. Interface Sci. 78*:271–273.

Bayerl, T. M., Thomas, R. K., Penfold, J., Rennie, A. and Sackmann, E. (1990). Specular reflection of neutrons at phospholipid monolayers. Changes of monolayer structure and headgroup hydration at the transition from expanded to the condensed phase. *Biophys. J. 57*:1095–1098.

Beastall, J., Hadgraft, J. and Washington, C. (1988). Mechanism of action of Azone as a percutaneous penetration enhancer: Lipid bilayer fluidity and transition temperature effects. *Int. J. Pharm. 43*:207–213.

Blume, A. (1979). A comparative study of the phase transitions of phospholipid bilayers and monolayers. *Biochim. Biophys. Acta 557*:32–44.

Born, M. and Wolf, E. (1980). *Principles of Optics*, 6th ed. Pergamon Press, New York.

Bouwstra, J. A., Gooris, G. S., Brussee, J., Salomons-de-Vries, M. A. and Bras, W. (1992). The influence of alkyl Azones® on the ordering of the lamellae in human stratum corneum. *Int. J. Pharm. 70*:141–148.

Champeney, D. C. (1973). *Fourier Transforms and Their Use in Physical Applications*. Academic Press, London.

Elias, P. (1990). The importance of epidermal lipids for the stratum corneum barrier.

In: Osbourne, D. and Amann, A., eds. *Topical Drug Delivery Formulations*. Dekker, New York, pp. 13–28.

Gray, D. E. (ed.) (1972). *American Institute of Physics Handbook*, 3rd ed. McGraw-Hill, New York, Section 8, pp. 230–231.

Grundy, M. J., Richardson, R. M., Roser, S. J., Penfold, J. and Ward, R. C. (1988). X-ray and neutron reflectivity from spread monolayers. *Thin Solid Films 159*:43–52.

Harrison, J. E., Brain, K. R. and Hadgraft, J. (1993). The effect of Azone on structured lipid monolayers. In: Brain, K. R., James, V. J. and Walters, K. A., eds. *Prediction of Percutaneous Penetration*. STS Publishing, Cardiff, U.K., Vol. 3b, pp. 174–182.

Hauser, H., Pascher, I., Pearson, R. H. and Sundell, S. (1981). Preferred conformation and molecular packing of phosphatidylethanolamine and phosphatidylcholine. *Biochim. Biophys. Acta. 650*:21–51.

Henderson, J. A., Richards, R. W., Penfold, J., Lu, J. R., and Thomas, R. K. (1993). The organization of polyethylene oxide monolayers at the air–water interface. *Macromolecules 26*:4591–4600.

Henderson, J. A., Richards, R. W., Penfold, J., Shackelton, C. and Thomas, R. K. (1991). Neutron reflectometry from stereotactic poly(methylmethacrylate) monolayers spread at the air–water interface. *Polymer 32*:3284–3293.

Hoogstraate, A. J., Verhoef, J., Brusse, J., Ijzerman, A. P., Spies, P. and Boddé, H. E. (1991). Kinetics, ultrastructural aspects and molecular modelling of transdermal peptide flux enhancement by *N*-alkylazacycloheptanones. *Int. J. Pharm. 76*:37–47.

Jain, M. K. (1983). Nonrandom lateral organization in bilayers and biomembranes. In: C. A. Roland, ed. *Membrane Fluidity in Biology* Academic Press, New York, Vol. 1, pp. 1–37.

Johnson, S. J., Bayerl, T. M., McDermott, D. C., Adam, G. W., Rennie, A. R., Thomas, R. K. and Sackmann, E. (1991a). Structure of an adsorbed dimyristoylphosphatidylcholine bilayer measured with specular reflection. *Biophys. J. 59*:289-294.

Johnson, S. J., Bayerl, T. M., Weihan, W., Noack, H., Penfold, J., Thomas, R. K., Kanaellas, D., Rennie, A. R. and Sackmann, E. (1991b). Coupling of spectrin and polylysine to phospholipid monolayers studied by specular reflection of neutrons. *Biophys. J. 60*:1017–1025.

Lee, E. M., Thomas, R. K., Penfold, J. and Ward, R. C. (1989). Structure of aqueous decyltrimethylammonium bromide solutions at the air/water interface studied by the specular reflection of neutrons. *J. Phys. Chem. 93*:381–388.

Lekner, J. (1987). *Theory of Reflection*, Martinus Nijhoff, Dordrecht, The Netherlands.

Lewis, D. and Hadgraft, J. (1990). Mixed monolayers of dipalmitoylphosphatidylcholine with Azone® or oleic acid at the air–water interface. *Int. J. Pharm. 65*:211–218.

Lewis, D., Hadgraft, J., and Boddé, H. E. (1990). Mixed monolayer studies of DPPC with *N*-alkyl-aza-cycloheptanones at the air–water interface, *Proceed. Intern. Symp. Control. Rel. Bioact. Mater. 17*:439–440.

Löfgren, H. and Pascher, J. (1977). Molecular arrangements of sphingolipids. The monolayer behavior of ceramides. *Chem. Phys. Lipids 20*:273–284.

Lu, J. R., Simister, E. A., Lee, E. M., Thomas, R. K., Rennie, A. R. and Penfold, J. (1992). Direct determination by neutron reflection of the penetration of water into surfactant layers at the air–water interface. *Langmuir 8*:1837–1844.

Luzzati, P. V., Mustacchi, H., Skoulious, A. and Husson, F. (1960). La structure des colloides d'association. I. Les phases-liquide-crystallines des systèmes amphiphie-eau, *Acta. Cryst. 13*:660–667.

Martel, P. and Ahmed, F. U. (1990). Neutron diffraction from cannabinoids in phospholipid membranes. *Chem. Phys. Lipids 53*:331–339.

Mitchell, M. L. and Dluhy, R. A. (1988). In situ FTIR investigations of phospholipid monolayer phase transitions at the air–water interface. *J. Am. Chem. Soc. 110*:712–718.

Ongpipattanakul, B., Burnette, R. R., Potts, R. O. and Francoeur, M. L. (1991). Evidence that oleic acid exists in a separate phase within the stratum corneum lipids. *Pharm. Res. 8*:350–354.

Penfold, J. and Thomas, R. K. (1990). The application of the specular reflection of neutrons to the study of surfaces and interfaces. *J. Phys.: Condens. Matter 2*:1369–1412.

Penfold, J., Ward, R. C. and Williams, W. G. (1987). A time-of-flight neutron reflectometer for surface and interfacial studies. *J. Phys E Sci. Instrum. 20*:1411–1423.

Presti, F. T. (1985). The role of cholesterol in regulating membrane fluidity. In: Aloia, A. C. and Boggs, J. M., eds. *Membrane Fluidity in Biology*. Academic Press, New York, Vol. 4, pp. 97–145.

Potts, R. O., Francoeur, M. L. and Guy, R. H. (1991). Lipid free-volume fluctuations, permeant size and stratum corneum permeability. In: Scott, R. C., Guy, R. H., Hadgraft, J. and Boddé, H., eds. *Prediction of Percutaneous Penetration*. IBC Technical Services, Vol. 2, pp. 148–155.

Richards, R. W. (1989). Neutron and x-ray scattering. In: Cooper, A. R., ed. *Determination of Molecular Weight*. Wiley, New York, pp. 87–116.

Ries, H. (1976). Electron micrographs of cholesterol monolayers. *J. Colloid Interface Sci. 57*:396–398.

Schuckler, F. and Lee, G. (1991). The influence of Azone on monomolecular films of some stratum corneum lipids. *Int. J. Pharm. 70*:173–186.

Shah, D. O. and Shiao, S. Y. (1975). The chain-length compatibility and molecular area in mixed alcohol monolayers. In: Goddard, E. D., ed. *Monolayers, Advances in Chemistry Series 144* Am. Chem. Soc., Washington, DC, pp. 153–164.

Simister, E. A., Lee E. M., Thomas, R. K. and Penfold, J. (1992). The structure of a tetradecyltrimethylammonium bromide layer at the air water interface determined by neutron reflection. *J. Phys. Chem. 96*:1373–1382.

Street, P. R. and Hadgraft, J. (1992). The squeeze-out of oleic acid esters from DPPC monolayers. *Proceedings of the 1st Annual UKAPS Conference*, York, U.K., p. 12.

Stubbs, C. D. and Smith, A. D. (1984). The modification of membrane polyunsaturated fatty acid composition in relation to membrane fluidity and function. *Biochim. Biophys. Acta* 779:89–137.

Tanford, C. (1972). Micelle shape and size. *J. Phys. Chem.* 76:3020–3024.

Vaknin, D., Kjaer, K., Als-Nielsen, J. and Losche, M. (1991). Structural properties of phosphatidylcholine in a monolayer at the air/water interface. Neutron reflection study and re-examination of x-ray reflection measurements. *Biophys. J.* 59:1325–1332.

Vaz, W. C., Melo, E. C. C., and Thompson, T. E. (1989). Translational diffusion and fluid domain connectivity in a two-component, two-phase phospholipid bilayer. *Biophysics J.* 56:869–876.

Watkinson, A. C., Street, P. R., Richards, R. W. and Hadgraft, J. (1991). Evidence for phase separation of oleic acid in liposomes of DPPC from a small angle neutron scattering (SANS) study. In: Scott, R. C., Guy, R. H., Hadgraft, J. and Boddé, H., eds. *Prediction of Percutaneous Penetration.* IBC Technical Services, Vol. 2, pp. 380–385.

Weis, R. M. (1991). Fluorescence microscopy of phospholipid monolayer phase transitions. *Chemistry and Physics of Lipids* 57:227–239.

Winter, R. and Pilgrim, W. C. (1989). A SANS study of high-pressure phase transitions in model biomembranes. *Ber. Bunsen. Ges. Phys. Chem.* 93:708–717.

8

Characterization of the Passive Transdermal Diffusional Route of Polar/Ionic Permeants

Kendall D. Peck
Abbott Laboratories, North Chicago, Illinois

William I. Higuchi
University of Utah, Salt Lake City, Utah

I. INTRODUCTION

The barrier properties of human skin, localized primarily in the stratum corneum, have been an area of focused research for approximately three decades. This research has originated from diverse scientific fields, including pharmaceutics, dermatology, physiology, toxicology, and biochemistry. The pharmaceutical community has recently shown particular interest in this area. A fundamental understanding of the microenvironment(s) encountered by drugs diffusing through the skin should aid in the rational design and optimization of transdermal drug delivery systems. Despite substantial interest in this area, however, the complex, heterogeneous structural properties of skin have prevented the development of a universally accepted model describing transdermal diffusion of molecules.

The early work of Scheuplein and his co-workers demonstrated that the primary transdermal diffusional pathway for moderately polar to nonpolar molecules is lipidlike, or lipoidal, in nature (Scheuplein, 1965, 1967; Scheuplein and Blank, 1971; Scheuplein et al., 1969). Since that time, numerous studies have confirmed this conclusion and gone further in characterizing the relationship between the physicochemical characteristics of permeant molecules and flux through the skin (Ackermann et al., 1987; Anderson et al., 1988; Anderson and Raykar, 1989; Cooper and Kasting, 1987; Guy and Hadgraft, 1988; Michaels et al., 1975; Morimoto et al., 1992; Raykar et al., 1988; Roberts et al., 1978). Flynn (1985) has reviewed much of the data that have led to the current understanding of the dependence of diffusional transport across skin upon the properties of the permeant molecules. Kasting et al. (1992) have gone further in attempting to establish a functional model to predict transdermal fluxes based upon the physicochemical properties of permeant molecules. The analyses of both Flynn (1985) and Kasting et al. (1992) included discussions of a porous/polar pathway in parallel with the lipoidal pathway. These analyses suggest ranges in what is expected for the contribution of the porous/polar route to the overall permeation, but further details, in terms of the characteristics of this pathway, were not discussed, since little has been done to characterize this pathway. The present chapter reviews the concept of a porous diffusional pathway through the stratum corneum and discusses recent findings of studies aimed specifically at understanding the nature of the porous permeation pathway through excised human epidermal membrane (HEM).

II. BACKGROUND

The concept of an alternative pathway, in parallel with the lipoidal pathway, has been in existence for several years. In analyzing the diffusional transport data for a series of steroid compounds, Scheuplein et al. (1969) attributed much of the observed presteady-state flux to diffusion through "shunt" routes. This aspect of their analysis was necessary in unifying the parameters estimated from the steady-state regions of experimental permeation profiles and the measured fluxes in the transient regions of these profiles. In discussing the transdermal permeation of polar permeants such as polyfunctional alcohols, Scheuplein and Blank (1971) noted that "a finite limiting permeability may be reached." A "limiting permeability" is expected, as the polarity of the permeants increases, for a membrane with a porous pathway in parallel with a lipoidal pathway (Kim et al., 1992a,b). One of the primary sources of evidence cited in support of a porous pathway has been a battery of hairless mouse skin permeation data for several permeants with a wide range of polarity and molecular weight (MW) (Flynn, 1985). The permeation characteristics of the moderately polar permeants within a homologous series of compounds (e.g., n-alkanols) are unquestionably consistent with transport through a lipoidal membrane. However, the more polar compounds show a positive deviation from expectations based upon transport through a lipoidal membrane and plateau at a permeability coefficient range of approximately 10^{-8} cm/sec (Flynn, 1985). This positive deviation from what is expected for permeability based strictly upon a lipid membrane partition/diffusion model has been viewed as evidence for a porous/polar pathway (Flynn, 1985, 1990). Recently, however, the validity of this interpretation has been questioned on the basis that the analysis did not consider the influence of permeant molecular volume (MV) upon permeation (Potts and Guy, 1992).

The strong MV dependence of permeation through lipid membranes is well established (Stein, 1986; Xiang and Anderson, 1994). Cooper and Kasting (1987) were the first to propose a model that included an MV dependence in describing the diffusion of molecules through the lipoidal regions in the skin. This model incorporated the standard oil/water partitioning behavior, with octanol as the reference oil phase, and proposed an exponential dependence upon MV of the solute with regard to skin permeation. This model can be represented by the following equation:

$$\log P_{\text{lipid}} = f \log (K_{\text{oct}}) - \phi MV + Y \tag{1}$$

where P_{lipid} is the lipid pathway permeability coefficient, K_{oct} is the octanol/water partition coefficient, and f, ϕ, and Y are constants. Potts and Guy (1992) have fit several data sets to a lipid pathway permeation model that, like the one proposed by Cooper and Kasting (1987), correlates permeability through skin with both the octanol/water partition coefficient of the solute and MV. One of the data sets they analyze is taken from Ackermann et al. (1987) and contains much of the data included in Flynn's (1985) initial analysis, described previously as supportive of a porous pathway. Potts and Guy (1992) claim that, even for the range in polarity of the compounds studied by Ackermann et al. (1987), fitting the data to a correlation that considers both MV and oil/water partitioning completely accounts for the permeation data based upon transport through a lipoidal membrane. They also fit human skin permeation data for 92 compounds, compiled by Flynn (1990), to a correlation similar to the one previously described, with the exception that MW was substituted for MV. Potts and Guy describe the fit of these data to their model ($r^2 = 0.67$) as adequate, considering the large variability in the data that results from independent laboratories. These authors conclude that it is not statistically necessary to include a porous pathway in their analysis to describe existing permeation data adequately.

Several authors have viewed their own experimental data, obtained under a variety of conditions, as consistent with permeation through a porous pathway. The views of Kasting et al. (1992) and Flynn (1985, 1990) have already been discussed. Higuchi and co-workers have extensively applied the dual-pathway model to account for hairless mouse skin permeation data from a number of chemical permeation enhancer systems, including the n-alkanols (Ghanem et al., 1987, 1992; Higuchi et al., 1987; Kim et al., 1992a,b) and N-alkyl-pyrrolidones (Yoneto et al., 1995). Hatanaka et al. (1993) studied the effect of polyethylene glycol–water and ethanol–water solvent systems upon the permeation of several lipophilic and hydrophilic permeants through hairless rat skin. Hatanaka et al. (1993) make the observation that their experimental data cannot be explained by a single-pathway model and also propose a dual-pathway model. Sznitowska et al. (1993) investigated the permeation of three amino acids as model multipolar ions and concluded that the data were "consistent with a weakly selective porous mechanism of transport." The hairless mouse skin permeation data originating from the University of Michigan laboratories were first presented by Flynn (1985). Along with the data later published by Ackermann et al. (1987), Flynn (1985) included the permeation data for vidarabine and three of its 5′ esters (acetate, valerate, and octanoate). As noted by Flynn, the ether/water partition coefficients (K_{eth}) for these compounds differ by four orders of magnitude, while the permeability coefficients differ by only a factor of 4. It is apparent that for vidarabine and its esters, even when appropriate MV considerations are applied, the permeation data cannot be accounted for by a model that considers only diffusion through lipoidal regions in the skin. Based upon his analysis of extensive transdermal diffusion data, Flynn (1990) considers the existence of a pore pathway through the skin as an "established fact." Because it is evident that several authors support the view that a complete description of transdermal diffusion must incorporate a porous pathway in parallel with the lipoidal pathway, a close examination of the permeants and data included in the analyses of Potts and Guy (1992) seems appropriate.

Of the human skin permeation data compiled by Flynn (1990) and analyzed by Potts and Guy (1992), only six of the 92 compounds have log K_{oct} values less than zero, and only two of those six have log K_{oct} values less than negative 1. Clearly, the regression performed by Potts and Guy (1992) for human skin data was weighted almost entirely by relatively lipophilic permeants. In light of this fact, it seems worthwhile to focus on the polar permeants included in the analyses of Potts and Guy (1992) to see how well the proposed correlations actually "predict" the permeability coefficients for these permeants. Of the permeants included in the human skin analysis, sucrose and water are the most polar (log $K_{oct} = -3.7$ and -1.4, respectively). The correlation that results from the fit of the compiled data to the equation proposed by Potts and

Guy predicts permeability coefficients for sucrose and water that are factors of 150 and 3 times lower than the experimental values reported in Flynn's (1990) compilation. The fit between predicted and experimental permeability of the permeants with log K_{oct} values between -1 and 0 is more satisfactory. Glucose is the most polar compound included in the data reported by Ackermann et al. (1987). The correlation resulting from the analysis of Potts and Guy for Ackermann's data set underestimates the permeability of glucose by a factor of 10. The magnitudes and direction of these discrepancies cause some doubt as to the adequacy of the proposed correlations in the polarity and MW range of sucrose and glucose.

Raising these issues illustrates that there is experimental evidence that a single lipoidal pathway cannot sufficiently account for all permeation data. An objective assessment of the existing data, however, also indicates that there is a definite need for additional systematic research focusing upon the porous/polar permeation pathway. As previously noted and evident from the compilation of permeation data by Flynn (1990), relatively little permeation data has been generated for "polar" permeants. The interest in performing permeation studies with polar and ionic solutes has been relatively limited due to the inherently low permeability of skin to polar permeants. Low permeabilities make polar drugs unlikely transdermal drug delivery candidates. Also, factors such as skin sample-to-sample variability make it difficult to obtain data from passive permeation experiments with polar permeants that lead to quantitative conclusions (Liu et al., 1993, Williams et al., 1992). Despite the obstacles associated with characterizing polar solute diffusion across skin, the importance of a fundamental understanding of transdermal permeation pathways should not be overlooked. The remainder of this chapter will focus primarily on recent results from studies aimed directly at elucidating the properties of the diffusional pathway followed by polar permeants.

III. EXPERIMENTAL METHODOLOGY AND SUCCESSIVE PERMEABILITY EXPERIMENTS

Characterization of the polar permeation pathway is dependent upon obtaining quantitative data from permeation studies with ionic and/or polar permeants. One major obstacle to overcome in such studies is the skin sample-to-sample variability observed when in vitro permeation studies are conducted, particularly with ionic and polar permeants (Liu et al., 1993; Williams et al., 1992). Since our goal was to obtain detailed information regarding the nature of the pathway followed by polar permeants through the skin, it became apparent that it would be necessary to develop an experimental protocol that facilitated quantitative analysis of the experimental data. One approach to eliminating uncertainty that results from sample-to-sample variability is to perform successive permeability experiments under a variety of experimental conditions with an individual HEM sample, thus maximizing the data obtained from each HEM sample and allowing each sample to serve as its own control (Peck et al., 1993). For such a protocol to be effective, however, it is also essential that an independent control be established to monitor the integrity of the barrier properties of the membrane throughout the protocol. It has also been recommended that skin samples intended for use in in vitro studies be prescreened based upon electrical resistance measurements (Kasting and Bowman, 1990a; Sims et al., 1991) or flux of tritiated water (Franz and Lehman, 1990) to ensure that the barrier properties have remained essentially intact through the sample-preparation and diffusion-cell-setup procedures. The feasibility of incorporating: (a) HEM sample prescreening, and integrity monitoring, via measuring electrical resistance; and (b) successive permeability experiments under a variety of conditions for a given HEM sample, into experimental HEM permeation protocols has been demonstrated (Peck et al., 1993). Initial studies indicated that the limitation of this approach, as one might expect, was due primarily to the length of time an HEM sample maintains its initial barrier properties under experimental conditions. This limitation can be largely overcome by supporting the HEM sample in the diffusion cell with a synthetic porous membrane to relieve physical stresses placed upon the HEM during sampling and washing phases of the protocol (Peck et al., 1993). The experimental studies described in the following sections were based upon successive permeation protocols. The source of the HEM was heat-separated cadaver skin prepared as described by Kligman and Christophers (1963). Electrical resistance was established as a criteria for acceptable membrane integrity. Successive permeability experiments were conducted for each HEM sample while the experimental conditions were varied. Each skin sample served as its own control. This approach made it possible to study systematically the diffusion of polar solutes across skin under a variety of conditions while minimizing the liability of skin-to-skin variability.

IV. EFFECT OF SOLUTION IONIC STRENGTH UPON IONIC PERMEANT PERMEATION

To obtain insights into the electrostatic properties of the ionic solute permeation pathway through HEM, the effect of changes in the ionic strength of the buffer solution in contact with the membrane upon the permeability of ionic permeants was investigated (Peck et al., 1993). The results of this study will be briefly summarized, including the findings that support the importance and effectiveness of supporting the HEM during successive permeation studies. The initial experimental protocol involved determining three permeability coefficients for each HEM sample, and a given permeant, over a 3-day period. The first and third permeability coefficients were to be determined in the same ionic strength medium to ensure that the HEM sample remained unchanged during the experiment. The second permeability coefficient was to be determined in a medium of different ionic strength than the first/third. The ionic strength was varied between 0.1 M and 0.004 M, with equivalent ionic strength maintained in the donor and receiver compartments of the diffusion cell. The electrical resistance of the HEM samples was also monitored during this protocol as a means of monitoring the condition of the HEM sample. For a porous membrane with a net surface charge density, it is expected that altering the ionic strength will affect the flux of ionic permeants through changes in the partitioning of the ions into the pores due to changes in the effective volume of the pore influenced by the electrical double layer next to the pore wall (Sims et al., 1993). Although there have been studies that indicate that HEM exhibits permselective properties under iontophoretic conditions (Burnette and Ongpipattanakul, 1987), and that, based upon the directionality of electroosmotic solvent flow, the effective surface charge density is negative (Pikal, 1990; Sims et al., 1991; Srinivasan et al., 1989), this study was aimed at addressing the electrostatic properties of the permeation pathway under passive conditions. There appeared to be an ionic-strength-dependent trend, with the permeability of the cationic permeant, tetraethylammonium (TEA), being enhanced by a reduction of ionic strength, and the anionic permeant, taurocholate, being inhibited by a reduction of ionic strength. The conclusions drawn from the initial studies, however, were softened due to drifting of the permeability coefficients determined on days 1 and 3 of the experiment (see Peck et al., 1993, Table 1). The increases in permeability correlated with proportional increases in the electrical conductance for each HEM sample. Both sodium azide (0.02%) and gentamicin sulfate (0.05 mg/ml) were evaluated as means to minimize membrane degradation caused by bacteria. Neither had a significant impact on the stability of HEM (unpublished results from our laboratory). Sodium azide was added to all buffers as a precautionary measure.

In an attempt to stabilize the HEM samples during the protocol, without changing the membrane properties being studied, a second set of experiments was conducted, with a synthetic porous membrane being placed next to the

HEM in the diffusion cell. Under these conditions, it was shown that the membrane barrier properties of the HEM samples remained constant in terms of TEA permeability, mannitol permeability, and electrical resistance for 5 days. The objective of establishing a protocol that enabled the determination of successive permeability coefficients over an extended period of time had been achieved. The effect of varying the ionic strength of the medium upon TEA permeability was investigated for HEM samples that were supported by a synthetic membrane. As a means of increasing the amount of data obtainable from a single HEM sample, dual-permeant experiments were conducted with tracer levels of ^{14}C-TEA and ^{3}H-mannitol to allow permeability coefficients to be determined simultaneously for these permeants. Representative results from one of these experiments are shown in Fig. 1. Note that the permeability of the neutral permeant, mannitol, and the electrical resistance at a given ionic strength are essentially constant over the 5-day protocol, while the permeability of TEA is dependent upon the ionic strength of the medium and consistent with expectations for a porous membrane with a net negative surface charge density (Sims et al., 1993). Since the intrinsic barrier properties of the membrane remained constant throughout the protocol, attributing changes in the permeability of TEA to changes in ionic strength is straightforward. Also note that the permeabilities of mannitol and TEA at the higher ionic strength are quite similar (within a factor of 2). This observation is also in agreement with expectations for diffusion through a porous membrane. It seems that this similarity in permeabilities would be quite difficult to rationalize, and a surprising coincidence, if the route of diffusion for these permeants were something other than a porous route.

V. TEMPERATURE DEPENDENCE STUDIES

The temperature dependence of transdermal permeability has been used to probe the barrier characteristics of the HEM, with the goal being to obtain information regarding the microenvironment for diffusion of compounds (Blank et al., 1967; Cornwell and Barry, 1993; Golden et al., 1987; Scheuplein, 1965). Although detailed mechanistic conclusions regarding permeation pathways drawn from this type of data should be viewed with caution due to the complex nature of the membrane (Michaels et al., 1975), definite conclusions can be drawn regarding the relative microenvironments for diffusion from temperature-dependence studies for different classes of permeant compounds. A test of the concept of HEM having parallel porous and lipoidal pathways is to measure the temperature dependence of the permeability of polar and

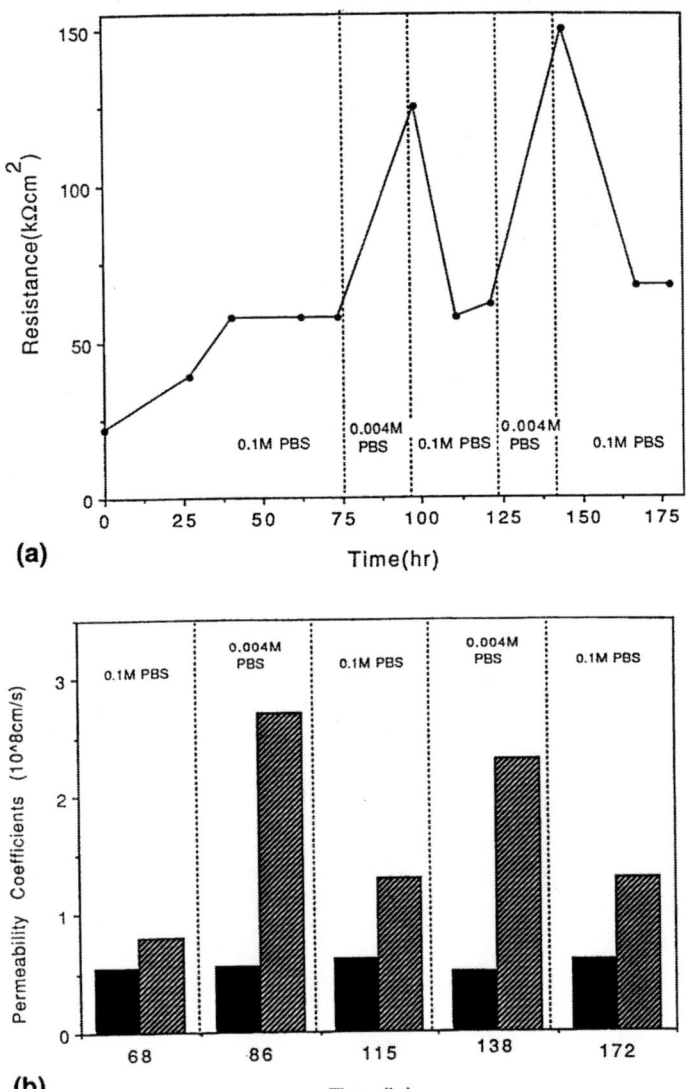

(a)

(b)

Figure 1 Representative results from Peck et al. (1993) for a 5-day protocol with HEM supported in the diffusion cell. (a) Resistance measurements taken throughout protocol. (b) Permeability coefficients determined simultaneously for TEA (hatched bars) and mannitol (filled bars). Times indicated are midpoints of permeability experiments corresponding to the time axis of panel (a). (Reprinted with kind permission of Elsevier Science, NL.)

nonpolar solutes through HEM. For the permeation of solutes through a porous membrane, this temperature dependence is expected to approach the temperature dependence for viscous flow. For the permeation of nonpolar solutes through lipoidal regions of the HEM, the temperature dependence is expected to approach that for lipid membranes. The initial goal of this study was to determine the degree that polar permeants approach, or deviate from, a temperature dependence for HEM permeability similar to that expected for a porous membrane (Peck et al., 1995). Studies were also conducted with a model lipophilic permeant to determine the extent that the temperature dependence of HEM permeability for this compound differed from that observed for the polar permeants.

The experimental philosophy for this study was as described previously. Each HEM sample acted as its own control. The temperature was varied while monitoring the permeability of a given solute through a given HEM sample. The effect of temperature upon the permeation of urea, mannitol, TEA, and corticosterone was determined (Peck et al., 1995). The electrical resistance of the HEM samples was also monitored to determine the effect of temperature upon the resistance properties of HEM as well as to monitor the stability of the HEM samples throughout the experimental protocol. The experimental protocol involved alternating the temperature between 27 and 39°C, and measuring permeability coefficients and electrical resistance at each temperature. Returning to, and measuring a permeability coefficient at, the original temperature ensured that membrane damage did not significantly affect the results of the study. The effect of temperature was quantitated as the ratio of the permeability coefficient determined at 39°C divided by the permeability coefficient determined at 27°C. For comparative purposes, the effect of temperature upon electrical resistance was quantitated as the resistance measured at 27°C divided by the resistance at 39°C.

In parallel with the HEM experiments, studies using a model porous membrane (Nuclepore®) system, with urea and mannitol as the permeants, were conducted. These studies showed that for these permeants, under experimental conditions identical to those of the HEM studies, the measured temperature dependence of permeation was in line with measured activation energies of bulk diffusion (Longsworth, 1953). The measured temperature-dependent ratios (P_{39}/P_{27}) were 1.34 ± 0.03 and 1.38 ± 0.02 ($N = 4$, ave. $\pm$ s.d.) for urea and mannitol, respectively (Peck et al., 1995). These ratios were viewed as a reference point to which the permeation temperature-dependence ratios determined for HEM could be compared.

Initial HEM studies with urea as the permeant showed that HEM samples with electrical resistance ≤ 20 kΩcm^2 approached a temperature dependence similar to that observed for Nuclepore®, while HEM samples with electrical resistance ≥ 20 kΩcm^2 showed temperature depedence ratios that were relatively independent of electrical resistance and in the range of 1.5 to 1.8 (Peck et al., 1995). Because it is possible that the lower-resistance HEM samples approached a temperature dependence similar to that of an ideal porous membrane due to defects in the stratum corneum, the majority of the data analysis dealt with the HEM samples that exhibited an electrical resistance ≥ 20 kΩcm^2. The average ratio (P_{39}/P_{27}) determined from the urea studies for which the HEM resistance was ≥ 20 kΩcm^2 was 1.66 ± 0.05 ($N = 22$, 95% confidence interval). The temperature-dependent ratios determined for mannitol and TEA were 1.76 ± 0.14 ($N = 9$, 95%) and 1.71 ± 0.11 ($N = 8$, 95%), respectively. In each case, N corresponds to the number of HEM samples studied. For these permeants, the protocol for an individual HEM sample extended over a 5-day period, from which four temperature-dependent ratios were determined. The ratio determined from the effect of temperature upon the electrical resistance for HEM samples with an electrical resistance ≥ 20 kΩcm^2 was 1.61 ± 0.09 ($N = 17$, 95%).

Corticosterone served as a model lipophilic permeant and demonstrated the difference observed between the temperature dependence of permeation for polar/ionic and lipophilic permeants. In the simplest view, a mechanistic interpretation of lipophilic permeant apparent activation energies, for HEM permeability, must consider the temperature dependence of solute partitioning from solution into the HEM, and the activation energy for diffusion through the bilayer regions of the stratum corneum. This summation of thermodynamic and kinetic effects complicates any attempt to make molecular-level interpretations based upon apparent activation energies. Also, the use of activation energies implies that no structural or morphological changes in the membrane properties have occurred as a result of the temperature change; for a heterogeneous membrane such as HEM, this may not be a valid assumption. For these reasons, interpretations based upon the temperature dependence of corticosterone have been kept to a macroscopic level and used only for comparative purposes. The average temperature dependence of corticosterone permeation through HEM, again measured by the ratio of permeability at 39°C divided by the permeability at 27°C, was 4.5 ± 0.4 ($N = 8$, 95%) (Peck et al., 1995). Figure 2 shows all of the temperature-dependence data collected for each of the four permeants using the two-temperature protocol.

The differences between the temperature dependence for permeation of the polar permeants and corticosterone suggest two distinct mechanisms of diffusion through HEM. Based upon comparisons with studies of model systems, the temperature dependence of the polar solutes approaches expecta-

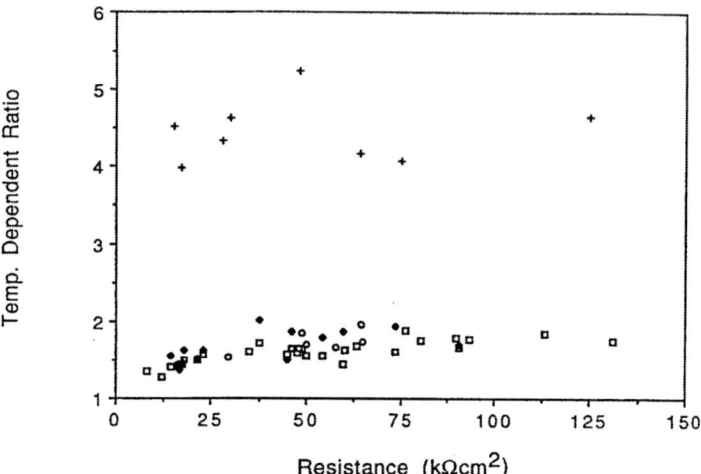

Figure 2   Permeation temperature-dependent ratios for urea (□), mannitol (◆), TEA (○) and corticosterone (+). Each point represents the average of data collected from an individual HEM sample. [Reprinted with permission from Peck et al. (1995). Copyright © 1995 by American Chemical Society.]

tions for a porous membrane, while the corticosterone temperature dependence is more consistent with the larger temperature dependence expected for diffusion through a lipid membrane (Stein, 1986).

VI. CORRELATION BETWEEN ELECTRICAL RESISTANCE AND POLAR PERMEANT PERMEATION

For an ideal porous membrane, an inverse proportionality is expected between solute permeability (P) and membrane electrical resistance (R_e). This proportionality can be expressed by the following relationship:

$$\log P = -\log R_e + \log Z \tag{2}$$

where Z is a proportionality constant. Sims et al. (1991) reported such a correlation between mannitol permeability and HEM electrical resistance. In the temperature-dependence studies just summarized, both the electrical resistance and urea permeability were determined for several HEM samples at two temperatures. For these data, Peck et al. (1995) reported a correlation between urea permeability and electrical resistance that is represented by Fig. 3. Several

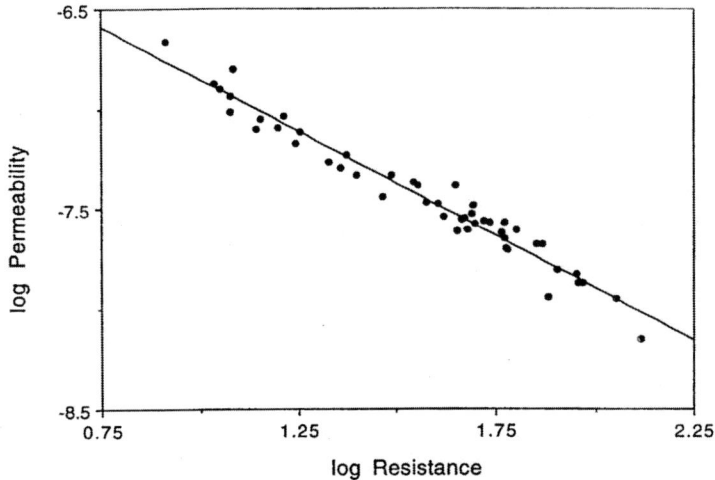

Figure 3 Correlation between urea permeability and electrical resistance. Each point represents the average of data collected at a given temperature for an individual HEM sample. Units of P are cm/sec, units of R are $k\Omega cm^2$. [Reprinted with permission from Peck et al. (1995). Copyright © 1995 by American Chemical Society.]

points regarding the correlation shown in Fig. 3 deserve special note: (a) the data are fit very well by a simple linear regression ($r^2 = 0.96$). (b) The slope of the linear regression is -1.04 ± 0.06 (95% univariate confidence interval), which is in quantitative agreement with predictions for a porous membrane model. (c) The data included in the regression represent the permeability and resistance data for both 27 and 39°C phases of the experiment protocol, indicating that the correlation is independent of temperature over the temperature range investigated. Of the data generated that support the existence of a porous permeation pathway through HEM, this correlation may be the most convincing. If transport of urea were dependent upon partitioning into and diffusion through lipid regions of the HEM, such a correlation would not be expected. The data shown in Fig. 3 indicate a high probability that the same pathway is responsible for urea diffusion and conduction of current-carrying ions. When the corticosterone permeation data from Peck et al. (1995) is plotted versus resistance in the same format as in Fig. 3, no correlation is observed. Again, to account for the urea and corticosterone permeation data coupled with HEM electrical resistances, parallel diffusional pathways must be invoked.

VII. SYSTEMATIC STUDY OF POLAR COMPOUND PERMEATION

With an experimental protocol in place that facilitated studies aimed at characterizing the porous permeation pathway, a systematic study of polar compound permeation through HEM was undertaken (Peck et al., 1994). As has already been described, there is a void in the literature with respect to the passive permeation of polar solutes through skin. The initial purpose of the studies outlined in this section was to add to the polar solute permeation database. An effort was again made to determine the degree to which the barrier characteristics of skin with respect to polar compounds approach, or deviate from, those of an ideal porous membrane.

Based upon the justification for the existence of a porous permeation pathway provided by the data outlined thus far in this chapter, a reasonable theoretical starting point for these studies is the simple equation that relates the permeability coefficient, P, of the solute through a porous membrane to its diffusion coefficient in the membrane, D_m:

$$P = \frac{\varepsilon D_m}{\tau h} \tag{3}$$

In Eq. 3, ε, τ, and h are the porosity, tortuosity, and membrane thickness, respectively. For a porous membrane, P is expected to be directly proportional to D_m, with a proportionality constant representative of the parameters that characterize the membrane. If the pore dimensions of a porous membrane are large relative to the solute radii, the diffusion coefficient of a solute within the membrane is essentially identical to the diffusion coefficient in the solution phase in contact with the membrane. Although the theory is very straightforward, applying Eq. 3 directly in analyzing skin permeation data is complicated by the fact that ε, τ, and h are essentially unknowns and may vary between HEM samples. For these reasons, the strategy for testing the concept of a porous membrane based upon Eq. 3 requires that the permeability coefficients of multiple permeants be determined through the same HEM sample, with the assumption that each permeant follows the same pathway. Based upon this assumption, the ratio of the permeability coefficients for two permeants through the same HEM sample leads to the elimination of the unknown parameters that characterize the membrane. The resulting ratio can then be expressed as (Peck et al., 1994)

$$\frac{P_x}{P_y} = \frac{D_{m,x}}{D_{m,y}} \tag{4}$$

where the subscripts x and y correspond to different permeants.

Based upon Eq. 4 a systematic study was performed with four polar permeants (urea, mannitol, sucrose, and raffinose) in an effort to characterize further the porous permeation pathway through HEM (Peck et al., 1994). Dual-labeled liquid scintillation counting and an experimental protocol that incorporated successive permeability experiments, as outlined in the previous sections, allowed the permeability coefficients for each permeant to be determined for each HEM sample studied. Again, Eq. 4 predicts that, for a porous membrane, the permeability coefficient ratio should be equal to the ratio of the diffusion coefficients for the solutes in the membrane. As a first approximation, if the relative radii of the solutes and the membrane pore radii R_p are such that hindrance considerations are negligible (Deen, 1987), then the ratio P_x/P_y should approach the ratio of the free diffusion coefficients D of the solutes in bulk solution.

The permeability data from 11 HEM samples for the four polar permeants studied are summarized in Table 1. The permeability coefficients for each HEM sample and each permeant are shown explicitly in the initial report (Peck et al., 1994). As expected, the permeability coefficients of a given solute varied significantly between HEM samples. The strength of the experimental protocol was evident, however, because the ratios of the permeability coefficients for the different solutes determined from a single HEM sample were reasonably constant between HEM samples. By determining the permeabilities of each

Table 1 Summary of HEM Polar Permeant Permeation Study

Ratio type (x/y)	D_x/D_y^a	P_x/P_y^b	$D_xH_x/D_yH_y^c$
Urea/mannitol	1.94	3.5 ± 0.9	3.0
Urea/sucrose	2.51	6.5 ± 1.1	5.4
Urea/raffinose	3.06	9 ± 3	9.1
Mannitol/sucrose	1.29	1.9 ± 0.4	1.8
Mannitol/raffinose	1.58	2.7 ± 0.5	3.0
Sucrose/raffinose	1.22	1.4 ± 0.3	1.7

[a]Ratios based upon free aqueous diffusion coefficients reported by Peck et al. (1994).
[b]Average ratios and standard deviations of permeability coefficients reported by Peck et al. (1994) determined from 11 HEM samples.
[c]Ratios based upon free aqueous diffusion coefficients corrected by diffusional hindrance factors that were calculated from Eq. 6 for each permeant based upon an R_p of 21 Å.

solute for each HEM sample, the difficulties generally associated with skin-to-skin variability were minimized, since each sample again served as its own control. The first column of Table 1 shows the ratio types obtained from the four permeants of this study. The second column shows the ratios of the free aqueous diffusion coefficients of these permeants, which were determined independently by a method described in the cited study (Peck et al., 1994). Column 3 shows the experimental HEM permeability-coefficient ratios. The differences between the permeability-coefficient ratios and the diffusion-coefficient ratios range from being indistinguishable for the sucrose/raffinose pair to approximately a factor of 3 for the urea/raffinose pair. Considering the range in the MW of the solutes studied and the complexity of the barrier properties of HEM, the agreement between the permeability-coefficient ratios and the diffusion-coefficient ratios indicates that there is validity to describing the diffusion of these molecules across HEM in terms of diffusion across a porous membrane. Systematic trends in the differences between D_x/D_y and P_x/P_y, however, indicate that these differences may be linked to not incorporating hindrance considerations into the data analysis. Examining the data in Table 1 shows that the P_x/P_y ratios are always larger than the D_x/D_y ratios. This would be expected if the dimensions of the pores were small enough to restrict the diffusion of the permeants within the membrane, necessitating appropriate hindrance corrections (Deen, 1987). The next level of analysis was an investigation into possible physical explanations for the observed differences between the permeability-coefficient and diffusion-coefficient ratios.

The basis for comparing the ratios of the free diffusion coefficients and permeability coefficients was the assumption that hindrance considerations could be ignored. In the instance that this assumption is valid (i.e., the case of large pore dimensions relative to solute radii), the free diffusion coefficients are a reasonable approximation to the diffusion coefficients of the solutes in the membrane. In the instance that hindrance considerations are not negligible, due to pore dimensions that lead to diffusion-restricting hydrodynamic interactions between the solute and the membrane, the diffusion coefficient of the solute in the membrane is a function of both the solute parameters and the properties of the membrane. In this case, the effective diffusion coefficient can be approximated by the product of the free diffusion coefficient and a diffusional hindrance factor, $H(\lambda)$ (Deen, 1987):

$$D_m = DH(\lambda) \tag{5}$$

For the idealized case of a cylindrical pore geometry, $H(\lambda)$ is a well-characterized function that was first proposed by Renkin (1954), later reviewed in detail by Deen (1987), and can be expressed as

$$H(\lambda) = (1 - \lambda)^2[1 - 2.1\lambda + 2.09\lambda^3 - 0.95\lambda^5] \qquad (6)$$

where λ is the ratio of the solute radius r to the pore radius R_p, $(\lambda = r/R_p)$. Substituting Eq. 5 into Eq. 4 leads to

$$\frac{P_x}{P_y} = \frac{H(\lambda_x)D_x}{H(\lambda_y)D_y} \qquad (7)$$

Through Eq. 7, the permeability-coefficient ratio for two solutes becomes a function of r and R_p. It therefore becomes possible to determine if there is an R_p value that will bring calculated $D_{m,x}/D_{m,y}$ values into agreement with experimental P_x/P_y ratios for a given HEM sample, considering R_p to be a fitted parameter with D and r obtainable from independent experiments. A detailed analysis of the HEM permeability-coefficient ratios, for the 11 HEM samples studied, led to R_p estimates of between 15 Å and 25 Å (Peck et al., 1994). Nonlinear least squares fitting of the permeation data in Table 1 to Eq. 7, with R_p as the variable parameter, resulted in an R_p of 21 ± 5 Å (95% univariate confidence interval). The final column of Table 1 shows that when the D_x/D_y ratios are corrected by diffusional hindrance factors based upon a 21-Å R_p and the appropriate parameters taken from Peck et al. (1994) for each permeant, the corrected ratios come into very close agreement with the experimental permeability-coefficient ratios. From this analysis, the permeability data for these polar permeants is consistent with diffusion through a porous membrane with relatively restrictive pore dimensions.

An alternative approach in analyzing the experimental data is to consider what might be expected in terms of the permeation characteristics for these polar molecules based upon proposed models for lipid membrane transport. As an example, the correlation represented by Eq. 7 taken from Potts and Guy (1992) can be used to "predict" the permeability of these compounds through HEM based upon the concept of partitioning into and diffusion through the lipid regions of the stratum corneum. The permeant parameters used in this analysis (MW and log K_{oct}) are the same as those previously reported for a similar analysis (see Table V in Peck et al., 1994). Figure 4 summarizes the results of this analysis. In Fig. 4, the permeability coefficients, normalized by the urea permeability coefficient, are shown for: (a) a fritted-glass system (Peck et al., 1994) for which the effective R_p is large relative to the solute r, thus making the permeability-coefficient ratios essentially equivalent to the ratios of the free diffusion coefficients; (b) HEM samples, and (c) permeability predictions made based upon the proposed correlation taken from Potts and Guy (1992).

The fritted-glass ratios and the HEM ratios plotted in Fig. 4 are equiva-

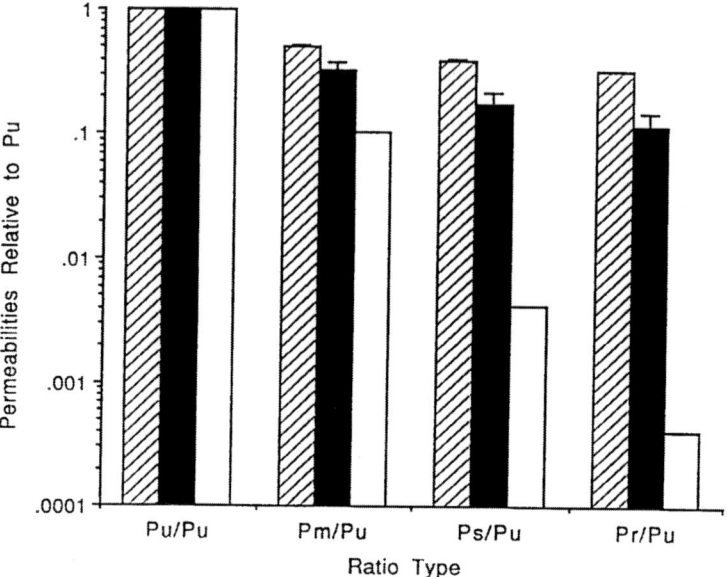

Figure 4 Permeability coefficients for each permeant (urea, mannitol, sucrose, and raffinose) normalized by urea permeability coefficient for: a fritted-glass membrane system [Peck et al., (1994)] (hatched bars); HEM (solid bars); and predictions based upon a correlation proposed by Potts and Guy (1992).

lent to the inverted forms of the first three D_x/D_y and P_x/P_y ratios shown in Table 1, respectively. As noted previously, the differences between the fritted-glass results and HEM results can be accounted for by modeling the HEM data according to diffusion through a porous membrane with a 21-Å R_p. The differences between the HEM results and the predictions of the correlation proposed by Potts and Guy, on the other hand, are much more substantial. The correlation proposed by Potts and Guy (1992) predicts over three orders of magnitude difference between the permeability coefficients of urea and raffinose, while the experimental permeability coefficients for these compounds differ by a factor of less than 10. The correlation also underestimates the permeability of these polar permeants, ranging from one order of magnitude for urea to over three orders of magnitude for raffinose. This result is consistent with the degree to which the "predicted" permeability coefficient for sucrose underestimates the actual sucrose permeability coefficient included in the data set from which the correlation was actually determined, as discussed in the background section of this chapter. Clearly, the predictive capabilities of this correlation, which is put forth by Potts and Guy as representative of the lipoidal permeation pathway, are limited for compounds with physicochemical parameters represented by the polar solutes of this study. This analysis shows that the permeation data for urea, mannitol, sucrose, and raffinose and fit much more adequately by a porous-membrane model than by a lipoidal-membrane model, even before hindrance corrections are applied.

The systematic study of polar permeant permeation served to confirm the existence of a porous permeation pathway through the HEM. It also led to the characterization of important properties of this pathway. The results of this study demonstrated that the diffusion of polar permeants through skin is limited by the low effective porosity of the HEM and by hindrance effects due to restrictive pore dimensions. Effectively enhancing the transport of polar drugs in the MW range of many therapeutic peptides may require increasing the effective R_p of the HEM as well as the effective porosity/tortuosity ratio. Perhaps novel combinations of chemical permeation enhancers and physical means such as an applied electrical field or ultrasound may be necessary to achieve this objective.

VIII. SUMMARY

For a number of years the existence of a porous or polar pathway through the stratum corneum, in parallel with the lipoidal pathway, has been hypothesized. Although there has been some criticism of this concept, it is our belief that the root of the lack of a common consensus among scientists in the field can be attributed largely to the limited number of systematic studies in the literature that directly address the issue of the diffusion of polar and ionic permeants across skin. Based upon recent studies that have focused upon this aspect of transdermal diffusion, the existence of a porous permeation pathway through HEM is clear (Hatanaka et al., 1993, 1994; Peck et al., 1993, 1994, 1995). At this point, we have made no attempt to correlate the findings from our studies with specific structural properties of the HEM. In some cases, authors have implicated "shunt" routes such as hair follicles and sweat ducts to account for permeation data not consistent with the concept of lipoidal membrane permeation (Cornwell and Barry, 1993; Scheuplein and Blank, 1971). Under iontophoretic conditions, such shunt routes have been shown to contribute to current conduction (Cullander and Guy, 1991; Scott et al., 1993). When efforts have been made to estimate the effective R_p of skin samples under iontophoretic conditions (Ruddy and Hadzija, 1992), osmotic conditions (Hatanaka et al.,

1994), and passive conditions (Peck et al., 1994), however, the results have been R_p estimates in the range of 20 Å. These observations are pointed out to discourage the assumption that the characteristics of a porous permeation pathway through skin must correspond to dimensions of the lumens of normal sweat ducts, hair follicles, etc. If the passive porous permeation pathway does correspond to diffusion through appendages, it is likely that the rate-limiting barrier is transport across the epithelial cell layers that line the appendages, as Kasting and Bowman (1990b) have suggested for sodium ion transport. Based upon studies aimed at visualizing the routes of penetration of mercuric chloride through human skin, Bodde et al. (1991) propose that the intercellular lipid regions of the stratum corneum provide a bicontinuous pathway for diffusion where small hydrophilic solutes diffuse via "interlamellar hydrophilic channels" (i.e., surface diffusion along the lipid polar headgroups). It is possible that such intercellular routes could also contribute to the penetration of the hydrophilic permeants discussed in this chapter. Although our studies have not been aimed at the localization of the porous permeation pathway, they have begun to characterize important aspects of this pathway based upon physically measurable permeation properties. Coupled with previous studies of the lipoidal properties of the stratum corneum, these studies have demonstrated that a comprehensive model describing transdermal diffusion of permeants through the HEM must include parallel lipoidal and porous permeation routes.

ACKNOWLEDGMENT

This research was supported by NIH Grant GM43181 and an American Foundation for Pharmaceutical Predoctoral Fellowship. TheraTech Inc. kindly provided the HEM samples used in these studies.

REFERENCES

Anderson, B. D. and Raykar, P. V. (1989). Solute structure–permeability relationships in human stratum corneum. *J. Invest. Dermatol. 93*:280–286.

Ackermann, C., Flynn, G. L. and Smith, W. M. (1987). Ether–water partitioning and permeability through nude mouse skin in vitro. II. Hydrocortisone 21-*n*-alkyl esters, alkanols and hydrophilic compounds. *Int. J. Pharm. 36*:67–71.

Anderson, B. D., Higuchi, W. I. and Raykar, P. V. (1988). Heterogeneity effects on permeability–partition coefficient relationships in human stratum corneum. *Pharm. Res. 5*:566–573.

Blank, I. H., Scheuplein, R. J. and MacFarlane, D. J. (1967). Mechanisms of percutaneous absorption. III. The effect of temperature on the transport of nonelectrolytes across the skin. *J. Invest. Dermatol. 49*:582–589.

Bodde, H. E., van der Brink, I., Koerten, H. K. and de Haan, F. H. N. (1991). Visualization of in vitro percutaneous penetration of mercuric chloride: Transport through the intercellular space versus cellular uptake through desmosomes. *J. Controlled Release 15*:227–236.

Burnette, R. R. and Ongpipattanakul, B. (1987). Characterization of the permselective properties of excised human skin during iontophoresis. *J. Pharm. Sci. 76*:765–772.

Cooper, E. R. and Kasting, G. (1987). Transport across epithelial membranes. *J. Controlled Release 6*:23–35.

Cornwell, P. A. and Barry, B. W. (1993). The routes of penetration of ions and 5-fluorouracil across human skin and the mechanisms of action of terpene skin penetration enhancers. *Int. J. Pharm. 94*:189–194.

Cullander, C. and Guy, R. H. (1991). Sites of iontophoretic current flow into the skin: Identification and characterization with the vibrating probe electrode. *J. Invest. Dermatol. 97*:55–64.

Deen, W. M. (1987). Hindered transport of large molecules in liquid-filled pores. *AIChE J. 33*:1409–1425.

Flynn, G. L. (1985). Mechanism of percutaneous absorption from physicochemical evidence. In: Bronaugh, R. L. and Maibach, H. I., eds. *Percutaneous Absorption*. Dekker, New York, pp. 17–52.

Flynn, G. L. (1990). Physicochemical determinants of skin absorption. In: Gerrity, T. R. and Henry, C. J., eds. *Principles of Route-to-Route Extrapolation for Risk Assessment*. Elsevier, New York, pp. 93–127.

Franz, T. J. and Lehman, P. A. (1990). The use of water permeability as a means of validation for skin integrity in in vitro percutaneous absorption studies. *J. Invest. Dermatol. 94*:525.

Ghanem, A. H., Mahmoud, H., Higuchi, W. I., Rohr, U. D., Borsadia, S., Liu, P., Fox, J. L. and Good, W. R. (1987). The effects of ethanol on the transport of β-estradiol and other permeants in hairless mouse skin. II. A new quantitative approach. *J. Controlled Release 6*:75–83.

Ghanem, A. H., Mahmoud, H., Higuchi, W. I., Liu, P. and Good, W. R. (1992). The effects of ethanol on the transport of lipophilic and polar permeants across hairless mouse skin: Methods/validation of a novel approach. *Int. J. Pharm. 78*:137–156.

Golden, G. M., Guzek, D. B., Kennedy, A. H., McKie, J. E. and Potts, R. O. (1987). Stratum corneum lipid phase transitions and water barrier properties. *Biochem. 26*:2382–2388.

Guy, R. H. and Hadgraft, J. (1988). Physicochemical aspects of percutaneous penetration and its enhancement. *Pharm. Res. 5*:753–758.

Hatanaka, T., Shimoyama, M., Sugibayashi, K. and Morimoto, Y. (1993). Effect of vehicle on the skin permeability of drugs: Polyethylene glycol 400-water and ethanol-water binary solvents. *J. Controlled Release 23*:247–260.

Hatanaka, T., Manabe, E., Sugibayashi, K. and Morimoto, Y. (1994). An application of the hydrodynamic pore theory to percutaneous absorption of drugs. *Pharm. Res. 11*:654–658.

Higuchi, W. I., Rohr, U. D., Burton, S. A., Liu, P., Fox, J. L., Ghanem, A. H., Mahmoud, H., Borsadia, S. and Good, W. R. (1987). The effect of ethanol on the transport of β-estradiol in hairless mouse skin: I. Comparison of experimental data with a pore model. In: Lee, P. I. and Good, W. R., eds. *Controlled Release Technology, Pharmaceutical Applications*, ACS Symp. Ser. 348. Am. Chem. Soc., Washington, DC, pp. 232–240.

Kasting, G. B. and Bowman, L. A. (1990a). DC electrical properties of frozen, excised human skin. *Pharm. Res. 7*:134–143.

Kasting, G. B. and Bowman, L. A. (1990b). Electrical analysis of fresh, excised human skin: A comparison with frozen skin. *Pharm. Res. 7*:1141–1146.

Kasting, G. B., Smith, R. L. and Anderson, B. D. (1992). Prodrugs for dermal delivery: Solubility, molecular size, and functional group effects. In: Sloan, K. B., ed. *Prodrugs: Topical and Ocular Drug Delivery*. Dekker, New York, pp. 117–161.

Kim, Y. H., Ghanem, A. H., Mahmoud, H. and Higuchi, W. I. (1992a). Short-chain alkanols as transport enhancers for lipophilic and polar/ionic permeants in hairless mouse skin: Mechanism(s) of action. *Int. J. Pharm. 80*:17–31.

Kim, Y. H., Ghanem, A. H. and Higuchi, W. I. (1992b). Model studies of epidermal permeability. *Seminars in Dermatology. 11*:145–156.

Kligman, A. M. and Christophers, E. (1963). Preparation of isolated sheets of human stratum corneum. *Arch. Dermatol. 88*:702–705.

Liu, P., Nightingale, J. A. S. and Kurihara-Bergstrom, T. (1993). Variation of human skin permeation in vitro: Ionic vs neutral compounds. *Int. J. Pharm. 90*:171–176.

Longsworth, L. G. (1953). Diffusion measurements, at 25°C, of aqueous solutions of amino acids, peptides and sugars. *J. Am. Chem. Soc. 75*:5705–5709.

Michaels, A. S., Chandrasekaran, S. K. and Shaw, J. E. (1975). Drug permeation through skin: Theory and in vitro experimental measurement. *AIChE J. 21*:985–996.

Morimoto, Y., Hatanaka, T., Sugibayashi, K. and Omiya, H. (1992). Prediction of skin permeability of drugs: Comparison of human and hairless rat skin. *J. Pharm. Pharmacol. 44*:634–639.

Peck, K. D., Ghanem, A. H., Higuchi, W. I. and Srinivasan, V. (1993). Improved stability of the human epidermal membrane during successive permeability experiments. *Int. J. Pharm. 98*:141–147.

Peck, K. D., Ghanem, A. H. and Higuchi, W. I. (1994). Hindered diffusion of polar molecules through and effective pore radii estimates of intact and ethanol treated human epidermal membrane. *Pharm. Res. 11*:1306–1314.

Peck, K. D., Ghanem, A. H. and Higuchi, W. I. (1995). The effect of temperature upon the permeation of polar and ionic solutes through human epidermal membrane. *J. Pharm. Sci.* *84*:975–982.

Pikal, M. J. (1990). Transport mechanisms in iontophoresis. I. A theoretical model for the effect of electroosmotic flow on flux enhancement in transdermal iontophoresis. *Pharm. Res.* *7*:118–126.

Potts, R. O. and Guy, R. H. (1992). Predicting skin permeability. *Pharm. Res.* *9*:663–669.

Raykar, P. V., Fung, M. C. and Anderson, B. D. (1988). The role of protein and lipid domains in the uptake of solutes by human stratum corneum. *Pharm. Res.* *5*:140–150.

Renkin, E. M. (1954). Filtration, diffusion and molecular sieving through porous cellulose membranes. *J. Gen. Physiol.* *38*:225–243.

Roberts, M. S., Anderson, R. A., Swarbrick, J. and Moore, D. E. (1978). The percutaneous absorption of phenolic compounds: The mechanism of diffusion across the stratum corneum. *J. Pharm. Pharmacol.* *30*:486–490.

Ruddy, S. B. and Hadzija, B. W. (1992). Iontophoretic permeability of polyethylene glycols through hairless rat skin: Application of hydrodynamic theory for hindered transport through liquid-filled pores. *Drug Design and Discovery* *8*:207–224.

Scheuplein, R. J. (1965). Mechanism of percutaneous absorption: I. Routes of penetration and the influence of solubility. *J. Invest. Dermatol.* *45*:334–346.

Scheuplein, R. J. (1967). Mechanism of percutaneous absorption: II. Transient diffusion and the relative importance of various routes of skin penetration. *J. Invest. Dermatol.* *48*:79–88.

Scheuplein, R. J. and Blank, I. H. (1971). Permeability of the skin. *Physiol. Rev.* *51*:702–747.

Scheuplein, R. J., Blank, I. H., Brauner, G. J. and MacFarlane, D. J. (1969). Percutaneous absorption of steroids. *J. Invest. Dermatol.* *52*:63–70.

Scott, E. R., Laplaza, A. I., White, H. S. and Phipps, J. B. (1993). Transport of ionic species in skin: Contribution of pores to the overall skin conductance. *Pharm. Res.* *10*:1699–1709.

Sims, S. M., Higuchi, W. I. and Srinivasan, V. (1991). Skin alteration and convective solvent flow effects during iontophoresis: I. Neutral solute transport across human skin. *Int. J. Pharm.* *69*:109–121.

Sims, S. M., Srinivasan, V., Higuchi, W. I. and Peck, K. D. (1993). Ionic partition coefficients and electroosmotic flow in cylindrical pores: Comparison of the predictions of the Poisson–Boltzmann equation with experiment. *J. Colloid Interface Sci.* *155*:210–220.

Srinivasan, V., Higuchi, W. I. and Su, M. H. (1989). Baseline studies with the four-electrode system: The effect of skin permeability increase and water transport on the flux of a model uncharged solute during iontophoresis. *J. Controlled Release* *10*:157–165.

Stein, W. D. (1986). *Transport and Diffusion Across Cell Membranes.* Academic Press, Orlando, FL.

Sznitowska, M., Berner, B. and Maibach, H. I. (1993). In vitro permeation of human skin by multipolar ions. *Int. J. Pharm. 99*:43–49.

Williams, A. C., Cornwell, P. A. and Barry, B. W. (1992). On the non-Gaussian distribution of human skin permeability. *Int. J. Pharm. 86*:69–77.

Xiang, T. X. and Anderson, B. D. (1994). The relationship between permeant size and permeability in lipid bilayer membranes. *J. Membrane Biol. 140*:111–122.

Yoneto, K., Ghanem, A. H., Higuchi, W. I., Peck, K. D. and Li, S. K. (1995). Mechanistic studies of the 1-alkyl-2-pyrrolidones as skin permeation enhancers. *J. Pharm. Sci. 84*:312–317.

9

Solute Structure as a Determinant of Iontophoretic Transport

Michael Stephen Roberts, Pamela M. Lai, and Sheree E. Cross
University of Queensland, Brisbane, Queensland, Australia

Nagahiro H. Yoshida
Bayer Yakuhin Ltd., Kyoto, Japan

I. INTRODUCTION

A range of solutes of differing charges and size and for different applications have been used in iontophoresis. In most cases, solutes are used for transdermal studies, but other sites, including ophthalmic, buccal, bladder, and ear, have also been studied.

The delivery of many ionized compounds across membranes is precluded by their inability to enter the membrane in sufficient concentration after topical application. Iontophoresis, which is normally used to indicate the process of transferring ionized drugs into the tissue by the use of a small electric current, offers a means of facilitating the transport of drugs unable to cross by diffusion alone. The basic mechanisms of drug delivery by iontophoresis have been appreciated since the turn of the century, when Ludec successfully demonstrated the transdermal iontophoretic delivery of strychnine sulfate and potassium cyanide into rabbits [1]. The principle of iontophoretic delivery is based on the fact that solute ions will be repelled by an electrode of like charge and migrate to an electrode of opposite charge under the influence of an electromotive force. Iontophoretic drug delivery is usually defined as "anodal," in which an anode electrode (positive charge) is placed in a solution on the membrane containing positively charged drug ions

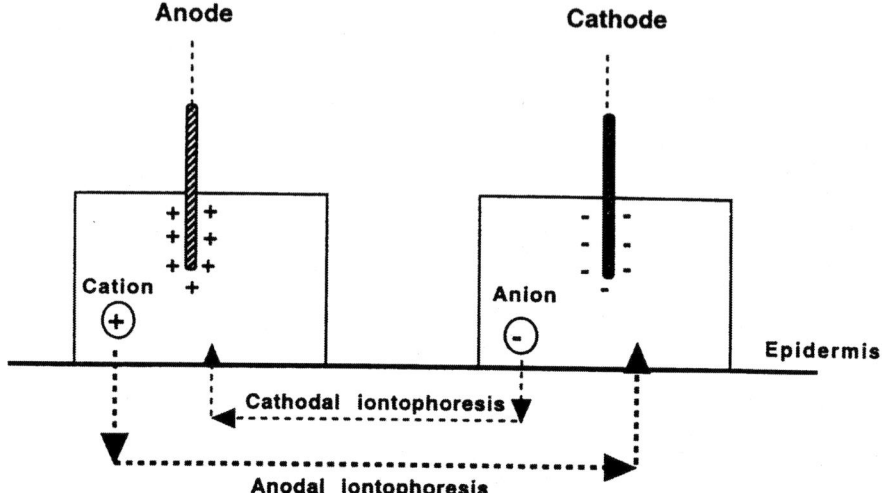

Figure 1 Schematic representation of the basis of anodal and cathodal iontophoretic drug delivery systems.

(cations) and the cathode (negative charge) is placed in a receptor solution in a nearby location (Fig. 1), or "cathodal," in which the electrode locations and drug ion charges are reversed.

In addition to solute structure, a number of factors affecting iontophoretic transport need to be gained for the development of useful optimal iontophoretic drug delivery systems. These include the behavior of solute ions in solution during iontophoresis, mechanisms of solute ion transport through the skin, the effect of different power sources, the choice of electrodes, the composition of vehicles, and the influence of other ions present in the process of drug delivery.

II. RANGE OF SOLUTES ADMINISTERED BY IONTOPHORESIS

Iontophoresis has the potential to overcome many of the physical barriers to topical drug absorption, and the literature is scattered with reports of the clinical use of iontophoresis for the application of drugs across a variety of epithelia, including the skin, eye, cervix, and buccal mucosa, with mixed success [2]. In general, as detailed below, a successful clinical application needs to meet at least three requirements: (a) The solutes must be relatively small; (b) the solutes must be predominantly ionized, and (c) an appropriate vehicle must be used for the iontophoresis. The types of solutes studied are now considered in more detail for each. The epithelia to which iontophoresis has been applied differ.

A. Transdermal

Table 1 shows the range of drugs used in transdermal clinical studies. It is to be noted that most solutes have a molecular weight (MW) around 1200 and are predominantly ionized under physiological pH conditions.

Table 1 Solute Iontophoretic Delivery in Clinical Studies

Solute	MW	Nature	Application	Ref.
Acetic acid	60	Anion	Calcium deposits	139
Acetic acid	60	Anion	Calcified tendonitis	140
Acetyl-*b*-methyl choline	195	Cation	Vasodilator, muscle relaxant; radiculitis, varicose ulcers, discogenic low-back arthritis	141
Acyclovir	225	Cation	Herpes simplex	18
Angiotensin II	1030	Cation	Predicting pre-eclampsia	142
Aspirin	180	Cation	Rheumatic diseases	143
Atropine	289	Cation	Hyperhidrosis	6
Bupivicane	288	Anion	Local skin anesthesia	144
Calcium	40	Cation	Myopathy, myospasm, frozen joints	145
Cisplatin	300	Cation	Carcinoma	146
Citrate	189	Anion	Rheumatoid arthritis	23
Clonidine	230	Cation	Skin response	147
Copper	63	Cation	Fungus infection	22
Dexamethasone	392	Cation		148
Dexamethasone	392	Cation	Tendonitis, bursitis, arthritis, tenosynovitis	24
Dexamethasone	392	Cation	Rheumatoid arthritis	25
Diphenhydramine	169	Cation		149
Gentamicin sulfate	477	Cation	Ear chondritis	150
Glycopyrronium	398	Cation	Hyperhidrosis	5
Histamine	111	Cation	Ulcers	151
Hyaluronidase	> 10,000	Cation	Scleroderma	152

Table 1 Continued

Solute	MW	Nature	Application	Ref.
Hyaluronidase	> 10,000	Cation	Lymphedema	153
Hydrocortisone phosphate	442	Cation	Peyronie's disease	154
Idoxuridine	354	Anion	Herpes simplex	21
Idoxuridine	354	Anion	Herpes simplex	155
Idoxuridine	354	Anion	Herpes simplex	156
Indomethacin	358	Anion	Rheumatic disease	157
Iodine	126	Anion	Scar tissue	158
Iron oxide	158	Cation	Pigment for dermabraded tattoos	159
Leuprolide acetate	1209	Cation		136
Leuprolide acetate	1209	Cation		137
Levamisole	204	Cation	Herpes simplex	155
Lidocaine	234	Cation	Local skin anesthesia	160
Lidocaine	234	Cation	Local skin anesthesia	161
Lidocaine	234	Cation	Local skin anesthesia	162
Lidocaine	234	Cation	Local skin anesthesia	46
Lidocaine	234	Cation	Local anesthesia of ear	48
Magnesium	24	Cation	Muscle relaxant, vasodilator, myalgias, neuritis, deltoid bursitis, low-back spasm	163
Meladinine	247	Anion	Vitiligo	164
Mepivicaine	246	Cation	Local skin anesthesia	161
Methyl-prednisolone	374	Anion	Lichen planus	21
Metoprolol	685	Cation	Hypertension	26
N-acetylcysteine	163	Anion	Otitis media	49
Noradrenaline	169	Cation		142
Penicillin	909	Anion	Infected burn wound	165
Phentolamine	281	Cation	Skin reaction	147
Phenylephrine	168	Cation	Skin reaction	147
Pilocarpine	208	Cation	Sweat test (cystic fibrosis)	166
Pirprofen	252	Anion	Rheumatic disease	143
Poldine methyl-sulfate	441	Anion	Hyperhidrosis	4
Potassium iodide	166	Anion	Scar tissue	167
Prazosin	383	Cation	Skin reaction	147
Prednisolone	360	Cation	Diseases of skin and nail	168
Propranolol	259	Cation	Skin reaction	147

Table 1   Continued

Solute	MW	Nature	Application	Ref.
Sodium salicylate	160	Anion	Plantar warts	15
Tetracaine	300	Anion	Local skin anesthesia	161
Titanium oxide	79	Cation	Pigment for dermabraded tattoos	159
Triamcinolone	394	Cation	Aphthous stomatitis	169
Vinblastine	881	Cation	Kaposi's sarcoma	170
Water	18	Anion/ Cation	Hyperhidrosis	7
Yohimbine	318	Cation	Skin response	147
Zinc oxide	81	Cation	Ischemic ulcer	11

There are a number of clinical studies in which iontophoresis has been employed. The key areas include the following.

Hyperhidrosis   Ichihashi [3] reported the possibility of reducing sweating by iontophoresis. Various compounds have been investigated, and anticholinergic compounds such as poldine methyl sulfate [4], glycopyrronium [5], and atropine [6] were found to be effective. Tap water has also been widely used, for it avoids any side effects associated with anticholinergics [7]. The mechanism of action in the treatment of hyperhidrosis remains unknown, although extensive investigations have been conducted and are shown to be effective. Shelly et al. [8] hypothesized that the sweating is reduced by the inhibition of the sweat ducts in the stratum corneum because the high current results in abnormal keratinization and hyperkeratonic plugging. However, Hill et al. [9], using light and electron microscopy techniques, found no changes in the appearance of the sweat ducts.

Ulcers   Histamine diphosphate has been administered to promote healing of chronic skin ulcers, with success [10,11] (Table 1).

Local anesthesia   Iontophoresis has been used to deliver local anesthetics, including for dentistry [12], ear surgery [13], and conjunctival surgery of the eye [14].

Warts   Iontophoresis of sodium salicylate has been used in the treatment of plantar warts with success [15].

Neurophysiology   Iontophoresis with microelectrodes has been utilized in the field of neuroscience to study the effects of drugs on a limited area, such as peripheral and central nervous systems and neuromuscular junctions, using a glass electrode filled with drug solution [16,17].

Infections Therapies exist for viral (*Herpes simplex*) [18–21], fungal [22], and bacterial infections.

Inflammatory conditions Iontophoresis has been used in conditions such as rheumatoid arthritis [23–25], tendonitis, bursitis, and tenosynovitis [24].

Systemic effects Little appears to be done at this stage. Metoprolol has been used for hypertension [26].

Animal studies Table 2 shows solutes that have been used in animal studies. As with the clinical studies, the solutes used are ionized and have small MW, with one exception, insulin. Srinivasan et al. [27] showed that in controlled experiments without ethanol pretreatment of human epidermis, insulin showed no measurable flux; however, with ethanol pretreatment, there was a significant increase in the permeability coefficients of insulin.

Excised epidermis Solutes used in excised epidermal studies are also predominantly low-MW polar solutes, as shown in Table 3. However, in a number of studies, the iontophoretic transport of uncharged solutes has also been demonstrated. The phenomenon of electro-osmotic flow will be discussed further in Section II.C. Excised skin used in transdermal studies includes hairless mouse, nude rat, shed snake skin, and human epidermis. The human epidermis is used in one of two forms, dermatomed [28,29] or heat separated [30].

B. Ophthalmology

Iontophoresis is a promising procedure for the localized delivery of intraocular drugs. Optimal penetration is achieved when molecules are ionized at the physiological pH of the eye and are water soluble, polar, and of a relatively small size (< 600 d) [31]. Table 4 shows the range of solutes used in ocular iontophoresis. The eye is an ideal iontophoretic delivery route because the aqueous and vitreous humor are good electrical conductors. In addition, the cornea is avascular, allowing the passage of ions without the removal by circulation of the blood [32]. Of relevance is the work of Cross and Roberts [33] in which higher tissue levels of solutes have been reported after transdermal iontophoresis in animal skin (sacrificed animals) than in normal skin, where the blood blow is intact.

Table 2 Solutes Used in In Vivo Transdermal Iontophoresis in Animal Studies

Solute	MW	Nature	Species	Refs.
Chromium	52	Cation	Guinea pigs	171
Dexamethasone	392	Cation	Guinea pigs	50
Dexamethasone	392	Cation	Monkey	148
Ethanolamine	61	Cation	Rats	33
Etidronate	206	Anion	Pigs	172
Fentanyl	529	Cation	Rats	88
Fosfomycin	138	Anion	Guinea pigs	50
Glucosamine	179	Cation	Rats	33
Growth hormone-releasing factor	5040	Cation	Hairless guinea pigs	135
Indomethacin	358	Anion	Pigs	157
Insulin	> 6000	Cation	Rabbits (diabetic)	133
Insulin	> 6000	Cation	Rabbits (diabetic)	134
Insulin	> 6000	Cation	Rats (diabetic)	83
KM-13[a]	337	Cation	Dogs	173
Lidocaine	234	Cation	Rats	63,33
Lidocaine	234	Cation	Pigs	55
Lidocaine	234	Cation	Guinea pigs	48
Mercuric chloride	272	Cation	Pigs	54
N-acetylcysteine	163	Anion	Guinea pigs	49
Phenylethylamine	121	Cation	Rats	33
Salicylic acid	138	Anion	Rats	63
Sodium	23	Cation	Guinea pigs	171
Sodium	23	Cation	Rats	33
Sodium cromoglycate	512	Anion	Excised hairless mouse skin	79
Sufentanil	387	Cation	Rats	88
Tetraethyl-ammonium bromide	210	Cation	Hairless mice	174
Vasopressin	1084	Cation	Rabbits	89

[a]N-1-methyl-1-3-propylamine

Transcorneal Iontophoresis

Transcorneal iontophoresis enhances the ocular penetration of solutes and is capable of delivering high concentrations of drug to the anterior segment of the eye. However, only small concentrations have been achieved in the vitreous humor using this method [34,35]. This is presumably because the lens–iris barrier impedes the movement of drug from the anterior to the

Table 3 Examples of In Vitro Transdermal Iontophoresis

Solute	MW	Species	Refs.
[^{14}C]alkanoic acid sodium salts	46–144	Nude rats	64
[^{14}C]alkanols	32–144	Nude rats	64
Antipyrine	188	Human cadaver skin	62
Aspirin	180	Human cadaver skin	115
Buserelin	1300	Human cadaver skin	175
Chloride	35	Human cadaver skin	62,176
Chlorpromazine HCl	355	Human cadaver skin	115
Chlorpheniramine maleate	391	Human cadaver skin	115
Cyclosporin A	1203	Human cadaver skin	62
Diclofenac sodium	318	Human cadaver skin	62
Ephedrine HCl	202	Human cadaver skin	115
Erythromycin	734	Hairless mouse skin	177
5-Fluorouracil	130	Human cadaver skin	62
Glucose	180	Human cadaver skin	62
Hydrocortisone	363	Hairless mouse skin	178
Hydrocortisone	363	Human cadaver skin	62
Insulin	> 6000	Human cadaver skin	121
Indomethacin	358	Human cadaver skin	62
Inulin	5000	Human cadaver skin	62
Leuprolide	1270	Human cadaver skin and Nuclepore™ membrane	138
Lignocaine	234	Human cadaver skin	62,115
Luteinizing hormone Releasing hormone	1182	Porcine skin flap	179
Melatonin	232	Hairless mouse skin	180
Methotrexate	454	Human cadaver skin	115
Metoprolol	685	Cellophane	28
Naproxen	230	Human cadaver skin	62
Phenol	94	Human cadaver skin	62
Phenylethylamine	121	Human cadaver skin	62,176
Pilocarpine HCl	245	Human cadaver skin	115
Propranolol	259	Human cadaver skin	62
Progesterone	314	Human cadaver skin	62
Salicylic acid	138	Human cadaver skin	62
Salicylic acid	138	Human cadaver skin	115
Salicylic acid	138	Human cadaver skin	67
Salicylic acid	138	Shed snake skin *Elaphe obsoleta*	67
Sodium	23	Human cadaver skin	62,176

Table 3 Continued

Solute	MW	Species	Refs.
Sotalol	272	Human cadaver skin	67
Sotalol	272	Shed snake skin *Elaphe obsoleta*	67
Spiperone	395	Human cadaver skin	62
Sucrose	342	Human cadaver skin	62
Terbutaline	452	Human cadaver skin	147
Verapamil	455	Hairless mouse skin	180
Water	18	Nude rats	64
Water	18	Human cadaver skin	62

Table 4 Iontophoresis of Solutes in the Ocular Region

Solute	MW	Animal	Location	Sample	Peak level ($\mu g/ml$)	Refs.
Cephazolin	477	Rabbit	Transscleral	Vitreous	119.0	40
Ciprofloxacin	331	Rabbit	Transscleral	Vitreous	0.1	181
Dexamethasone	392	Rabbit	Transscleral	Vitreous	140.0	182
Fluorescein	332	Rabbit	Transcorneal	Aqueous	1.0	37
Fluorescein	332	Rabbit	Transscleral	Vitreous	0.2	183
Fluorouracil	130	Rabbit	Transscleral	Conjunctiva sclera	480.0 ug/g 165.0 ug/g	184
Foscarnet	192	Rabbit	Transscleral	Vitreous	200.0	185
Gentamicin	477	Rabbit	Transcorneal (aphakic)	Aqueous Vitreous	77.8 10.4	36
Gentamicin	477	Rabbit	Transcorneal	Aqueous	9.0	37
Gentamicin	477	Rabbit	Transscleral	Vitreous	10.0–20.0	186
Gentamicin	477	Rabbit	Transscleral	Vitreous	207.0	40
Gentamicin	477	Monkey	Transscleral	Vitreous	28.0	39
Gentamicin	477	Rabbit	Transcorneal Transscleral	Aqueous Vitreous	54.8 53.4	187
Ketoconazole	531	Rabbit	Transcorneal Transscleral	Aqueous Vitreous	1.4 0.1	188
Reactive black 5		Rabbit	Transscleral	Conjunctiva		185
Ticarcillin	428	Rabbit	Transscleral	Vitreous	94.0	40
Tobramycin	468	Rabbit	Transcorneal	Aqueous	312.8	189,190
Vancomycin		Rabbit	Transcorneal Transscleral	Aqueous Vitreous	20.2 13.4	31
Vidarabine monophosphate	285	Rabbit	Transcorneal	Aqueous	0.5	191

posterior chamber, since one study achieved peak vitreal concentrations of about 10 g/ml in the aphakic rabbit eye [36].

Transcorneal iontophoresis is superior to subconjunctival injection and simple immersion in drug solutions in producing earlier and higher peak levels in the aqueous humor and in the cornea [31,37].

Transscleral Iontophoresis

Transscleral iontophoresis has been tried as an alternative method to intravitreal injection of antibiotics such as cephalosporins, penicillins, and aminoglycosides [38–40]. Barza et al. [39] reported that the technique of transscleral iontophoresis was a safe, effective, noninvasive way of producing high concentration of antibiotics in the vitreous humor, when gentamicin sulfate iontophoresis was applied to the eyes of monkeys.

C. Bladder

Iontophoresis of mepivacaine and lidocaine with epinephrine have been reported in human cadaver bladders and in clinical trials by Lugnani et al. [41]. The study reported that the active electrode must be sited close to the geometric center of the bladder cavity in order to anesthesize the entire bladder. Siting the electrode close to the wall resulted in anesthesia of only that section of the bladder.

Several studies have described methods and devices involving the internal placement of iontophoretic electrodes into body cavities [42,43]. Stephen et al. [42] described a method and apparatus specifically for the placement of an iontophoretic electrode in the form of a tubular catheter into hollow body cavities containing ion-rich physiological fluids, such as the bladder and vagina. The purpose of their invention was to introduce a technique whereby the selection of the active electrode material and drug counterion would be such as to produce ionic species that interact with one another to minimize or reduce the number of water hydrolysis products produced by electrode decay as a result of the iontophoretic process. Zimmer et al. [43] also described electrodes designed for implantation into fluid-containing hollow body cavities, specifically the bladder, for the local treatment of bladder cancer by iontophoresis. In the patent, the receptor electrode was enclosed in a type of girdle worn around the lower part of the body and connected to the electrode placed in the bladder. The electrode placed in the bladder comprised a tubular rigid probe having a peripheral wall and opposed rows of delivery apertures in the peripheral wall. The inserted end of the probe was sealed and a conductor passed down the hollow interior of the probe and was connected to a source of current at an outer end. Davis et al. [44] also referred to electrode placement in the bladder to prevent infection. In this case both donor and receptor electrodes, in the form of the rigid metal probes, were inserted into the bladder, and the surrounding bladder contents were sterilized by the ions generated by the decomposition of the electrode when the current was passed. All of the above-mentioned studies relied upon the presence of a fluid environment around their donor electrodes for the passage of drug solution or the generation of heavy metal ions.

D. Buccal

Iontophoresis has been used to deliver local anesthetics in the field of dentistry. Gangarosa [45] reported the iontophoresis of a 2% solution of lidocaine, with epinephrine (1:100,000) for the local anesthesia for extraction of retained deciduous teeth. Iontophoresis has also been used to desensitize teeth [46].

E. Ear (Otology)

Iontophoresis in the ear to relieve pain was reported by Albrecht in 1911 [47]. He used cocaine in high concentrations (20%–40%), copper electrodes, and uncontrolled high current (1.5–2 mA) on perforated tympanic membranes. Despite excellent anesthesia, many of his patients were vertiginous during and after treatment, with some patients suffering permanent loss of hearing. However, relatively recent studies have demonstrated that the use of lidocaine [48], N-acetylcysteine [49], or dexamethasone and fosfomycin [50] in iontophoresis to the ear has no adverse effects in either animal or clinical trials. Echols et al. [51] confirmed that lidocaine could be iontophoresed in the middle ear for at least 30 minutes at 1 mA without any adverse effects.

III. MOLECULAR SIZE AND PATHWAYS FOR TRANSPORT

A. Pathways of Iontophoretic Transport Through Epidermis

The application of an iontophoretic current to solute ions on the surface of the skin causes solute ions to traverse the skin along pathways that offer the least electrical resistance. These pathways may or may not be the same as those used during the passive diffusion of solutes through the skin, because the imposition of an exogenous transdermal potential may cause changes in the skin's permeability and create new routes of permeation. Figure 2 shows three

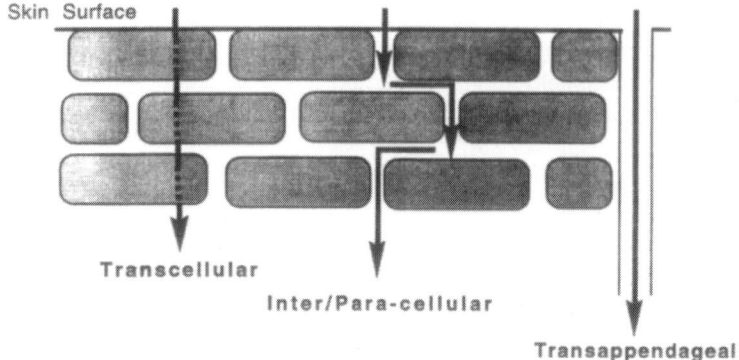

Figure 2 Three possible routes of solute ion transport through epidermis during iontophoresis.

possible routes of solute transport through the epidermis during iontophoresis: (a) transcellular, which involves the sequential partitioning of the solute ion between cells and intercellular lipids as it moves vertically down through the skin; (b) inter- or paracellular, which involves the movement of solute ions through the lipid pathways between cells in the skin; and (c) transappendageal, which involves the movement of ions through skin appendages, such as hair follicles and sweat ducts.

Presently, the literature contains evidence to support the existence of paracellular and transappendageal pathways, with the transcellular route remaining unlikely and only speculative. Based on their studies revealing pore patterns following the iontophoresis of basic and acidic dyes and metallic ions, Abramson and Gorin [10] suggested that appendages, most likely sweat glands, acted as the primary channel for iontophoretic solute transport through the skin. It has been suggested that since the estimated area of invaginated appendageal epithelium is less than 0.1% of the total body surface area, most transdermal transport does not occur via this route [52]. Scheuplein [53] suggested that appendageal transport was important only during the initial stages of percutaneous penetration. Recent evidence supporting the existence of the paracellular route of iontophoretic transport includes the studies of Monteiro-Riviere [54], who examined the ultrastructural patterns of staining of mercuric chloride in pig skin following iontophoresis. In earlier studies she had also implied that transport took place over the whole skin surface area by showing that a uniform alteration in epidermal morphology, rather than at many focal points, occurred secondary to the iontophoresis of lidocaine through pig skin [55]. The visualization of fluorescent ions using confocal microscopy as they permeate through the skin has also demonstrated the presence of charged polar ions in paracellular and follicular spaces during iontophoretic permeation through mouse skin [56]. Although it can be accepted that ionic flow is associated with transappendageal routes, Cullander and Guy [57], using a vibrating probe electrode, have detected the movement of ions in the skin at locations where no appendageal structures or skin injuries are apparent, further suggesting a role of paracellular transport through the skin during iontophoresis. The present state of mind concerning routes of iontophoretic transport was neatly stated by Cullander in his review of iontophoretic pathways through mammalian skin [58] that "iontophoretic currents flow through skin via pores, and that not all pores are associated with appendages."

The contribution of pores to the overall skin conduction of iontophoresis was examined by Scott et al. [59], using scanning electrochemical microscopy (SECM) to image the ionic flux of $Fe(CN)_6^{4-}$ through hairless mouse skin. They reported that initially, pores contribute little to the total conductance, but within 5–30 min, the pores are the primary routes of ionic transport. The rate and number of pores that are activated during iontophoresis is dependent mainly on the magnitude of applied current and correlates directly with a decrease in skin resistance; however, the conductance of individual pores is not a function of the current [59]. The opening of pores suggests that shunts result from the modulation of endogenous skin structures rather than from the current-induced creation of artificial holes [59]. When the iontophoretic current was removed, the impedance increased, but did not return to the pre-iontophoresis value [60,61].

Further evidence for pore transport is presented by Yoshida and Roberts [62] in terms of the temperature dependence of iontophoretic flux for solutes of differing size. They showed that the iontophoretic flux for sodium (MW = 23) and cyclosporin (MW = 1203) were relatively temperature insensitive (Fig. 3). The activation energies for iontophoretic transport are similar to activation energies observed for differences of solutes in aqueous solution and indicate that the iontophoretic transport of both solutes is through the pores [62].

Singh and Roberts [63] have shown that iontophoretic delivery through intact epidermis yields deeper tissue concentrations, identical to that after dermal delivery. Figure 4 shows similar tissue concentrations for lidocaine and salicylate after iontophoretic delivery through intact skin and passive application of these solutes to the dermis. It is therefore concluded that iontophoresis

(A)

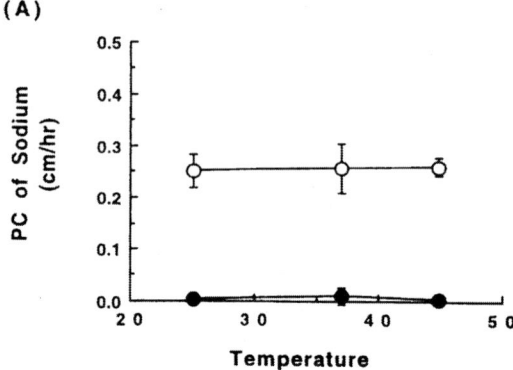

(B)

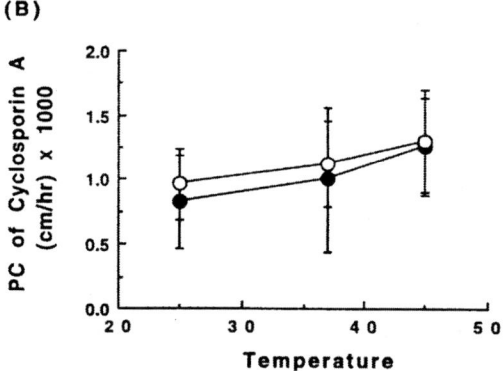

Figure 3 (A) Effect of temperature on sodium permeability coefficient across excised human skin in passive (●) and anodal iontophoresis (○) at 0.38 mA/cm². (B) Effect of temperature on cyclosporin A permeability coefficient across excised human skin in passive (●) and anodal iontophoresis (○) at 0.38 mA/cm². (From Ref. 62.)

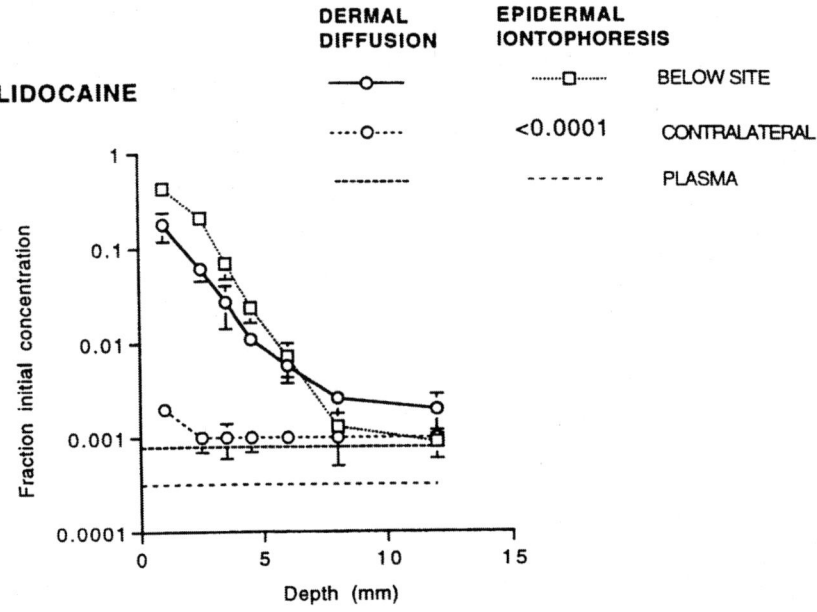

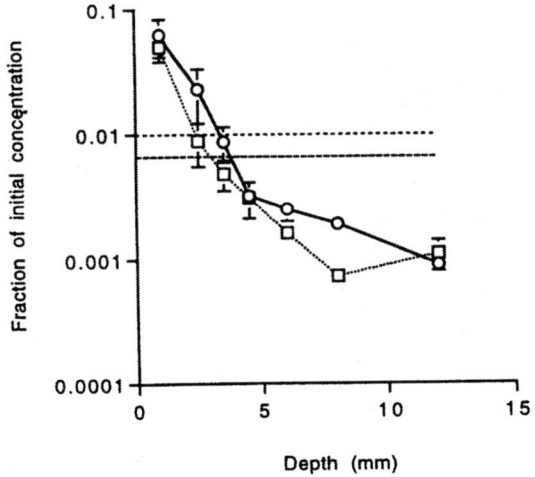

Figure 4 Comparison of dermal diffusion and epidermal iontophoresis in tissues of lidocaine and salicylic acid after 2 hours' application.

simply facilitates transport of ions through the epidermis and not necessarily to deeper tissues.

B. Type of Epidermis

Del Terzo et al. [64] compared the iontophoretic permeation enhancement of a homologous series of ionized (*n*-alkanoic acids) and nonionized (*n*-alkanols) compounds in furry rat skin and nude rat skin. The furry rat skin provided a higher enhancement than nude rat, although the effect was moderate. It was further noted that the advantage of the furry rat skin declined as the permeants became more lipophilic. Furthermore, Siddiqui et al. [65] reported that in vivo iontophoretic delivery of insulin through hairless rat skin was found to be comparable to that through the furry rat skin.

      Shed snake skin has been proposed as a relatively good model for human skin in transdermal permeation studies [66]. Hirvonen et al. [67] compared the transdermal iontophoresis of sotalol and salicylate in shed snake skin, *Elaphe obsoleta*, and human cadaver skin. They advised that snake skin should be used with caution as a model for human skin because snake skin has anion-selective properties while human skin has cation-selective properties.

C. Theoretical Considerations on Iontophoretic Flux

The measured flux of a charged ion across a membrane during iontophoresis is the result of a combination of the following transport mechanisms: (a) simple "passive" diffusion; (b) the electric potential difference across the membrane induced by the presence of the charged electrode, the so-called "direct effect"; (c) electroosmotic or convective flow, which occurs when charged mobile solvent molecules move through the membrane and induce the movement of uncharged or less mobile molecules; and (d) alterations in the permeability of the stratum corneum induced by the presence of the electric field. Each of these transport mechanisms is further related to (a) the mobility of the individual solute molecules in question, u_i, (b) the concentration of solute molecules, c_i, and (c) the electrical force acting on those molecules, f_i.

$$J_i = c_i u_i f_i \tag{1}$$

      The Nernst–Planck equation is conventionally applied to measure iontophoretic flux and arises from the theoretical development of Eq. 1 to define the flux of an ionic solute J_i across a membrane (a) by simple diffusion due to the solute concentration gradient and (b) as a result of the electric potential difference across the membrane (electrochemical transport) [68–70].

$$J_i = -D_i \frac{\partial C_i}{\partial x} \quad - \quad D_i \frac{C_i z_i F}{RT} \frac{\partial \phi}{\partial x} \tag{2}$$

Passive   **Electrochemical**
diffusion   **transport**

where D_i is the diffusion coefficient of the solute, C_i is the concentration of the solute ion, z_i is the charge of the solute, F is the Faraday constant, R is the gas constant, T is the absolute temperature, and $\partial \phi / \partial x$ is the electric potential difference across the membrane. The Nernst–Planck equation now appears in many texts in a modified form that includes an extra term to account for the contribution of electroosmotic or convective flow to the transport of the ion [33,68,71,72].

$$J_i = -D_i \frac{\partial C_i}{\partial x} \quad - \quad D_i \frac{C_i z_i F}{RT} \frac{\partial \phi}{\partial x} \quad \pm \quad C_i J_v (1 - s)$$

Passive   **Electrochemical**   **Convective**
diffusion   **transport**   **flux**

where J_v is the convective flow rate and s is the reflection coefficient. Integration of Eq. 3, assuming a constant electric field and sink conditions below the epidermis, yields a modified Goldman–Hodgkin–Katz equation [68,72].

$$J_i = -P_i C_{is} \frac{(z_i F \, \Delta \phi / RT) \pm J_v (1 - \sigma)(h/D_i)}{1 - \exp\,[(z_i F \, \Delta \phi / RT) \pm J_v (1 - \sigma) h / D_i]} \tag{4}$$

where the passive permeability coefficient $P_i = D_i \beta_i / h$, with β_i the apparent partition coefficient for the ion between the interface of the membrane of thickness h and the adjacent solution, $\partial \phi$ is the electric potential difference across the epidermis, and C_{is} is the concentration of ion in the donor solution. Equation 4 is frequently expressed in the form of an enhancement ratio (ER) [68,72]:

$$\mathrm{ER} = \frac{J_i}{Jp_i} = \frac{\alpha}{1 - \exp\,(-\alpha)} \tag{5}$$

where Jp_i is the passive flux of the solute ion through the membrane ($= P_i C_s$) and α is $-(z_i F \, \Delta \phi / RT) \pm J_v (1 - \sigma) h / D_i$. When the convective component of the iontophoretic flux is negligible, accumulation of solute in the dermis (C_{dermis}) is more likely to arise and affect the observed flux. The flux in this situation may be re-expressed as [68]

$$J_i = -P_i \frac{(z_i F \, \Delta\phi/RT)[C_i - C_{\text{derm}} \exp (z_i F \, \Delta\phi/RT)]}{1 - \exp (z_i F \, \Delta\phi/RT)} \qquad (6)$$

Transient solutions for the Nernst–Einstein equation have been derived assuming a constant source concentration [69]. An approximate solution may be obtained when the decline in source concentration is small over the time period of the study by assuming: (a) a constant iontophoretic permeability coefficient P_{iont}; (b) the donor iontophoretic compartment is a well-stirred solution; (c) sink conditions exist; and (d) the solute concentration in the donor solution C_s of volume V_s changes at a rate equal to the total flux $J_i A$ out of the compartment into the outer layer of the epidermis:

$$V_s \frac{dC_s}{dt} = -J_i A = -P_{\text{iont}} A C_s \qquad (7)$$

where A is the surface area of the epidermis and P_{iont}, the iontophoretic permeability coefficient, is defined as

$$P_{\text{iont}} = P_i \frac{(z_i F \, \Delta\phi/RT) \pm J_v(1 - \sigma)h/D_i}{1 - \exp [(z_i F \, \Delta\phi/RT) \pm J_v(1 - \sigma)h/D_i]} \qquad (8)$$

When the contribution to iontophoretic flux due to convection is small and accumulation in the dermis occurs, Eq. 7 should be expressed as

$$V_s \frac{dC_s}{dt} = -J_i A = -P_{\text{iont}}^* A \left[C_s - C_{\text{derm}} \exp \left(\frac{z_i F \, \Delta\phi}{RT} \right) \right] \qquad (9)$$

where P_{iont}^* is defined as

$$P_{\text{iont}}^* = K_m P_i \frac{z_i F \, \Delta\phi/RT}{1 - \exp (z_i F \, \Delta\phi/RT)} \qquad (10)$$

Separating variables and integrating Eq. 7 between time 0 and time t yields

$$C_i = C_0 \exp -kt = C_0 \exp -\frac{\text{Cl}_t}{V_S} = C_0 \exp -\frac{P_{\text{iont}} At}{V_S} \qquad (11)$$

where C_0 is the concentration of ion in donor compartment at time 0, k is the apparent first-order disappearance-rate constant for the ion from the donor compartment, and Cl is the clearance from that compartment.

Various models have been suggested to describe the interdependence of an ion's ionic mobility, its size, and its charge. Three of these models are described later: (a) the Stokes–Einstein model, (b) the free-volume, or sieving, model, and (c) the pore-restriction model. It is of note here that the modeling and determination of the factors affecting the mobility of an ion in solution has been described as one of the oldest unsolved questions in physical chemistry [73].

The iontophoretic flux of an ion J_i can also be defined in terms of the transport number of the solute, t_i, by

$$J_i = \frac{t_i I_T}{z_i F} \tag{12}$$

where I_T is the total current density, z_i is the charge of the ion, and F is the Faraday constant. The transport number of an ion in solution reflects the proportion of the current carried by concentration c_i of an ion with charge z_i and mobility u_i relative to the current produced by the summation of the contribution of all ions in the solution:

$$t_i = \frac{F c_i z_i u_i}{F \sum_{i=0}^{n} c_i z_i u_i} \tag{13}$$

When a trace amount of solute, i.e., radiotracer, is used, then $c_i z_i u_i \ll \sum_{i=0}^{n} c_i z_i u_i$ and Eq. 13 can be re-expressed as

$$t_i = A c_i z_i u_i \tag{14}$$

where A is a proportionality constant that is dependent on the buffer composition used and the type of solute molecules present. Hence, it is expected that A would differ between anions and cations. Substituting Eq. 14 into Eq. 12, an alternative expression for the iontophoretic permeability coefficient P_{iont} (see Eqs. 7–11) is generated:

$$P_{iont} = \frac{J_i}{c_i} = A u_i I_T \tag{15}$$

Equation 15 shows that P_{iont} is dependent on the ionic mobility, u_i, of a given solute molecule.

Pikal and Shah [74] suggested that the enhanced iontophoretic flux of uncharged low molecular weight solutes (glycine, glucose, and tyrosine) are accounted for by electroosmotic flow from the anode to the cathode. Gangarosa et al. [75] demonstrated an increase in the penetration of non-electrolytes into mouse skin during iontophoresis, with cathodal iontophoresis resulting in the absorption of 0.077% of water applied, anodal iontophoresis accounting for 0.114%, and passive diffusion accounting for 0.003%. Srinivasan and Higuchi [72] found that electroosmotic flow was dependent on the charge of the solute, with the flux of a positively charged solute being increased and that of a negatively charged solute decreased with increasing water flow. However, Pikal [76] reported that the delivery of carboxy inulin, a large anion, was more effective during anodal than cathodal iontophoresis as a consequence of electroosmotic flow.

The above findings are consistent with electroosmotic flow being dependent on the direction of iontophoresis. Pikal and Shah [74] used an electroosmotic flow cell to demonstrate that water flow due to electroosmosis was higher during anodal than during cathodal iontophoresis over a given pH range. We have suggested that the apparent water flow across excised human skin accounts for about 5% of the ion transported during iontophoresis of tritiated water [77]. Solute molecular size and skin thickness appear to be major factors in modifying iontophoresis of nonelectrolytes. The effect of electroosmotic flow may be expected to become dominant for solutes whose relative ionic mobility is negligible. The mechanisms involved in electroosmotic flow can be affected by a number of factors, including the charge density of the pore, the magnitude of the applied current density, the extent of membrane hydration, and the ionic strength of the solution applied [72]. As the size of the solute increases, the importance of electroosmotic flow increases; for monovalent ions with Stokes radii larger than approximately 1 nm, electroosmotic flow is the dominant flow mechanism [76]. The extent to which electroosmotic flow affects transport of different solutes remains unclear.

Del Terzo et al. [64] compared the iontophoretic and passive diffusion profiles of n-alkanols and reported an enhanced iontophoretic transport of the small-MW solutes (methanol, ethanol, and butanol) over passive diffusion, equivalent transport of hexanol, and a decreased iontophoretic transport of the longer-chained solutes (octanol and decanol). In terms of electroosmosis, the hydrophobic molecules have greater difficulty in associating with water molecules, which form the hydration shells of ions in solution. Therefore, the iontophoretic transport of alkanols with increasing chain lengths should decrease [64].

D. Skin Capacitance and the Use of Direct and Depolarizing Pulsed Currents

An electric potential difference can be generated across the skin due to the low conductivity of the stratum corneum and the presence of highly conductive electrolytes (e.g., Cl^-, Na^+) within extracellular fluids below the stratum corneum [78]. This potential difference is responsible for the driving force exerted on ions during iontophoretic transport. Figure 5 shows the typical placement of electrodes on the skin surface and electrical pathways involved in the iontophoretic delivery of cationic drug ions (D^+) in solution with their corresponding counterions (A^-). The iontophoretic current is carried through the skin by the movement of the drug cations toward the cathode and the simultaneous movement of a negatively charged ion from beneath the cathode toward the anode. Other ions present not shown in this simplified diagram, either in the iontophoretic solutions or below the skin surface, are equally capable of using a fraction of the iontophoretic current for transport and thereby reducing the transport of drug ions in a competitive manner.

The iontophoretic flux of solute ions through membranes has been shown experimentally, using several different solutes, to be related to the current density applied across that membrane [28,79]. Lawler et al. [80] suggested that the use of direct currents conventionally used in iontophoresis may have the problem of creating a polarizing current that will decrease the efficiency of the direct current applied, relative to the duration of application of that current, due to the capacitance properties of the skin. The polarization of skin aqueous pores can markedly reduce the iontophoretic flux of a solute by hindering both the entry of that solute into the pore and its passage along it (Fig. 6).

The capacitance of the skin relates to its ability to store electric charge flowing into it in the form of a current. Figure 7 shows the electric potential

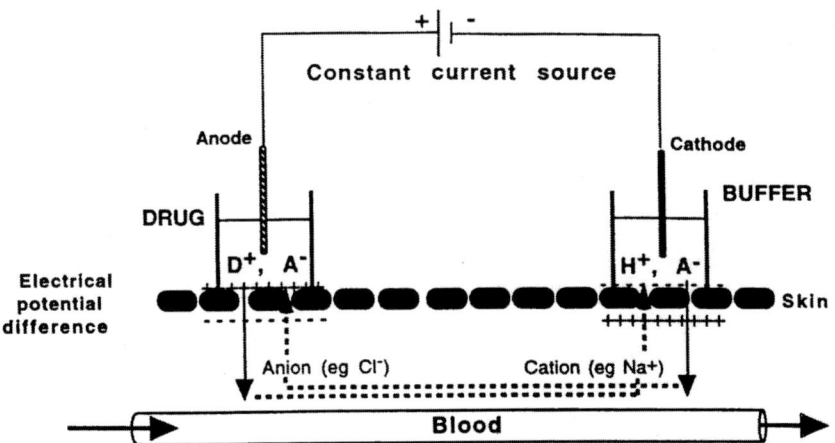

Figure 5 Arrangement of a typical constant-current iontophoretic delivery device on the skin.

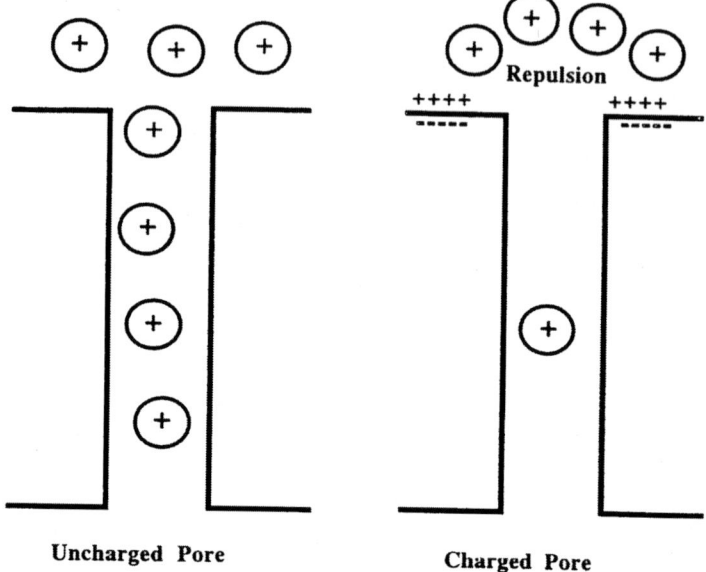

Uncharged Pore   Charged Pore

Figure 6 The effect of pore polarization, caused by the capacitance properties of the skin, on the transport of monovalent solute cations.

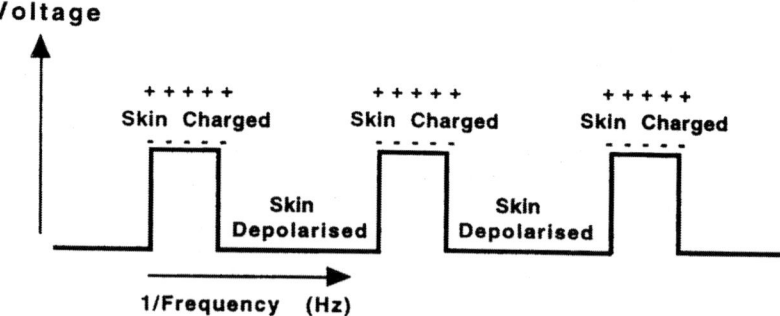

Figure 7 Demonstration of the changes in skin polarization anticipated with the application of a pulsed current.

difference created across the skin by the iontophoretic current that, it is suggested, builds up with the duration of the current. The use of pulsed currents, a direct current that is delivered periodically within a cycle of only microseconds, has been proposed to minimize the capacitor effect of the skin and to increase iontophoretic transport efficiency. A pulsed current would give the skin a chance to depolarize during the time of no current flow before the next segment of current is applied (Fig. 7); with the correct selection of current intensity and frequency it should therefore be possible to start each current cycle with no polarization present in the skin from the previous charge.

Thysman et al. [81] studied solute transport through hairless rat skin with both direct and pulsed currents and found, contrary to the thinking above, that direct currents were much more potent than pulsed currents in the delivery of the cation fentanyl. These authors also noted that after the application of a direct current for only 1 hour, the flux of fentanyl remained higher than that measured during passive diffusion for up to 6 hours compared to that after pulsed current, when no alterations in skin permeability were seen. Other authors have failed to show any significant alteration in skin permeability after the application of direct current for shorter time durations [82,83]. Thysman et al. [81] concluded that pulsed current was more effective than direct current in promoting the transdermal delivery of large drugs like peptides [83–85], whereas direct current may be more potent at inducing transdermal penetration of smaller molecules, such as sodium and glucose [86,87], similarly a solute molecular-weight dependence on the effects of applied direct and pulsed currents has been eluded to by Pikal and Shah [74] and Thysman and Préat [88]. In agreement with these reports, we found that the observed iontophoretic flux of salicylic acid for continuous dc was approximately twofold higher than for pulsed dc ("on–off" ratio of 1:1 for 5 min, at 0.38 mA/cm^2) (Fig. 8).

A pulsed depolarizing iontophoretic system has been developed by Advance Co. [26] that delivers a current of frequency 40 Hz and an on–off duty of 30% to deliver a significant amount of metoprolol into the blood without any observed skin irritation or erythema at the site of application. Okabe et al. [26] hypothesized that the high-frequency pulses provided low skin impedance; in addition, the capacitance of the skin was restored to its initial state at the start of each pulse cycle. Chien et al. [89] reported that a sine waveform induced a faster hypoglycemic effect with insulin, with the peak at approximately 2 hours, than either a trapezoidal (7 hours) or a square waveform (12 hours); however, the duration of the hypoglycemia was also shorter (11 hours) compared with the other two waveforms [89].

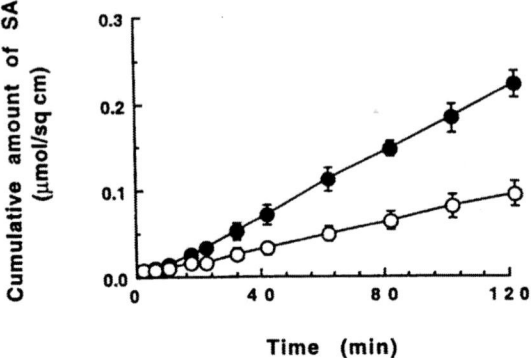

Figure 8 The cumulative amount of salicylate delivered through excised human skin using continuous (●) and pulsed (○) dc currents.

IV. MODELS FOR STRUCTURE-EPIDERMAL PENETRATION RELATIONSHIPS

A. Theoretical Models to Describe the Interdependence of Solute Ionic Mobility, Molecular Size, and Charge

Initially, Roberts et al. [77] assumed a free-volume model. The results for different sets of data are analyzed by Yoshida and Roberts [68] and reproduced in Figure 9. Despite scatter, the slopes are similar. Yoshida and Roberts [62,68] have also compared three models that may describe the interdependence of solute ionic mobility molecular size and charge. These are the Stokes–Einstein, free-volume, and pore-restriction models. We now examine each of these models in more detail.

Stokes–Einstein Model

When a solute ion, i, with z_i elementary charges of an electron (valence), e (1.602×10^{-19} coulombs) is placed in an electric field of intensity E (Vm^{-1}), it will be accelerated until the force F_e is balanced by the drag force F_d exerted on the ion by the hydrodynamic medium in which it is placed [73].

$$F_e = F_d \tag{16}$$

where $F_e = z_i e E$ and F_d are given by Stokes law when the ion is of spherical radius r_i and laminar flow conditions apply in a medium of viscosity h:

$$F_d = 6\pi\eta r_i v_i \tag{17}$$

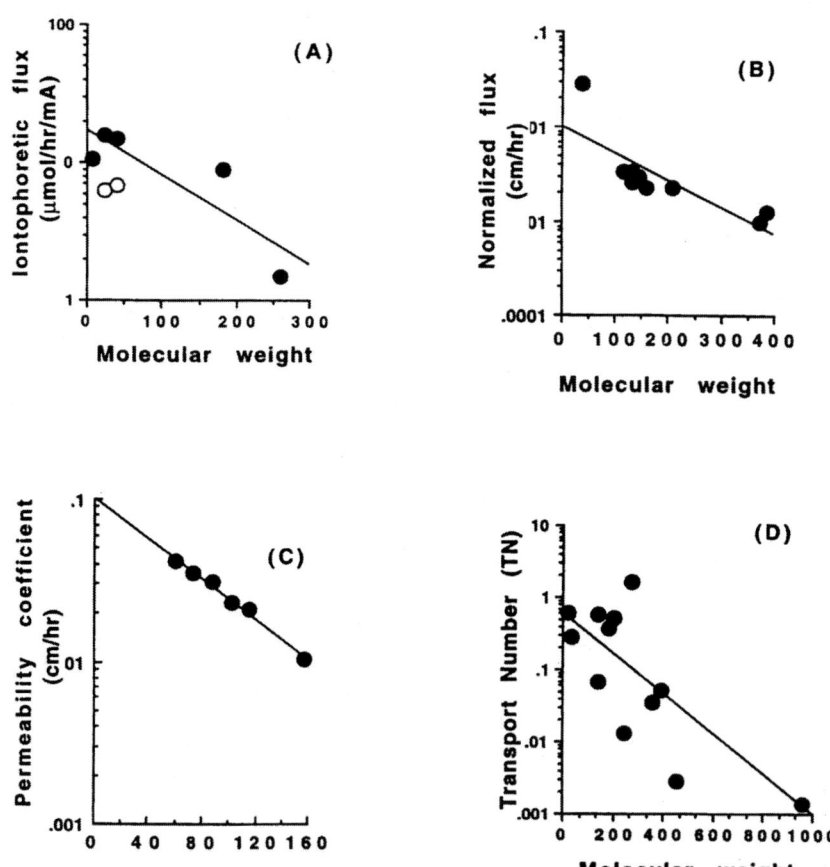

Figure 9 (A) Iontophoretic flux of various cations across excised pig skin versus molecular weight. The donor concentration was 1.0 M of drug as chloride salt. (Data from Ref. 108.) *Key*: (●) monovalent ions, (○) divalent ions. (B) Normalized cathodal iontophoretic flux of anionic solutes across hairless mice versus molecular weight. (Data from Ref. 109.) (C) Cathodal iontophoretic permeability coefficient of alkanoic acid across nude rat skin versus molecular weight. (From Ref. 64.) (D) Comparison of transport number and molecular weight in human epidermis.

where v_i is the constant velocity resulting at the equilibrium of the force. Re-expressing Eqs. 16 and 17 in terms of v_i and u_i yields

$$v_i = u_i E = \frac{z_i e}{6\pi\eta r_i} E \tag{18}$$

The ionic radius r_i is that of the hydrodynamically equivalent sphere consisting of both the molecular ion and its attached hydration shell. Given that the volume of a sphere is $(4/3)\pi r^3$, Eqs. 15 and 18 predict that the logarithm of the iontophoretic permeability coefficient, P_{iont}, for a given solute should be linearly related to the logarithm of its molal volume (MV) with a slope of $-1/3$:

$$\log_{10} P_{iont} = \log_{10} I_T + \log_{10} \frac{z_i e}{6\pi\eta} - \frac{1}{3}\log_{10}\frac{0.75}{\pi} - \frac{1}{3}\log_{10} MV \tag{19}$$

There are, however, a number of inconsistencies in the application of Stokes law to ion conductivity in electrolytes [90]. Of particular concern is the presence of electrical interactions between the charged solute ion and the solvent molecules present that result in a larger-sized hydrated solute ion. It has been suggested that solvated solute ions move through the solvent from one "cage" of solvent molecules to an adjacent "cage" [90], a model originally proposed by Glasstone et al. [91].

Free-Volume, or Sieving, Model

The theoretical basis of the transport of solute ions during iontophoresis can be compared to electrophoresis through a gel network. When the ionized solute has a mean Stokes radius smaller than the average mesh size (hole in the network), the solute is considered as a rigid sphere undergoing Brownian movement, with a mobility dependent on the frequency of solute interaction with the porous network. The sphere mobility is assumed to be proportional to the fractional volume of the pore that is accessible to the sphere [92]. The electrophoretic mobility, u, of such a solute sphere has been shown to be directly related to the molecular weight of the solute [93]:

$$\log_{10} u = A + B \times MW \tag{20}$$

where A and B are empirical constants.

A similar theoretical basis for such a relationship can be deduced from the work of Cohen and Turnbull [94], which introduces the concept of a dynamic "free volume" with a low activation energy that is created and into which solute ions move to and fro. The model is valid when solute movement is not restricted by the dimensions of the pore or gel network, and it appears to be consistent with the "cage" model of Glasstone et al. [91]. Cohen and Turnbull [94] suggested that no energy exchange is associated with redistribution of the free volume, the total free volume in the system being constant. The probability of finding a hole of volume V^* or larger can be expressed by

$$P_f = \frac{1}{V_i} \exp \frac{-V^*}{V_i} \tag{21}$$

where P_f is the probability of finding a hole produced by the redistribution of the free volume and V_i is the average free volume. Since the diffusion coefficient is related to P_f, Eq. 21 can be rewritten as

$$D = B \exp \frac{-V^*}{V_i} \tag{22}$$

where B is a constant. This model has been modified to describe the diffusion of solutes in liquids and is often expressed as the "Macedo–Litovits" equation [95]:

$$D = D_0 \exp \frac{E}{RT} \exp \frac{-\partial V^*}{V_i} \tag{23}$$

where D_0 is the pre-exponential factor, ∂ is the overlap factor introduced because the same free volume is available to more than one solute ion, and E is the energy per mole that an ion needs to overcome the attractive forces that hold it to neighboring molecules.

The free-volume model has been used to describe the rapid decrease in solute diffusivity through human red cell membranes with increases in molecular size [96]. A statistical thermodynamic model for size distribution can then be employed to show that the diffusion coefficient of a solute is related to its MV:

$$D = B \exp \frac{-MV}{V_{av}} \tag{24}$$

where V_{av} is the average free volume. Other investigators have attempted to correlate conductivity in polymer membranes with the free-volume model using the concept of *fluidity* [97,98]. Application of the free-volume model to iontophoretic transport requires that the ionic mobility, u_i, be expressed as a function of the diffusion coefficient:

$$u_i = \frac{|z_i|FD_i}{RT} \tag{25}$$

Substituting Eqs. 24 and 25 into Eq. 15 yields

$$\log_{10} P_{\text{iont}} = \log_{10} B' - \frac{MV}{2.3V_{\text{av}}} \tag{26}$$

where V_{av} can be obtained from the slope of a plot of the logarithm of iontophoretic flux against MV and $B' = |z_i| FB / RT$. The average free volume gives a measure of the size of the hole into which a solute can enter readily. When the solute ions move into a neighboring hole or create a new hole, a certain activation energy is required [99]. A temperature dependence of the average free volume in polymer transport has been expressed in the following form [100]:

$$V_{\text{av}} = V_0 \, g(T - T_0) \tag{27}$$

where g is the coefficient of the thermal free-volume expansion and T_0 is the temperature at which the free-volume disappears (close to the equilibrium glass transition temperature) and V_0 is the volume of the liquid at T_0. If the free volume is formed by the creation of a new hole, as suggested by Eyring and Hirschfelder [99], a low activation energy, corresponding to viscous drag of water molecules, could be anticipated.

Pore-Restriction Model

A third model of iontophoretic flux arises from the idea of a retardation in the entry of solute ions into, and movement via, pores in the skin. Renkin [101] described a pore-restriction model for the diffusion of uncharged molecules through water-filled cylindrical pores. He suggested that diffusion would be restricted relative to the movement in aqueous solution by (a) steric hindrance inhibiting the entry of solute ions into the pore, and (b) hindrance due to frictional forces during the movement of solute ions through the pore. According to this model, P_{iont} may be expressed by

$$\frac{P_{\text{iont}}}{PC_s} = \left(1 - \frac{r_i}{r_p}\right)^2 \left(1 - 2.10\frac{r_i}{r_p} + 2.09\frac{r_i^3}{r_p} - 0.95\frac{r_i^5}{r_p}\right) \tag{28}$$

Pore　　**Movement in pore**
entry

where PC_s is the permeability coefficient in solution, r_i is the radius of the solute ion, and r_p is the radius of the pore. When $r_i/r_p < 0.2$, Eq. 28 approximates to

$$\frac{P_{iont}}{PC_s} = \left(1 - \frac{r_i}{r_p}\right)^4 \tag{29}$$

Though this model has been used widely in membrane absorption studies, difficulties in applying the model to iontophoresis arise when: (a) solute ions are nonspherical, (b) a heterogeneity in pore sizes exists, or (c) interactions occur with the pore surface. Expressing Eq. 29 in logarithms and noting that for small x, $\log_{10}(1 - x)$ approximates to $-(x/2)$, then:

$$\log_{10}\left(1 - \frac{r_i}{r_p}\right)^4 = -2\frac{r_i}{r_p}$$

and

$$\log_{10} P_{iont} = -2\frac{r_i}{r_p} + N \tag{30}$$

where N is a constant. The free-volume and pore-restriction models become comparable when the radius of the ion is much less than that of the pore, since restriction will be evident if the ratio of iontophoretic flux through the skin divided by the solute's ionic mobility in solution is not constant with increasing solute size. Equation 30 suggests that a linear relationship should exist between the logarithm of P_{iont} and the radius, r_i, rather than r_i^3.

A second commonly used pore-restriction model is defined by the permeability of a solute ion through a membrane relative to water, using the reflection coefficient, σ. It was pointed out by Davson [102] that the reflection coefficient, with limits $\sigma = 1$, no entry, and $\sigma = 0$, no restriction on entry, correlates well with the Renkin model. In the present context, $1 - \sigma$ is simply P_{iont}/P_{water}, where P_{water} is the iontophoretic permeability coefficient of water [68]. Plots of $\log(1 - \sigma)$ versus r_i, $\log MV$, or MV should give slopes identical to plots based on P_{iont}. The reflective coefficient, σ, is often now used to correct for differences in the extent of solute ion transport with convective flow during iontophoresis [68,103,104].

B. Application of Theoretical Models in In Vitro Iontophoretic Studies

Yoshida and Roberts [62,68] have expressed the size dependence of P_{iont} in terms of the Stokes–Einstein, free-volume, and pore-restriction models and suggested that the free-volume model may be most appropriate for epidermal transport.

However, discrimination among the three models is not straightforward, as is evident in the regressions reported for cations (Fig. 10) and anions (Fig. 11). The slope of the free-volume model relationship for anions (negative charge), 0.0035 (Fig. 10B), appeared to be steeper than that for cations (positive charge), 0.002 (Fig. 10B). Yoshida and Roberts [62] suggested that a difference in the slopes could have been anticipated due to the fixed negative charge on the stratum corneum. At pH 7.4, the amino acid residues of proteins in the stratum corneum are negatively charged [105], and hence positively charged solutes should be transported through a pore more readily than a negatively charged solute [106]. An intermediate situation may be anticipated for the slope of the free-volume relationship as observed in Fig. 12. In their comparison of iontophoretic models, Yoshida and Roberts [62] also looked at the data of Ruddy and Hadjiza [104]. These data appear to be described best by the free-volume model (Fig. 13). Yoshida and Roberts [62] suggest that these relationships will not apply to the iontophoretic transport of larger solutes, whose mechanism of transport is likely to be mainly by electroosmotic flow.

Combining regressions for the free-volume relationships (Eq. 26) obtained for cations, anions, and uncharged solutes, Yoshida and Roberts [62] were able to estimate that the average free volume of the holes required for a solute to migrate was equivalent to an ionized solute with a MV of 155 (MW approximately 200). Fluctuations in the local density would of course be expected to occur, depending on the nature of the diffusion medium used. Yoshida and Roberts [62] suggested that solutes with a MV greater than 155 will show limited iontophoretic transport due to restriction by the volume of a solvent hole. Crank and Park [107], from their work examining diffusion in polymers, suggested that even though the hole may not be large enough to accommodate a diffusion molecule, the cooperative motion of several neighboring molecules may allow two or more holes to merge into one hole large enough for a diffusional jump to occur. Examination of other work in the literature revealed that the logarithm of transport numbers (Fig. 14), iontophoretic fluxes, and permeability coefficients for solute data reported by Roberts et al. [77], Phipps et al. [108], Green et al. [109], and Del Terzo et al. [64] were linearly related to MW. These data can be interpreted to give a free volume corresponding to an ionized solute with MW approximately 180, which is similar to that predicted by the study of Yoshida and Roberts [62].

(A)

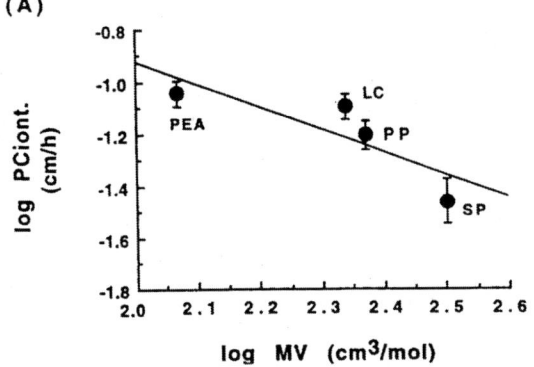

(B)

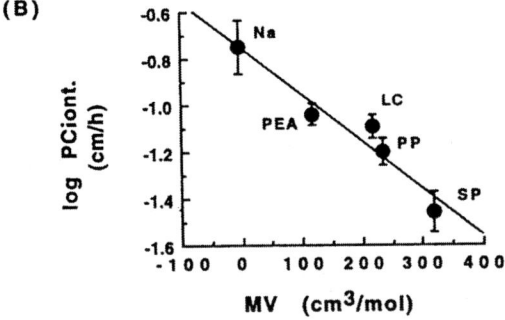

(C)

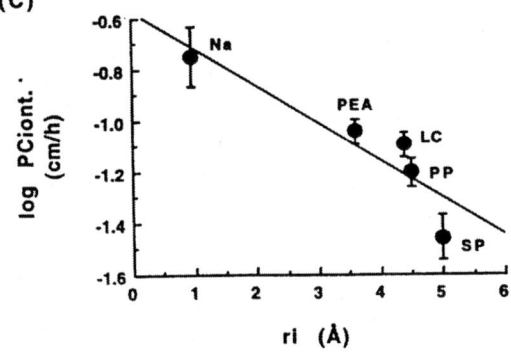

Figure 10   Iontophoretic permeability coefficient ($PC_{iont.}$) of various positively charged solutes in anodal iontophoresis at 0.38 mA/cm^2. (A) log $PC_{iont.}$ versus log MV. (B) log $PC_{iont.}$ versus MV. (C) log $PC_{iont.}$ versus radius. (Redrawn from Ref. 62.)

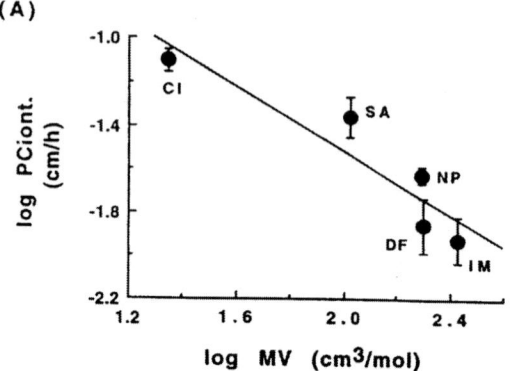

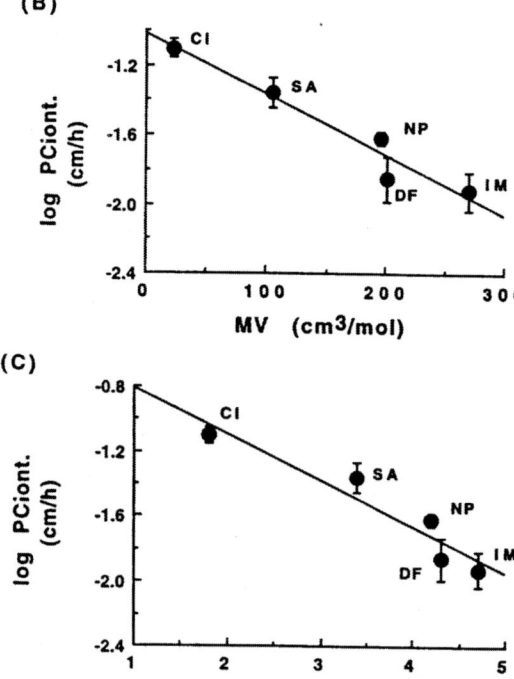

Figure 11 Iontophoretic permeability coefficient ($PC_{iont.}$) of various negatively charged solutes in cathodal iontophoresis at 0.38 mA/cm². (A) log $PC_{iont.}$ versus log MV. (B) log $PC_{iont.}$ versus MV. (C) log $PC_{iont.}$ versus radius. (Redrawn from Ref. 62.)

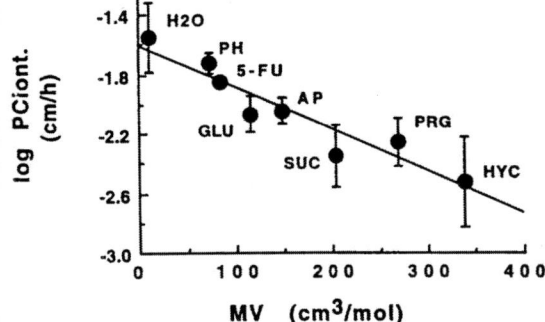

Figure 12 Logarithm of iontophoretic permeability coefficient of various non-electrolytes during anodal iontophoresis through excised human skin versus molecular volume according to the free-volume model.

Amphoteric Molecules

Roberts et al. [77] examined the flux of amphotericin, a large (MW = 960) amphoteric (pK_{aS} 5.5 and 10) molecule. Figure 15 shows the graph plotted for the iontophoretic transport of para-aminobenzoic acid (MW = 137) and amphotericin at the pHs of 3.5, 7.5, and 12. At the higher pH of 12, the higher flux may be due to skin damage. At pH 3.5, para-aminobenzoic acid and amphotericin both exist as cations and require anodal iontophoretic transport. It is to be noted that at pH 4.7 and pH 7.75, respectively, for para-amino-benzoic acid and amphotericin, these solutes exist as zwitter ions and allow anodal and cathodal transport to be compared for a single solute with a defined size and identical solution conductivity. Figure 15 shows that the relative cation and anion fluxes are approximately in accordance with the observed 0.6:0.4 ratio of total cation to total anion flux [106].

V. ROLE OF BLOOD SUPPLY AND DEPTH OF PENETRATION IN VIVO

The determinants of in vivo iontophoretic delivery and subsequent tissue distribution have been studied to only a limited extent. The concentrations of solute in a given tissue below the epidermis will be dependent on the flux of solute into that tissue and on the clearance of solute from the tissue [62,110]. Clearance of a solute by the local blood supply is an important concern, given

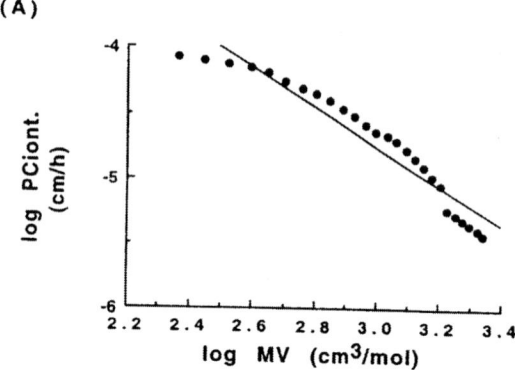

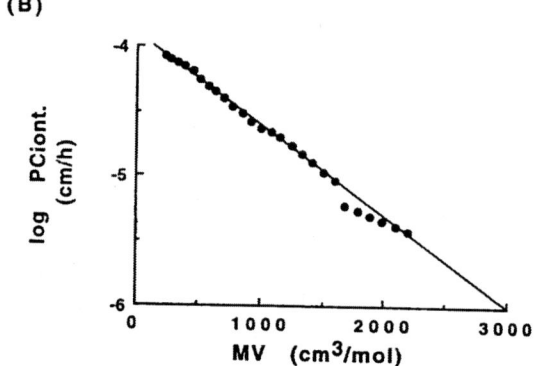

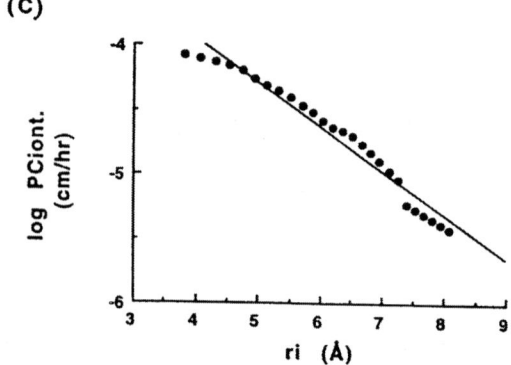

Figure 13 Iontophoretic permeability coefficient ($PC_{iont.}$) of a homologous series of polyethylene glycols solutes in cathodal iontophoresis at 0.38 mA/cm^2. (A) log $PC_{iont.}$ versus log MV. (B) log $PC_{iont.}$ versus MV. (C) log $PC_{iont.}$ versus radius. (Data from Ref. 104.)

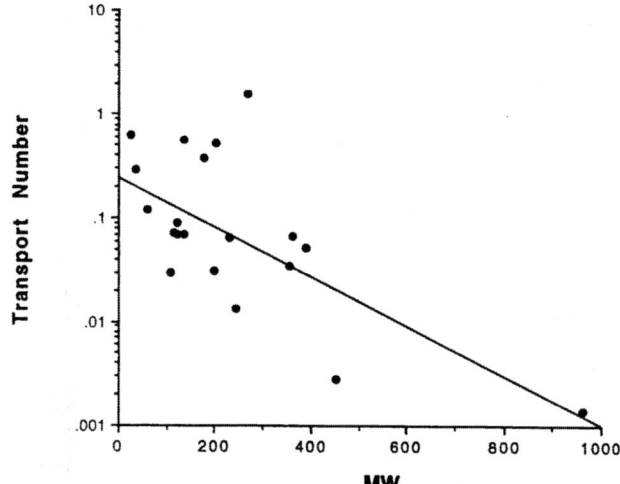

Figure 14 Relationship between transport number and solute molecular weight (MW) for human epidermis. (Data from Refs. 106, 115, and 118.)

that iontophoresis often leads to erythema [111]. In the absence of any solute accumulation in the dermis due to recirculation, and making the simplistic assumption that the dermis can be approximated by a compartment model [63], the concentrations in the dermis C_{derm} is defined by Eq. 31 for an epidermal flux defined by Eqs. 7 and 9 [33].

$$V_{derm} \frac{dC_{derm}}{dt} = P_{iont}AC_s - Cl_B C_{derm} - Cl_{derm \to sc} C_{derm} \tag{31}$$

$$V_{derm} \frac{dC_{derm}}{dt} = P^*_{iont}A\left(C_s - C_{derm}\exp\frac{z_i F \Delta\phi}{RT}\right) - Cl_B C_{derm} - Cl_{derm \to sc} C_{derm} \tag{32}$$

where V_{derm} is the volume of the dermis for the cross-sectional area of penetration, Cl_B is the clearance by the blood supply, and $Cl_{derm \to sc}$ is the clearance of the solute from the dermis into the subcutaneous tissue. At steady state, $V_{derm}(dC_{derm}/dt) = 0$ and Eqs. 31 and 32 can be reexpressed as Eqs. 33 and 34, respectively:

$$C_{derm,ss} = \frac{P_{iont}AC_s}{Cl_B + Cl_{derm \to sc}} \tag{33}$$

(A)

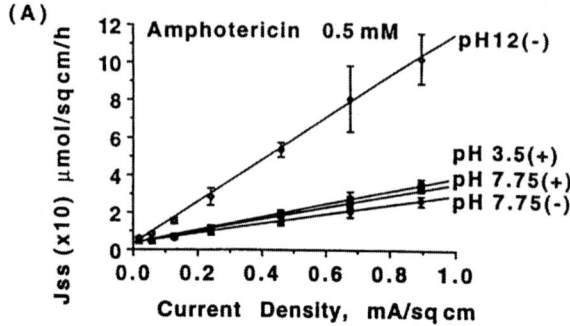

(B)

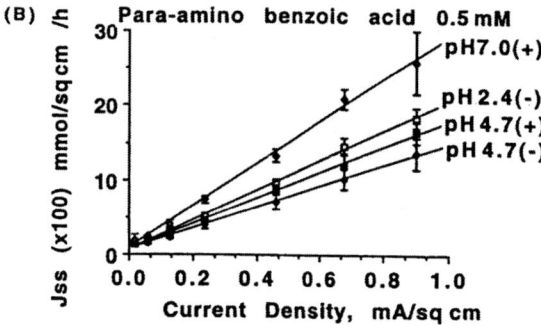

Figure 15 (A) Effect of current strength on the iontophoresis of amphotericin B at pH 12 (–), pH 3.5 (+), pH 7.75 (+), and pH 7.75 (–). (B) Effect of current strength on the iontophoresis of para-aminobenzoic acid at pH 12 (–), pH 3.5 (+), pH 7.75 (+), and pH 7.75 (–).

$$C_{\text{derm},ss} = \frac{P^*_{\text{iont}}AC_s}{P^*_{\text{iont}}A \exp{(z_iF\,\Delta\phi/RT)} + \text{Cl}_B + \text{Cl}_{\text{derm}\rightarrow sc}} \tag{34}$$

According to Eqs. 34 and 35, a higher dermal concentration $C_{\text{derm},ss}$ is anticipated if the dermal blood supply is compromised, but a higher concentration will be apparent only when $\text{Cl}_B \gg \text{Cl}_{\text{derm}\rightarrow sc}$ in Eq. 34 and $\text{Cl}_B \gg P_{\text{iont}}A \exp{(z_iF\,\Delta\phi/RT)} + \text{Cl}_{\text{derm}\rightarrow sc}$ in Eq. 34. The corresponding steady-state concentrations for a solute in the subcutaneous tissue are

$$C_{sc,ss} = \frac{Cl_{derm \to sc} P_{iont} A C_s}{(Cl_B + Cl_{derm \to sc})(Cl_{derm \to sc} + Cl_B + Cl_{sc \to fascia})} \qquad (35)$$

$$C_{sc,ss} = \frac{Cl_{derm \to sc} P_{iont} A C_s}{[P_{iont} A \exp(z_i F \Delta\phi/RT) + Cl_B + Cl_{derm \to sc}](Cl_{derm \to sc} + Cl_B + Cl_{sc \to fascia})} \qquad (36)$$

Again, a higher concentration may be anticipated in the subcutaneous tissue if the clearance due to the blood flow Cl_B is significantly higher than that due to transport of the solute between the tissues. The expressions for deeper tissues are similar in form to those just described.

A. Experimental Evidence for the Dependence of Iontophoretic Tissue Distribution on Blood Supply

Riviere et al. [112,113] have shown that the iontophoretic transport rate of lidocaine in the isolated perfused porcine skin flap (IPPSF) preparation is modified by the coadministration of vasoactive drugs. The authors suggested that discrepancies arising between in vitro and in vivo data may be due to the lack of sink conditions available in vitro without a viable dermal blood supply, leading to significant underestimates of drug flux achievable in the in vivo situation [114]. A number of studies have shown that the in vivo rate of passive solute diffusion through the dermis is significantly dependent on the dermal blood supply and that the subsequent extent of tissue absorption of a solute can be related to the lipophilicity of the solute [110,114–118]. A more recent study of Cross and Roberts [33] showed that the iontophoretic flux of five monovalent cations delivered by anodal iontophoresis in rats was independent of dermal blood supply (Table 5). In contrast, they showed that during iontophoresis, the depth of transdermal absorption and the extent of tissue distribution were dependent on dermal blood supply (Fig. 16). The blood flow interdependence of solute absorption from the donor solutions in that study was consistent with the effective sink conditions existing below the epidermis. Cross and Roberts [33] noted that, in accordance with Eqs. 6 and 9, the iontophoretic flux and disappearance rate from the donor solution increase only when the dermal concentration of the solute becomes significant, if all other conditions are kept identical.

The higher concentrations of iontophoresed solutes in tissues below the epidermis had also been expected, in accordance with Eqs. 32 and 34, when $Cl_B > Cl_{dermis \to sc}$ and $Cl_B > Cl_{sc \to fascia}$. Singh and Roberts [118] have previously shown, in passive diffusion studies of solutes, that $Cl_B > Cl_{dermis \to sc}$ and $Cl_B > Cl_{sc \to fascia}$ for salicylic acid and lidocaine.

Table 5 Iontophoretic Permeability Coefficients Measured During Iontophoresis of Monovalent Cations in Rats

Solute	MW	PC_{iont} (ml/hr/cm^2)	
		Anaesthetised	Sacrificed
Sodium	23	0.910 ± 0.115	0.838 ± 0.058
Ethanolamine	61	0.326 ± 0.007	0.330 ± 0.030
Phenylethylamine	121	0.312 ± 0.015	0.366 ± 0.046
Glucosamine	179	0.145 ± 0.025	0.255 ± 0.042
Lignocaine	234	0.332 ± 0.040	0.296 ± 0.016

Mean $\pm$ s.e., $n = 3$.
Modified from Ref. 33.

VI. OTHER CONSIDERATIONS

Table 6 outlines the factors affecting iontophoresis.

A. Solute Ionization, Buffer Composition, and Vehicle pH

The pH of the donor solution used during iontophoresis is critical, for it controls the degree of ionization of the solutes contained within it. Siddiqui et

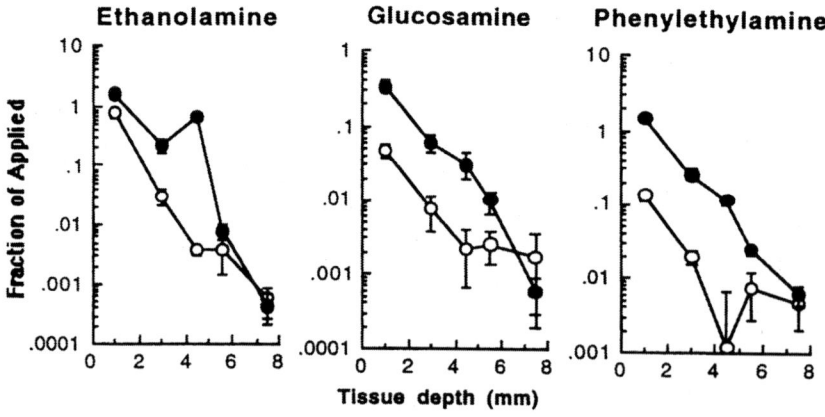

Figure 16 Tissue concentrations of three monovalent cations measured as a fraction of the applied concentration following iontophoresis in rats in the presence (O) or absence (●) of blood flow. Mean $\pm$ s.e., $n = 3$. (Reproduced from Ref. 33.)

Table 6 Factors Influencing Iontophoretic Transdermal Delivery

Physiochemical factors	Physiological factors	Electrical factors
Ionic charge	Region (density of append-ages)	Current density
Extraneous	Age	Electrodes
pH in the donor solution	Sex	Duration of treatment
Ionic strength	Race	Nature of current
Solute concentration	Hydration of the skin	
Buffer constituents	Delipidization (ethanol pretreatment)	
Chemical structure of the solute	Fluidization of lipids (en-hancer)	

al. [110,115] demonstrated that iontophoretic flux increases with the degree of ionization of solutes, and particularly reflects the permselectivity of the skin for positively charged ions. The ionization of amino acid groups on proteins within the skin may also be induced by pH changes and lead to changes in solute iontophoretic flux. Increases in the iontophoretic flux of verapamil over the pH range 4–6, in which its degree of ionization is relatively constant, were suggested to arise from increases in the negative charge on the skin [85]. We have also observed changes in pH-affected phenylethylammonium (PEA) flux during anodal iontophoresis (Fig. 17A) and salicylate during cathodal iontophoresis (Fig. 18A). The change is, however, most likely a consequence of the altered ionic composition of the buffer constituents, since the solution conductivity also increased with pH. Roberts et al. [77] and Phipps and Gyory [119] have suggested that iontophoretic drug delivery is dependent on the ionic composition of the vehicle and that the transport may be predicted from the concentrations, charge, and ionic mobility of ions present, using development of Eq. 13. Consistent with the addition of buffer ions, resulting in greater competition for transport for the ion of interest both PEA (Fig. 17B) and salicylate (Fig. 18B) have lower iontophoretic fluxes at higher buffer concentrations. Buffer constituents also affect solute iontophoretic fluxes, as shown for salicylic acid in Figure 18C. Both the flux for PEA (Fig. 17C and D) and salicylate (Fig. 18C) can be related directly to the ratio of specific conductivity for various vehicles in which the pH, buffer constituents, and buffer concentrations have been altered. Hence, the ionic composition of a vehicle is a major determinant of the iontophoretic delivery of any ion.

The ionic mobility of ions is also a determinant of iontophoretic trans-

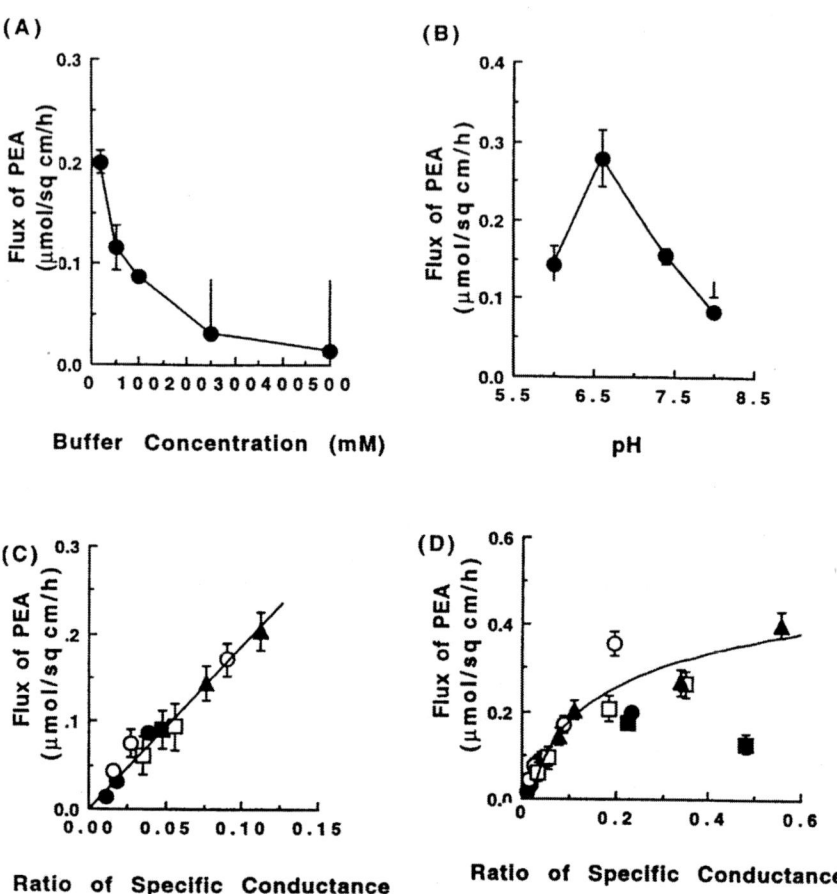

Figure 17 (A) Effect of pH in the donor compartment on PEA anodal iontophoresis at 0.38 mA/cm^2. Donor solution contained 1 mM PEA and 50 mM HEPES buffer. (B) Effect of pH in the donor compartment on PEA anodal iontophoresis at 0.38 mA/cm^2. Donor solution contained 1 mM PEA and 50 mM HEPES buffer. (C) Relationship between PEA flux and the ratio of specific conductance on anodal iontophoresis 0.38 mA/cm^2. (D) Relationship between PEA flux and the ratio of specific conductance on anodal iontophoresis 0.38 mA/cm^2.

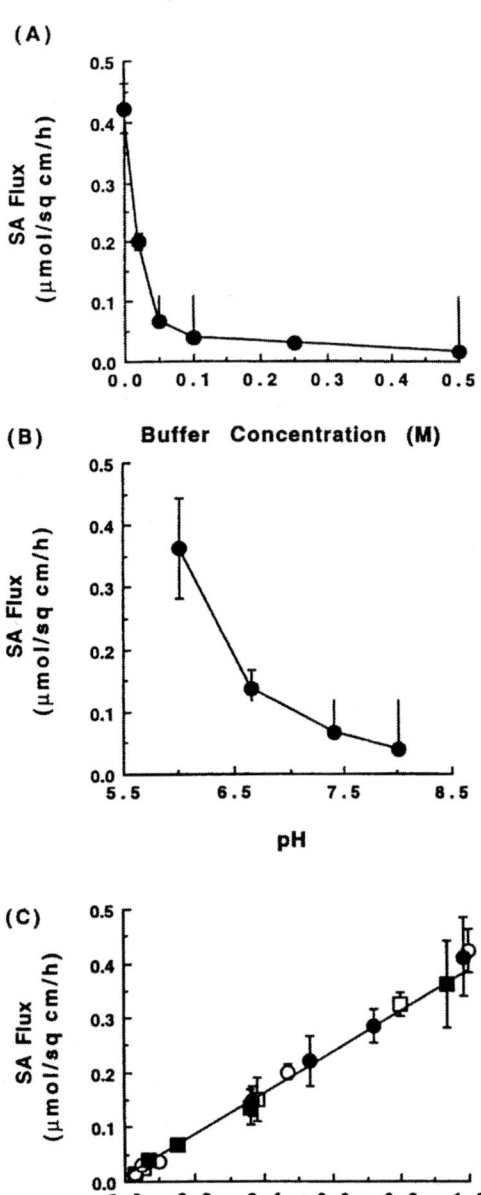

(A)

(B)

(C)

Ratio of Specific Conductance

Figure 18 (A) Effect of pH in the donor compartment on salicylic acid (SA) anodal iontophoresis at 0.38 mA/cm^2. Donor solution contained 1 mM SA and 50 mM HEPES buffer. (B) Effect of pH in the donor compartment on SA anodal iontophoresis at 0.38 mA/cm^2. Donor solution contained 1 mM SA and 50 mM HEPES buffer. (C) Relationship between SA flux and the ratio of specific conductance on anodal iontophoresis 0.38 mA/cm^2.

port. Yoshida and Roberts [62] found a direct relationship between ionto-phoretic permeability coefficients for a range of solutes of different sizes and their mobilities. Bellantone et al. [120], in observing that benzoate ion flux decreased following the addition of extraneous ions to the donor solution, suggested the avoidance of small mobile ions of the same charge as solute ions to be delivered in the donor vehicle. Del Terzo et al. [64] also commented that (a) dissociation of mixed valance salts provided greater numbers of competi-tive ions in solution, and their use in iontophoresis studies should be avoided, and (b) electrolytes having multivalent cations (e.g., Mg^{2+}) appear to be superior to those with monovalent cations (e.g., Na^+, K^+).

B. Clinical Considerations

Candidates for Iontophoretic Delivery

The nature of iontophoretic delivery restricts its clinical usefulness to ex-tremely potent drugs and to those active at the immediate site of delivery, due to the relatively small concentrations capable of being driven through the skin without causing skin damage. The theoretical maximum flux, J_{max}, can be estimated from the following equation [77], assuming that the maximum current that can be applied to the skin is 1 mA cm^{-2}:

$$J_{max} = \frac{I_T}{F}$$

where I_T is the total current applied and F is the Faraday constant.

$$J_{max} = \frac{\text{current flux } (10^{-3}\text{A, C sec}^{-1}\text{ cm}^{-2}) \text{ per hour } (\times 3{,}600 \text{ sec hr}^{-1})}{\text{charges per mole } (96{,}490 \text{ C, 1 Faraday})}$$

$$= 37.3 \text{ }\mu\text{mol cm}^{-2}\text{ hr}^{-1}$$

Assuming a solute MW of 200 and a 24-hr dose, a maximum dose of 180 mg cm^{-2} ($37.3 \times 24 \times 200$) can be achieved. Solutes containing ions other than sodium and chloride appear to have an upper limit transport number of around 0.2; therefore, the previous figure needs to be adjusted to account for a transport number of this degree. Assuming a dosing area of 10 cm^2, the estimated daily maximum dose is 360 mg ($180 \times 0.2 \times 10$) [77].

Figures 9 through 13 suggest that as the solute size increases, the transport number decreases, so for a solute of MW 1000, a transport of 0.001 is anticipated, yielding a maximum daily dose equivalent of 0.18 mg. Thus, large solutes will be usable by iontophoresis only if they are quite potent.

Penetration Enhancers

Penetration enhancers work by changing the structure of lipophilic bilayers or the keratinized domains in the stratum corneum, thus increasing the flux of the permeants. Rao and Misra [121] reported that the use of 30% DMSO (dimethylsulfoxide) increased the flux of penetration by 9.8%. The increase in penetration is due to the ability of DMSO to disrupt the stratum corneum [122] slightly and thus to enhance the rate of pore formation. Ten percent urea increases the penetration of solute by 33%, due to the ability of urea to hold water, resulting in better conductivity. Of the surfactants used, the nonionic Pluronic F68 contributed the least (63.55%) to the conductivity and therefore offers the least enhancement in flux value. The bile salts sodium taurocholate (STC) and sodium tauroglycocholate (STGC) significantly enhanced conductivity of the system; hence, the rate of flux enhancement is greater than that obtained for control [122]. As stated earlier, ethanol pretreatment of human epidermis increased the flux of insulin, compared with no ethanol pretreatment [27].

Hirvonen et al. [67] used dodecyl *N,N*-dimethyl amino acetate (DDAA) and Azone as penetration enhancers in the transdermal iontophoresis of sotalol and salicylate. They compared the action of both enhancers in passive diffusion studies and iontophoretic studies and found no significant difference between the two, with the permeability of sotalol in the passive diffusion studies increasing to the order of magnitude found in the iontophoretic studies. The main mechanism of action of DDAA and Azone is the disordering of the lipids and the closing of iontophoretic penetration routes [123,124].

Problems of Iontophoresis in Clinical Practice

Despite the many advantages of iontophoresis in the delivery of ionized drug molecules through the skin, it is not without its disadvantages or without potential for injury if not used correctly. The major danger in all iontophoretic treatments is the occurrence of skin irritation, burns, or excessive destruction of mucous membranes as a consequence of excessive current densities applied between electrodes. Pain sensation has in many cases been relied upon as a criterion for the prevention of skin burns. Current density, the relationship between the current strength and the size of the electrodes, should always be evaluated and kept below 0.5 mA/cm^2, which is the reported current density before discomfort is felt in humans [10].

Another common cause of iontophoretic burns is the touching of the skin surface by the exposed electrode metal. If the electrode metal touches the skin, burns are caused by a much lower current, due to the excessive current density at the site of contact. Skin irritation can also be caused by the properties of the solute ions being delivered or by delivery from buffer solutions with a pH much above or below physiological levels. Sanderson et al. [125] examined the mechanisms behind the side effects of iontophoresis and reviewed ways in which the therapeutic dose or optimal infusion rate of solutes can be achieved with the minimum current and therefore the minimum number of side effects. The suggestions of Sanderson et al. [125] included (a) the use of unbuffered donor solutions to minimize competition from nondrug cations, (b) the use of weak acid salts to control pH in the boundary layer, and thereby to minimize proton transport, and to increase the solubility of the drug in the donor solution to maximize transport, depending on which drug is the primary positive-current-carrying species in the donor solution, and (c) to modify the perm-selectivity of the skin to reduce resistance to certain ions.

Zelter et al. [126] compared iontophoretic and subcutaneous delivery of lidocaine and reported that although cutaneous burns were observed in two of the 13 patients for iontophoretic delivery, the majority of the subjects suffered only blanching or mild erythema of the treated site. Other studies also reported blanching and erythema of the skin [127], mild skin irritation [128], sensations of localized heat or cold [111], tingling and itching [126], and allergic contact dermatitis and virus activation [111].

C. Noninvasive Sampling of Biological Fluids

The use of iontophoresis in the noninvasive sampling of biological fluids is based on the idea that the solvent flow generated toward the electrode during iontophoresis could be used to convect molecules in a reverse direction through the skin to the surface. Glikfeld et al. [129] described an in vitro iontophoretic "back-extraction" procedure to sample [^{3}H]clonidine hydrochloride and [^{14}C]theophylline and [^{14}C-U]glucose, an uncharged solute, through the skin. Each solute in solution was perfused through a specially designed cell, and current was applied for 2 hours. For [^{3}H]clonidine hydrochloride and [^{14}C]theophylline, the authors reported a linear correlation between drug concentration in the perfusate and the amount back-extracted by iontophoresis. The ratio of glucose extracted in the sample was found to be related to the ratio of glucose in the perfusing solution. In both cases, if no current was applied, then no radioactivity was detected. In a followup study, Rao et al. [130] monitored [^{14}C]glucose using a similar technique. Surprisingly, they found that the radioactivity in the anode chamber was much higher than that in the cathode chamber. The authors hypothesized that the high level of radioactivity present at the anode was due to the metabolism of glucose by enzymes present in the dermis to negatively charged metabolites (e.g., lactate and pyruvate), which were then drawn to the anode. In conclusion, they noted that reverse iontophoresis, in conjunction with an appropriate analytical biosensor, has the potential to provide a noninvasive approach to glucose monitoring; however, the extraction time of 2 hours would have to be decreased for a more practical application.

Lactic acid ions have also been measured in vitro by noninvasive sampling, using chloride ions as internal standard and a constant, pulsed direct current (frequency 40 kHz; on–off duty 30%), to decrease damage to the skin [131]. When the concentration of lactic acid applied in the dermal side was increased, the flux of lactic acid and chloride ions increased and decreased, respectively. When the skin membrane resistance decreases at a constant current, the potential gradient, which is the driving force of the ion across the skin membrane, also decreases. The flux ratio of lactic acid/chloride ion was constant and independent of the potential gradient. For this reason, the noninvasive sampling technique with chloride ion as an internal standard can be used to estimate the lactic acid concentration whenever the skin is damaged or the applied current is changed.

D. Peptides and Proteins

The use of iontophoresis for the delivery of "difficult" drugs by the transdermal route, such as those based on peptide and protein structures, is being increasingly investigated. Several biotechnology-produced peptide-based pharmaceuticals have been approved for medical use (e.g., factor VIII:C for hemophilia, hepatitis B vaccine, human growth hormone, human insulin, interferon, monoclonal antibodies, somatotropin, and tissue plasminogen activator [132]). These preparations are extremely potent and often require daily doses of only a few micrograms. Unfortunately, the delivery of peptide molecules is particularly "difficult," because they are highly susceptible to degradation by proteolytic enzymes in the gastrointestinal tract and have a large "first-pass" metabolism and notoriously short biological half-lives; therefore they usually require parenteral administration. Although transdermal delivery would be an advantageous route for delivery of these preparations, it was often ruled out due to the additional obstacles of large molecular sizes and hydrophobicity. However, the possibility of administering peptides by iontophoresis has been investigated in vivo with some encouraging results. Kari [133] and Meyer et al. [134] have been able to demonstrate therapeutic concentrations of insulin (MW > 6000) administered by iontophoresis in diabetic rabbits; Chien et al. [89] demonstrated antidiuretic activity of iontophoretically administered vasopressin (MW = 1084) in rabbits; and Kumar et al. [135] have been able to deliver growth-hormone-releasing factor to hairless guinea pigs. To date the only demonstration of the use of iontophoresis to deliver peptides in human volunteers is that of Meyer et al. [136,137], who suggested that iontophoretic delivery of leuprolide acetate (MW = 1209) achieved levels similar to subcutaneous injection. Hoogstraate et al. [138] studied the iontophoresis of leuprolide and reported that leuprolide adsorbs onto negatively charged membranes, leading to a change in the net membrane charge and therefore changing the direction of electroosmotic flow, resulting in the convective solvent flow impeding the flux of positively charged solutes and assisting the flux of negatively charged solutes.

VII. FUTURE PERSPECTIVES

Iontophoresis has gained a great deal of attention during the last decade, and the knowledge available on the transport mechanism in iontophoresis has exploded. The technique has been of particular interest as an alternative to the parenteral delivery of peptide drugs because of their instability in the gastrointestinal tract. Iontophoresis may also offer many opportunities in the re-examination of existing oral drug therapy, in terms of avoiding first-pass effect in the liver, improving patient compliance, and reducing the risk of side effects when only local effects are required. Although iontophoretic drug delivery presents formidable challenges to the development of safe, effective, and commercializable delivery not only for peptides but also for a wide variety of drugs, the enormous market potential and patient compliance offered by such a system has generated much of the activity in this area.

The pharmaceutical industry has been aware of the advantages of iontophoretic drug delivery since the technique was first introduced in the field of pharmaceutical sciences. The probability of creating a safe, effective, and commercializable iontophoretic delivery system most likely will depend on three main issues: iontophoretic device design, drug applied, and vehicle.

Iontophoretic Device Design

A number of iontophoretic devices have been developed over the years. Consistent with the technological advances in other areas, iontophoretic devices have become more sophisticated and compact, with recent products using paper batteries and time-controllable films. Recently, Japanese university scientists have utilized a photo-etching technique in an iontophoretic device to deliver insulin [192]. They reported a 70% decrease in blood glucose levels in diabetic rats after iontophoretic application (1.5 V); this is consistent with results obtained from a 5-U/kg intravenous injection of insulin. Although further investigations are still required in order to limit skin damage, their new device is interesting in that the earlier animal work of Kari [133] reported successful iontophoretic delivery of insulin after scratching the skin.

Drug Applied

Given that molecular size limits iontophoretic transport flux of drugs, the potential of iontophoretic delivery is increasing with the advent of smaller peptides and active protein fragments. Given the nature of iontophoretic delivery, the delivery of certain drugs for systemic effects would be limited to extremely potent drugs, due to the relatively small concentrations capable of being driven through the skin without causing skin damage.

Vehicle

A wide range of vehicles can be used in iontophoretic drug delivery, giving consideration to drug solubility in the donor delivery site, protection of the skin from irritation or burns, and the maximum release of drug.

VIII. CONCLUSION

The use of constant-current iontophoresis in transdermal drug delivery appears to be most useful for solutes of a low MW (< 1000). Iontophoretic delivery with such solutes has been used in a number of clinical applications and applied to a range of epithelia, including skin, eye, buccal, bladder, and ear. Models have been developed to describe the iontophoretic transport of different-sized and -charged solutes through the epidermis, the main models being the Stokes–Einstein, free-volume, and pore-restriction models. Drug delivery into deeper tissues appears to be related not to iontophoretic delivery but rather to the diffusivity of solutes and the effect of the local blood supply in those tissues. The role of solute size in iontophoretic transport is also dependent on codeterminants for transport such as solute ionization, buffer composition, vehicle pH, and the presence of enhancers. It seems to us that the commercialization of iontophoresis is about to explode, with the clinical acceptability of the process, in terms of skin irritation and erythema, being actively resolved. Future developments are emerging and include reverse iontophoresis for sampling blood and tissues, protein and peptide delivery, and the use of alternative electric fields.

ACKNOWLEDGMENTS

The authors wish to acknowledge the financial support of the National Health and Medical Research Council of Australia, the Princess Alexandra Hospital Foundation, and the Queensland and Northern New South Wales Lions Kidney and Medical Research Foundation.

REFERENCES

1. Leduc, S. *Electric Ions and Their Use in Medicine*. London, Robman Ltd, 1908.
2. Singh, J. and Roberts, M. S. Transdermal delivery of drugs by iontophoresis: A review. *Drug Design Delivery 4*:1, 1989.
3. Ichihashi, T. Effect of drugs on the sweat glands by cataphoresis, and an effective method for suppression of local sweating. Observation on the effect of diaphorectics and adiaphoretics. *J. Orient. Med. 25*:101, 1936.
4. Hill, B. M. R. Poldine iontophoresis in the treatment of plantar and palmar hyperhidrosis. *Aust. J. Dermatol. 17*:92, 1976.
5. Abell, E. and Morgan, K. The treatment of idiopathic hyperhidrosis by glucopyrronium bromide and tap water iontophoresis. *Br. J. Dermatol. 91*:87, 1974.
6. Gibinski, K., Giec, L., Zmudzinski, J. et al. Transcutaneous inhibition of sweat gland function by atropine. *J. Appl. Physiol. 34*:850, 1973.
7. Shrivastava, S. and Singh, G. Tap water iontophoresis for palmar hyperhidrosis. *Brit. J. Dermatol. 96*:189, 1977.
8. Shelly, W. B., Horwath, P., and Weidman, F. Experimental milaria in man. Production of sweat retention anhidrosis and vesicles by means of iontophoresis. *J. Invest. Dermatol. 11*:275, 1948.
9. Hill, A. C., Baker, G. F., and Jansen, G. T. Mechanism of action of iontophoresis in the treatment of palmar hyperhydrosis. *Curtis 28*:69, 1981.
10. Abramson, H. A. and Gorin, M. H. Skin reactions. IX. The electrophoretic demonstration of the patent pores of the living human skin. *J. Phys. Chem. 44*:1094, 1940.
11. Cornwall, M. W. Zinc iontophoresis to treat ischemic skin ulcers. *Phys. Ther. 61*:359, 1981.
12. Gangarosa, L. P. Iontophoresis for surface anesthesia. *J. Am. Dent. Assoc. 88*:125, 1974.
13. Echols, D. F., Norris, C. H., and Tabb, H. G. Anesthesia of the ear by iontophoresis of lidocaine. *Arch. Otolaryngol. 101*:353, 1977.

14. Sisler, H. A. Iontophoretic local anesthesia for conjunctival surgery. *Ann Ophthalmol. 10*:597, 1978.

15. Gordon, A. H. and Weinstein, M. V. Sodium salicylate iontophoresis in the treatment of plantar warts. *Phys. Ther. 49*:869, 1968.

16. West, M. O. and Woodward, D. J. A technique for microiontophoretic study of single neurons in a freely moving rat. *J. Neurosci. Methods 11*:179, 1984.

17. Neuman, R. S. and White, S. R. A simple inexpensive circuit to add balance to microiontophoresis apparatus. *Electroencephalogr. Clin. Neurophysiol. 47*:507, 1979.

18. Henley-Cohn, J. and Hausfeld, J. N. Iontophoretic treatment of oral herpes. *Laryngoscope 94*:118, 1984.

19. Gangerosa, L. P., Park, N.-H., and Hill, J. M. Iontophoretic assistance of 5-iodo-2'-deoxyuridine penetration into neonatal mice skin and effect of DNA synthesis. *Proc. Soc. Exp. Biol. Med. 154*:439, 1977.

20. Gangerosa, L. P., Merchant, H. W., Park, N.-H., and Hill, J. M. Iontophoretic application of idoxuridine for recurrent herpes labialis: Report of Preliminary clinical findings. *Methods Find. Exp. Clin. Pharmacol. 1*:105, 1979.

21. Gangarosa, L. P. *Iontophoresis in Dental Practice.* Quintessence, Chicago, 1983, pp. 40–52.

22. Haggard, H., Strauss, M., and Greenberg, I. Fungus infections of hand and feet treated by copper iontophoresis. *J. Am. Med. Assoc. 112*:1229, 1939.

23. Coyer, A. Citrate iontophoresis in rheumatoid arthritis of the hands. *Ann. Phys. Med. 2*:16, 1954.

24. Harris, P. Iontophoresis: Clinical research in musculoskeletal inflammatory conditions. *J. Orthopaed. Sports Phys. Ther. 4*:109, 1982.

25. Hasson, S. M., English, S. E., Daniels, J. C. and Reich, M. Effect of iontophoretically delivered dexamethasone on muscle performance in a rheumatoid arthritic joint. *Arthritis Care Res. 1*:177, 1988.

26. Okabe, K., Yamaguchi, H., and Kawa, Y. New iontophoretic transdermal administration of the beta-blocker metoprolol. *J. Controlled Rel. 4*:79, 1986.

27. Srinivasan, V., Higuchi, W. I., Sims, S. M., Ghanem, A. H., and Behl, C. R. Transdermal iontophoretic drug delivery and application to polypeptide delivery. *J. Pharm. Sci. 78*:370, 1989.

28. Thysman, S., Préat, V., and Roland, M. Factors affecting iontophoretic mobility of metoprolol. *J. Pharm. Sci. 81*:670, 1992.

29. Petelenz, T. J., Buttke, J. A., Bonds, C., Lloyd, L. B., Beck, J. E., Stephen, R. L., Jacobsen, S. C., and Rodriguez, P. Iontophoresis of dexamethasone: laboratory studies. *J. Controlled Rel. 20*:55, 1992.

30. Anderson, B. D., Higuchi, W. I., and Raykar, P. V. Heterogeneity effects of permeability-partition coefficient relationships in human stratum corneum. *Pharm. Res. 5:566*, 1988.

31. Choi, T. B. and Lee, D. A. Transscleral and transcorneal iontophoresis of vancomycin in rabbit eyes. *J. Ocul. Pharmacol. 4*:153, 1988.

32. Duke-Elder, S. Iontophoresis. In: *The Foundation of Ophthalmology*. Mosby, St. Louis, 1962, Vol. VII, pp. 507–513.
33. Cross, S. E. and Roberts, M. S. The importance of dermal blood supply and the epidermis on the transdermal iontophoretic delivery of monovalent cations. *J. Pharm. Sci. 84*:584, 1995.
34. Von Sallman, L. Penetration of penicillin into the eye; further studies. *Arch. Ophthalmol. 34*:195, 1945.
35. Von Sallman, L. and Meyer, K. Penetration of penicillin into the eye. *Arch. Ophthalmol. 31*:1, 1944.
36. Fishman, P. H., Walter, M. J., Rissing, J. P. et al. Iontophoresis of gentamicin into aphakic rabbit eyes. *Invest. Ophthalmol. Vis. Sci. 25*:343, 1984.
37. Hughes, L. and Maurice, D. M. A fresh look at iontophoresis. *Arch. Ophthalmol. 102*:1825, 1984.
38. Barza, M., Peckman, C., and Baum, J. Transscleral iontophoresis as an adjunctive treatment for experimental endophthalmitis. *Arch. Ophthalmol. 105*:1418, 1987.
39. Barza, M., Peckman, C., and Baum, J. Transscleral iontophoresis of gentamicin in monkeys. *Invest. Ophthalmol. Vis. Sci. 28*:1033, 1987.
40. Barza, M., Peckman, C., and Baum, J. Transscleral iontophoresis of cefazolin, ticarcillin, and gentamicin in the rabbit. *Ophthalmology 93*:133, 1986.
41. Lugnani, F., Mazza, G., Cerulli, N., Rossi, C., and Stephen, R. Iontophoresis of drugs in the bladder wall: Equipment and preliminary studies. *Artif. Org. 17*:8, 1993.
42. Stephen, R. L., Lugnani, F., Rossi, C., and Eruzzi, S. Intracorporeal Iontophoretic Method. U.S. Patent 5,222,936, 1993.
43. Zimmer, P., Thiel, K. H., Fay, H., and Kziewior, J. In einem Körperhohlraum einführbare Innenelektrode. German patent 3809815A1, 1989.
44. Davis, C. P. and Warren, M. M. Iontophoretic Device and Method. U.S. Patent 4,411,648, 1983.
45. Gangarosa, L. P. Iontophoresis for surface local anesthesia. *JADA 88*:125, 1974.
46. Jensen, A. L. Hypersensitivity controlled by iontophoresis: Double blind clinical investigation. *J. Am. Dent. Assoc. 68*:217, 1964.
47. Albrecht, W. Neue versuche sur lokalen anasthesierung des trommielfells. *Arch. Ohren 85*:198, 1911.
48. Comeau, M., Brummett, R., and Vernon, J. Local anesthesia of the ear by iontophoresis. *Arch. Otolaryngol. 98*:114, 1973.
49. Passali, D., Bellussi, L., and Masieri, S. Transtympanic iontophoresis: Personal experience. *Laryngoscope 94*:802, 1984.
50. Sato, H., Takahashi, H., and Honjo, I. Transtympanic iontophoresis of dexamethasone and fosfomycin. *Arch. Otolaryngol. Head Neck Surg. 114*:531, 1988.
51. Echols, D. F., Norris, C. H., and Tabb, H. G. Anesthesia of the ear by iontophoresis of lidocaine. *Arch. Otolaryngol. 101*:418, 1975.

52. Tregar, R. T. *Physical Functions of Skin.* Academic Press, London, 1966, Vol. 5, pp. 22–23.

53. Scheuplein, R. J. Mechanism of percutaneous absorption. I. Routes of penetration and the influence of solubility. *J. Invest. Dermatol.* 45:334, 1965.

54. Monteiro-Riviere, N. A. Identification of the pathway of transdermal iontophoretic drug delivery: Ultrastructural studies using mercuric chloride in vivo in pigs. *Pharm. Res.* 8:S-141, 1991.

55. Monteiro-Riviere, N. A. Altered epidermal morphology secondary to lidocaine iontophoresis: in vivo and in vitro studies in porcine skin. *Fundam. Appl. Toxicol.* 15:174, 1990.

56. Cullander, C. and Guy, R. H. Visualizing the pathways of iontophoretic current flow in real time with laser-scanning confocal microscopy and the vibrating probe electrode. In: R. C. Scott, R. H. Guy and J. Hadgraft, eds. *Prediction of Percutaneous Penetration*, Vol. 2, IBC Technical Services, London, 1991.

57. Cullander, C. and Guy, R. H. Sites of iontophoretic current flow into the skin: Identification and characterisation with the vibrating probe electrode. *J. Invest. Dermatol.* 97:55, 1991.

58. Cullander, C. What are the pathways of iontophoretic current flow through mammalian skin? *Adv. Drug Deliv. Rev.* 9:119, 1992.

59. Scott, E. R., Laplaza, A. I., White, H. S., and Phipps, J. B. Transport of ionic species in skin: Contribution of pores to the overall skin conductance. *Pharm. Res.* 10:1699, 1993.

60. Foley, D., Corish, J., and Corrigan, O. I. Iontophoretic delivery of drugs through membranes including human stratum corneum. *Solid State Ionics* 53–56:184, 1992.

61. Burnette, R. R. Iontophoresis. In: J. Hadgraft and R. H. Guy, eds. *Transdermal Drug Delivery Developmental Issues and Research Initiatives.* Dekker, New York, 1988, pp. 247–292.

62. Yoshida, N. H. and Roberts, M. S. Solute molecular size and transdermal iontophoresis across excised human skin. *J. Cont. Rel.* 25:177, 1993.

63. Singh, P. and Roberts, M. S. Iontophoretic transdermal delivery of salicylic acid and lidocaine to local subcutaneous structures. *J. Pharm. Sci.* 82:127, 1993.

64. Del Terzo, S., Behl, C. R., and Nash, R. A. Iontophoretic transport of a homologous series of ionized and non-ionized model compounds: influence of hydrophobicity and mechanistic interpretation. *Pharm. Res.* 6:85, 1989.

65. Siddiqui, O., Sun, Y., Liu, J. C., and Chien, Y. W. Facilitated transdermal transport of insulin. *J. Pharm. Sci.* 76:341, 1987.

66. Itoh, T., Xia, J., Magavi, R., Nishihata, T., and Rytting, J. H. Use of shed snake skin as a model membrane for in vitro percutaneous penetration studies: Comparison with human skin. *Pharm. Res.* 7:1042, 1990.

67. Hirvonen, J., Kontturi, K., Murtomäki, L., Paronen, P., and Urtti, A. Transdermal iontophoresis of sotalol and salicylate: The effect of skin charge and penetration enhancers. *J. Controlled Rel.* 26:109, 1993.

68. Yoshida, N. H. and Roberts, M. S. Structure–transport relationships in transdermal iontophoresis. *Adv. Drug Deliv. Rev. 9*:239, 1992.
69. Keister, J. C. and Kasting, G. B. Ionic mass transport through a homogenous membrane in the presence of a uniform electric field. *J. Memb. Sci. 29*:155, 1986.
70. Schultz, S. G. *Basic Principles of Membrane Transport.* Cambridge University Press, New York, 1980, pp. 21–30.
71. Sims, S. M., Higuchi, W. I., and Srinvasan, V. Skin alteration and convective solvent flow effects during iontophoresis. II. Monovalent anion and cation transport across human skin. *Pharm. Res. 9*:1402, 1990.
72. Srinivasan, V. and Higuchi, W. I. A model for iontophoresis incorporating the effect of convective solvent flow. *Int. J. Pharm. 60*:133, 1990.
73. Evans, D. F., Tominaga, T., Hubbard, J. B., and Wolynes, P. G. Ionic mobility. Theory meets experiment. *J. Phys. Chem. 83*:2669, 1979.
74. Pikal, M. and Shah, S. Transport mechanisms in iontophoresis III. An experimental study of the contributions of electro-osmotic flow and permeability change in transport of low and high MW solutes. *Pharm. Res. 7*:222, 1990.
75. Gangerosa, L. P., Park, N.-H., Wiggins, C. A., and Hill, J. M. Increased penetration of non-electrolytes into mouse skin during iontophoretic water transport (Iontohydrokinesis). *J. Pharm. Exp. Ther. 212*:377, 1980.
76. Pikal, M. J. The role of electroosmotic flow in transdermal iontophoresis. *Adv. Drug Deliv. Rev. 9*:201, 1992.
77. Roberts, M. S., Singh, J., Yoshida, N. H., and Currie, K. I. In: R. C. Scott, R. H. Guy and J. Hadgraft, eds. *Prediction of Percutaneous Penetration.* IBC Technical Services, London, 1989, Vol. 1, pp. 231–241.
78. Yamamoto, T. and Yamamoto, Y. Electrical properties of the epidermal stratum corneum. *Med. Biol. Engl. 14*:151, 1976.
79. Li, L. C., Vu, N. T., and Allen, L. V. Iontophoretic permeation of sodium cromoglycate through synthetic membrane and excised hairless mouse skin. *J. Pharm. Pharmacol. 44*:444, 1992.
80. Lawler, J. C., Davis, M. J., and Griffith, E. Electrical characteristics of the skin: The impedance of the surface sheath and deep tissues. *J. Invest. Dermatol. 34*:301, 1960.
81. Thysman, S., Tasset, C., and Préat, V. Transdermal iontophoresis of fentanyl: Delivery and mechanistic analysis. *Int. J. Pharm. 101*:105, 1994.
82. Tyle, P. Iontophoretic devices for drug delivery. *Pharm. Res. 3*:318, 1986.
83. Liu, J. C., Sun, Y., Siddiqui, O., Shi, W. M., and Li, J. Blood glucose control in diabetic rats by the transdermal delivery of insulin. *Int. J. Pharm. 44*:197, 1988.
84. Lelawangs, P., Liu, J. C., Siddiqui, O., and Chien, Y. W. Transdermal iontophoretic delivery of arginine-vasopressin: I. physicochemical considerations. *Int. J. Pharm. 56*:13, 1989.
85. Wearley, L. and Chien, Y. W. Enhancement of the in vitro skin permeability of azidothymine (AZT) via iontophoresis and chemical enhancer. *Pharm. Res. 7*:34, 1990.

86. Bagniefski, T. and Burnette, R. R. A comparison of pulsed and continuous current iontophoresis. *J. Controlled Rel. 11*:113, 1990.

87. Pikal, M. and Shah, S. Study of the mechanisms of flux enhancement through hairless mouse skin by pulsed dc iontophoresis. *Pharm. Res. 8*:365, 1991.

88. Thysman, S. and Préat, V. In Vivo iontophoresis of fentanyl and sufentanil in rats: Pharmacokinetics and acute antinociceptive effects. *Anesth. Analg. 77*:61, 1993.

89. Chien, Y. W., Lelawongs, P., Siddiqui, O., and Shi, W. M. Facilitated transdermal delivery of therapeutic peptides and proteins by iontophoretic delivery devices. *J. Contr. Release 13*:263, 1990.

90. Pau, P. C., Berg, J. O., and McMillan, W. G. Application of Stokes law to ions in aqueous solution. *J. Phys. Chem. 94*:2671, 1990.

91. Glasstone, S., Laidler, K., and Eyring, H. *The Theory of Rate Processes.* McGraw-Hill, New York, 1941, pp. 477–599.

92. Smisek, D. L. and Hoagland, D. A. Electrophoresis of flexible macromolecules: Evidence for a new mode of transport in gels. *Science 248*:1221, 1990.

93. Kleparnik, K. and Bocek, P. Theoretical background for clinical and biomedical applications of electromigration techniques. *J. Chromatogr. 569*:3, 1991.

94. Cohen, M. H. and Turnbull, D. Molecular transport in liquids and glasses. *J. Chem. Phys. 31*:1164, 1959.

95. Vrentas, J. S., Duda, J. L., and Ling, H. C. Free volume theories for self-diffusion in polymer-solvent systems. I. Conceptual differences in theories. *J. Polym. Sci. 23*:275, 1985.

96. Lieb, W. R. and Stein, W. D. Non-Stokian nature of transverse diffusion within human red cell membranes. *J. Membr. Biol. 92*:111, 1986.

97. Miyamoto, T. and Shibayama, W. D. Free volume model for ionic conductivity in polymers. *J. Appl. Phys. 44*:5372, 1973.

98. Chand, N. Free volume and dc conductivity in polymers. *J. Appl. Polym. Sci. 27*:4889, 1982.

99. Eyring, H. and Hirschfelder, J. O. Theory of the liquid state. *J. Phys. Chem. 41*:249, 1937.

100. Kawamura, J. and Shimoji, M. Ionic conductivity and glass transition in superionic conducting glasses II. Structural relaxation and excess free volume theory. *J. Non-Cryst. Solids 88*:295, 1986.

101. Renkin, E. M. Filtration, diffusion and molecular sieving through porous cellular membranes. *J. Gen. Physiol. 38*:225, 1954.

102. Davson, A. *A Textbook of General Physiology*, 4th ed. 1970, Vol. 1, pp. 395–507.

103. Kasting, G. B. Theoretical models for iontophoretic delivery. *Adv. Drug Deliv. Rev. 9*:177, 1992.

104. Ruddy, S. B. and Hadzija, B. W. Iontophoretic permeability of polyethylene glycols through hairless rat skin: Application of hydrodynamic theory for hindered transport through liquid filled pores. *Drug Design Discovery 8*:207, 1992.

105. Rosendal, T. Studies on the conducting properties of human skin to direct current. *Acta Physiol. Scand. 5*:130, 1942.

106. Burnette, R. R. and Ongpipattanakul, B. Characterization of permselective properties of excised human skin during iontophoresis. *J. Pharm. Sci. 76*:765, 1987.

107. Crank, J. and Park, G. S. *Diffusion in Polymer*, Academic Press, London, 1968, Chap. 4, pp. 107–140.

108. Phipps, J. B., Padmanabham, R. V., and Lattin, G. A. Iontophoretic delivery of model inorganic drug ions. *J. Pharm. Sci. 78*:365, 1989.

109. Green, P. G., Hinz, R. S., Kim, A., Scoba, F. C., and Guy, R. H. Iontophoretic delivery of a series of tripeptides across the skin in vitro. *Pharm. Res. 8*:1121, 1991.

110. Siddiqui, O., Roberts, M. S., and Polack, A. The effect of iontophoresis and vehicle pH on the in vitro permeation of lignocaine through human stratum corneum. *J. Pharm. Pharmacol. 37*:732, 1985.

111. Ledger, P. W. Skin biological issues in electrically enhanced transdermal delivery. *Adv. Drug Del. Rev. 9*:289, 1992.

112. Riviere, J. E., Monteiro-Riviere, N. A., and Inman. A. Determination of lidocaine concentrations in skin after transdermal iontophoresis: Effects of vasoactive drugs. *Pharm. Res. 9*:211, 1992.

113. Riviere, J. E., Sage, B., and Williams, P. L. Effects of vasoactive drugs on transdermal lidocaine iontophoresis. *J. Pharm. Sci. 80*:615, 1991.

114. Sage, B. H. and Riviere, J. E. Model systems in iontophoresis-transport efficacy. *Adv. Drug Deliv. Rev. 9*:265, 1992.

115. Siddiqui, O., Roberts, M. S., and Polack, A. E. Percutaneous absorption of steroids: Relative contributions of epidermal penetration and dermal clearance. *J. Pharmacokin. Biopharm. 17*:405, 1989.

116. Roberts, M. S. In: R. C. Scott, R. H. Guy and J. Hadgraft, eds. *Structure–Permeability Considerations in Percutaneous Penetration*. IBC Technical Services, London, 1991, Vol. 2, pp. 210–228.

117. Cross, S. E., Wu, Z.-Y., and Roberts, M. S. In: R. C. Scott, R. H. Guy and J. Hadgraft, eds. *Predictions of Percutaneous Penetration*. IBC Technical Services, London, 1993, Vol. 3b, pp. 93–101.

118. Singh, P. and Roberts, M. S. Effects of vasoconstriction on dermal pharmacokinetics and local tissue distribution of compounds. *J. Pharm. Sci. 83*:783, 1994.

119. Phipps, J. B. and Gyory, J. R. Transdermal ion migration. *Adv. Drug Deliv. Rev. 9*:137, 1992.

120. Bellantone, N. H., Rim, S., Francoeur, M. L., and Rasadi, B. Enhanced percutaneous absorption via iontophoresis. I. Evaluation of an in vitro system and transport of model compounds. *Int. J. Pharmacol. 30*:63, 1986.

121. Rao, V. U. and Misra, A. N. Enhancement of iontophoretic permeation of insulin across human cadaver skin. *Pharmazie 49*:538, 1994.

122. Flynn, G. L., Yalkowsky, S. H., and Roseman, T. J. Mass transport phenomena and models: Theoretical concepts. *Pharm. Sci. 63*:479, 1974.

123. Barry, B. W. Mode of action of penetration enhancers in human skin. *J. Controlled Rel. 6*:85, 1987.

124. Kontturi, K., Murtomaki, L., Hirvonen, J., Paronen, P., and Urtti, A. Electrochemical characterization of human skin by impedance spectroscopy: The effect of penetration enhancers. *Pharm. Res. 10*:381, 1993.

125. Sanderson, J. E., de Riel, S., and Dixon, R. Iontophoretic delivery of non-peptide drugs: Formulation optimisation for maximum skin permeability. *J. Pharm. Sci. 78*:361, 1989.

126. Zelter, L., Regalado, M., Nichter, L. S., Barton, D., Jennings, S., and Pitt, L. Iontophoresis versus subcutaneous injection: a comparison of two methods of local anesthesia delivery in children. *Pain 44*:73, 1991.

127. Arvidsson, S. B., Ekroth, R. H., Hansby, A. M. C., Lindholm, A. H., and William-Olsson, G. Painless venipuncture. A clinical trial of iontophoresis of lidocaine for venipuncture in blood donors. *Acta Anaesthesiol. Scand. 28*:209, 1991.

128. Hölzle, E. and Alberti, N. Long-term efficacy and side effects of tap water iontophoresis of palmoplantar hyperhidrosis—The usefulness of home therapy. *Dermatologica 175*:126, 1987.

129. Glikfeld, P., Hinz, R. S., and Guy, R. H. Noninvasive sampling of biological fluids by iontophoresis. *Pharm. Res. 6*:988, 1989.

130. Rao, G., Glikfeld, P., and Guy, R. H. Reverse iontophoresis: Development of a noninvasive approach for glucose monitoring. *Pharm. Res. 10*:1751, 1993.

131. Numajiri, S., Sugibayashi, K., and Morimoto, Y. Non-invasive sampling of lactic acid ions by iontophoresis using chloride ion in the body as an internal standard. *J. Pharm. Biomed. Anal. 11*:903, 1993.

132. Chien, Y. W., Siddiqui, O., Shi, W.-M., Lelawongs, P., and Liu, J. C. Direct current iontophoretic transdermal delivery of peptide and protein drugs. *J. Pharm. Sci. 78*:376, 1989.

133. Kari, B. Control of blood glucose levels in alloxan-diabetic rabbits by iontophoresis of insulin. *Diabetes 35*:217, 1986.

134. Meyer, B. R., Katzeff, H. L., Eschbach, J., Trimmer, J., Zacharias, S. B., Rosen, S., and Sibalis, D. Transdermal delivery of insulin to albino rabbits using electrical current. *Am. J. Med. Sci. 297*:321, 1989.

135. Kumar, S., Char, H., Patel, S., Piemontese, D., Malick, A. W., Iqbal, K., Neugroschel, E., and Behl, C. R. In vivo transdermal iontophoretic delivery of growth hormine-releasing factor GRF (1-44) in hairless guinea pigs. *J. Contr. Rel. 18*:213, 1992.

136. Meyer, B. R., Kreis, W., and Eschbach, J. Successful transdermal administration of therapeutic doses of a polypeptide to normal human volunteers. *Clin. Pharmacol. Ther. 44*:607, 1988.

137. Meyer, B. R., Kreis, W., Eschbach, J., O'Mara, V., Rosen, S., and Sibalis, D.

Transdermal versus subcutaneous leuprolide: A comparison of acute pharmacodynamic effect. *Clin. Pharmacol. Ther.* *48*:340, 1990.

138. Hoogstraate, A. J., Srinivasan, V., Sims, S. M., and Higuchi, W. I. Iontophoretic enhancement of peptides: Behavior of leuprolide versus model permeants. *J. Controlled Rel.* *31*:41, 1994.

139. Kahn, J. Acetic acid iontophoresis for calcium deposits. *Phys. Ther.* *57*:658, 1977.

140. Psaki, C. and Carroll, J. Acetic acid ionization: A study to determine the absorptive effects upon calcified tendonitis of the shoulder. *Phys. Ther. Rev.* *35*:84, 1955.

141. Macht, M. B. and Bader, M. E. Iontophoresis with acetyl-*b*-methylcholine and blood flow through the hand at low environmental temperature. *J. Appl. Physiol.* *1*:205, 1948.

142. Eneroth-Grimfors, E., Lindblad, L.-E., Westgren, M., Etzell, B.-M., and Bevegard, S. Iontophoresis of vasoactive drugs: Effect on peripheral blood flow during pregnancy. *Acta Obstet. Gynecol. Scand.* *70*:25, 1991.

143. Garagiola, U., Dacatra, U., Braconaro, F., Porretti, E., Pisetti, A., and Azzolini, V. Iontophoretic administration of pirprofen or lysine soluble aspirin in the treatment of rheumatic diseases. *Clin. Ther.* *10*:553, 1988.

144. Gangerosa, L. P. Defining a practical solution for iontophoretic local anaesthesia of skin. *Meth. Find. Exp. Clin. Pharmacol.* *3*:83, 1981.

145. Kahn, J. Calcium iontophoresis in suspected myopathy. *Phys. Ther.* *55*:376, 1975.

146. Chang, B. K., Guthrie, T. H., Hayakawa, K., and Gangerosa, L. P. A pilot study of iontophoretic cisplatin chemotherapy of basal and squamous cell carcinomas of the skin. *Arch. Dermatol.* *129*:425, 1993.

147. Hornqvist, R., Back, O., and Henrikson, R. Adrenoreceptor-mediated responses in human skin studied by iontophoresis. *Br. J. Dermatol.* *111*:561, 1984.

148. Glass, J. M., Stephen, R. L., and Jacobsen, S. C. The quantity and distribution of radiolabeled dexamethasone delivered to tissue by iontophoresis. *Int. J. Dermatol.* *19*:519, 1980.

149. Groning, R. Electrophoretically controlled dermal or transdermal application systems with electronic indicators. *Int. J. Pharm.* *36*:37, 1987.

150. LaForest, N. and Cofrancesco, C. Antibiotic iontophoresis in the treatment of ear chondritis. *Phys. Ther.* *53*:32, 1978.

151. Abramson, D. I., Tuck, S., Chu, L. S. W., and Buso, E. Physiologic and clinical basis for histamine by ion transfer. *Arch. Phys. Med. Rehabil.* *48*:583, 1967.

152. Popkin, R. J. The use of hyaluronidase by iontophoresis in the treatment of generalized scleroderma. *J. Invest. Dermatol.* *16*:97, 1951.

153. Schwartz, H. S. Use of hyaluronidase by iontophoresis in treatment of lymphedema. *Arch. Intern. Med.* *95*:662, 1955.

154. Rothfeld, S. H. and Murray, W. The treatment of Peyronie's disease by iontophoresis of C21 esterified glucocorticoids. *J. Urol.* *97*:874, 1967.

155. Gangarosa, L. P., Park, N. H., and Hill, J. M. Iontophoretic assistance of 5-iodo-2′-deoxyuridine penetration into neonatal mouse skin and effects on DNA synthesis (39689). *Proc. Soc. Exp. Biol. Med. 154*:439, 1977.

156. Boxhall, M. and Frost, J. Iontophoresis and *Herpes labialis. Med. J. Aust. 140*:686, 1984.

157. Pratzel, H., Dittrich, P., and Kukovetz, W. Spontaneous and forced cutaneous absorption of indomethacin in pigs and humans. *J. Rheumatol. 13*:1122, 1986.

158. Tannenbaum, M. Iodine iontophoresis in reducing scar tissue. *Phys. Ther. 60*:792, 1980.

159. Batner, H. B. Cataphoresis in dermabrasion tattooing. *Plast. Reconstr. Surg. 27*:613, 1961.

160. Irsfeld, S., Klement, W., and Lipfert, P. Dermal anaesthesia: Comparison of Emla cream with iontophoretic local anaesthesia. *Br. J. Anaesth. 71*:375, 1993.

161. Gangarosa, L. P. Defining a practical solution of iontophoretic local anesthesia of skin. *Meth. and Find. Exptl. Clin. Pharmacol. 3*:83, 1981.

162. Maloney, J. M., Bezzant, J. L., Stephen, R. L., and Petelenz, T. J. Iontophoretic administration of lidocaine anaesthesia in office practice. *J. Dermatol. Surg. Oncol. 18*:937, 1992.

163. Weinstein, M. and Gordon, A. The use of magnesium sulfate iontophoresis in the treatment of deltoid bursitis. *Phys. Ther. Rev. 38*:96, 1958.

164. Moawad, M. B. Treatment of vitiligo with 1% solution of the sodium salt of meladine using the iontophoresis technique. *Dermatol. Monatsschr. 155*:338, 1969.

165. Rapperport, A. S., Larson, D. L., Henges, D. F. et al. Iontophoresis—A method of antibiotic administration in the burn patient. *Plast. Reconstr. Surg. 36*:547, 1965.

166. Gibson, L. E. and Cooke, R. E. A test for concentration of electrolytes in sweat in cystic fibrosis of the pancreas utilizing pilocarpine by iontophoresis. *Pediatrics 23*:545, 1959.

167. Puttemans, F. et al. Iontophoresis: Mechanism of action studied by potentiometry and x-ray fluorescence. *Arch. Phys. Med. Rehabil. 63*:176, 1982.

168. James, M. P., Graham, R. M., and English, J. Percutaneous iontophoresis of prednisolone—A pharmacokinetic study. *Clin. Exp. Dermatol. 11*:54, 1986.

169. Lekas, M. D. Iontophoresis treatment. *Otolaryngol Head Neck Surg. 87*:292, 1977.

170. Smith, K. J., Konzelman, J. L., Lombardo, F. A., Skelton, H. G., Holland, T. T., Yeager, J., Wagner, K. F., Oster, C. N., and Chung, R. Iontophoresis of vinblastine into normal skin for treatment of Kaposi's sarcoma in human immunodeficiency virus-positive patients. *Arch. Dermatol. 128*:1365, 1992.

171. Wahlberg, J. E. Skin clearance of iontophoretically administered Chromium (^{51}Cr) and Sodium (^{22}Na) ions in the guinea pig. *Acta Dermatovener (Stockholm) 50*:255, 1970.

172. Slough, C. L., Spinelli, M. J., and Kasting, G. B. Transdermal delivery of etidronate (EHDP) in the pig via iontophoresis. *J. Membr. Sci. 35*:161, 1986.

173. Sanderson, J. E., Caldwell, R. W., Hsaio, J., Dixon, R., and Tuttle, R. R. Noninvasive delivery of a novel inotropic catecholamine: iontophoretic versus intravenous infusion in dogs. *J. Pharm. Sci. 76*:215, 1987.

174. Su, M.-H., Srinivasan, V., Ghanem, A.-H., and Higuchi, W. I. Quantitative in vivo iontophoretic studies. *J. Pharm. Sci. 83*:12, 1994.

175. Knoblauch, P. and Moll. F. In vitro pulsatile and continuous transdermal delivery of buserelin by iontophoresis. *J. Controlled Rel. 26*:203, 1993.

176. Yoshida, N. H. and Roberts, M. S. The role of conductivity in iontophoresis 2. Anodal iontophoretic transport of phenylethylamine and sodium across excised human skin. *J. Pharm. Sci. 83*:344, 1994.

177. Kislalioglu, M. S., Sethi, P. K., Malick, A. W., and Behl, C. R. In vitro iontophoretic permeation of a weak base erythromycin from different buffer solutions using hairless mouse skin. *Pharm. Pharmacol. Lett. 2*:85, 1992.

178. Wang, Y., Allen, Jr., L. V., Li, L. C., and Tu, Y.-H. Iontophoresis of hydrocortisone across hairless mouse skin: investigation of skin alteration. *J. Pharm. Sci. 82*:1140, 1993.

179. Heit, M. C., Monteiro-Riviere, N. A., Jayes, F. L., and Riviere, J. E. Transdermal iontophoretic delivery of luteinizing hormone releasing hormone (LHRH): Effect of repeated administration. *Pharm. Res. 11*:1000, 1994.

180. Santi, P., Catellani, P. L., Massimo, G., Zanardi, G., and Colombo, P. Iontophoretic transport of verapamil and melatonin. I. Cellophane membrane as a barrier. *Int. J. Pharm. 92*:23, 1993.

181. Yoshizuma, M. O., Cohen, D., Verbukh, I. et al. Experimental transscleral iontophoresis of ciprofloxacin. *J. Ocul. Pharmacol. 7*:163, 1991.

182. Lam, T. T., Edward, D. P., Zhu, X., and Tso, M. O. M. Transscleral iontophoresis of dexamethasone. *Arch. Ophthalmol. 107*:1368, 1989.

183. Maurice, D. M. Iontophoresis of fluorescein into the posterior segment of the rabbit eye. *Ophthalmology 93*:128, 1986.

184. Kondo, M. and Araie, M. Iontophoresis of 5-fluorouracil into the conjunctiva and sclera. *Invest. Opthalmol. Vis. Sci. 30*:583, 1989.

185. Sarraf, D. and Lee, D. A. Iontophoresis of reactive black 5 for pulsed dye laser sclerostomy. *J. Ocul. Pharmacol. 9*:25, 1993.

186. Burstein, N. L., Leopold, I. H., and Bernachi, D. B. Transscleral iontophoresis of gentamicin. *J. Ocul. Pharmacol. 1*:363, 1985.

187. Grossman, R., Chu, D. F., and Lee, D. A. Regional ocular gentamicin levels after transcorneal and transscleral iontophoresis. *Invest. Ophthalmol. Vis. Sci. 31*:909, 1990.

188. Grossman, R. and Lee, D. A. Transscleral and transcorneal iontophoresis of ketoconazole in the rabbit eye. *Ophthalmology 96*:724, 1989.

189. Rootman, D. S., Hobden, J. A., Jantzen, J. A. et al. Iontophoresis of tobramycin

for the treatment of experimental *Pseudomonal keratitis* in the rabbit. *Arch. Ophthalmol. 106*:262, 1988.

190. Rootman, D. S., Jantzen, J. A., Gonzales, J. R. et al. Pharmacokinetics and safety of transcorneal iontophoresis of tobramycin in the rabbit. *Invest. Ophthalmol. Vis. Sci. 20*:1397, 1988.

191. Hill, J. M., Park, N.-H., Gangarosa, L. P., Hull, D. S. et al. Iontophoresis of vidarabine monophosphate into rabbit eyes. *Invest. Ophthalmol. Vis. Sci. 17*:473, 1978.

192. Haga, M., Akatani, M., Kikuchi, J., Uneo, Y., and Hayashi, M. Transdermal iontophoretic delivery of insulin using a photoelectrode microdevice. *J. Controlled Release 43*:139, 1997.

Index